Deciding Who Lives

Deciding
Who Lives

*Fateful Choices
in the Intensive-Care
Nursery*

Renée R. Anspach

UNIVERSITY OF CALIFORNIA PRESS
Berkeley · Los Angeles · Oxford

University of California Press
Berkeley and Los Angeles, California

University of California Press, Ltd.
Oxford, England

Library of Congress Cataloging-in-Publication Data

Anspach, Renée R.
    Deciding who lives : fateful choices in the intensive-care nursery / Renée R. Anspach.
      p.   cm.
    Includes bibliographical references and index.
    ISBN 0-520-05268-4
    1. Neonatal intensive care—Decision making. 2. Neonatal intensive care—Moral
    and ethical aspects. I. Title.
    RJ253.5.A58 1993
    174'.24—dc20   91-44245
                                                                   CIP

Printed in the United States of America
9 8 7 6 5 4 3 2 1

The paper used in this publication meets the minimum requirements of American
National Standard for Information Sciences—Permanence of Paper for Printed Library
Materials, ANSI Z39.48-1984. ∞

*To the memory of my father, Raymond Anspach,
and for my mother, Celine Anspach*

Contents

Figures and Tables

Figures

Tables

Acknowledgments

I would like to thank the *Journal of Health and Social Behavior* and Westview Press for permission to reprint portions of several of my articles. I am grateful to five of the nine campuses of the University of California for providing a superb education that I could also afford. However, it is a particular pleasure to be able to acknowledge some of the many people who, over the years, participated in the creative process.

I could not have had better mentors than Aaron Cicourel, Fred Davis, Joseph Gusfield, Kristin Luker, Roy D'Andrade, and Albert Jonsen, who showed unflagging support and unfailing generosity. By encouraging good writing and clear thinking, they made this project possible.

Two former teachers, Arlie Hochschild and the late Nancy Tanner, believed in my abilities and taught me to believe in them. Without having read this book, they nonetheless shaped the character of my thinking. Steven Segal introduced me to the theory and practice of research. Oscar Grusky and Richard Lempert provided helpful comments on earlier drafts of this manuscript.

Three fellow medical sociologists, Diane Beeson, Sydney Halpern, and the late Marcine Cohen—friends and intellectual "soul mates"— listened patiently to jumbled paragraphs and embryonic ideas. Other friends—Donna Levy and Irving Cohen—also physicians, patiently translated medicalese and provided tests of "subjective adequacy."

Peter and Patti Adler, Virginia Forrest, Candace West, Charlane Brown, Gail Hall, Irving Feurst, Lee Quevedo, and David Gilmartin provided support that was less tangible but no less significant. Jane Sparer's contributions to my life over the last two decades cannot be summarized in a single sentence.

Paul Weisser painstakingly edited my manuscript with consummate skill and good humor. Katherine Bischoping helped me prepare the graphics, and Ravishankar provided valuable technical assistance. I am also grateful for the support of Naomi Schneider at the University of California Press, whose superb editorial judgment improved the quality of the manuscript. I thank Erika Büky, also at the University of California Press, for her patience.

My mother, Celine Anspach, in ways that cannot be enumerated fully, single-handedly rescued this book from the trash bin on more than one occasion.

Above all, I wish to thank the physicians, nurses, social workers, and parents at the two newborn intensive-care units I studied. With exceptional patience, generosity, and candor, they gave of their time, their insights, and themselves.

The road has been long, steep, and winding. My heartfelt thanks to those who shared the journey with me.

CHAPTER I

Introduction

The Dilemmas and Their Dimensions

The visitor who enters an intensive-care unit for newborn infants for the first time may have what seems to be a surrealistic encounter with the twenty-first century. The diffuse din of the monitors, the many incubators and intravenous lines, the eerie glow of the ultraviolet lights used to combat jaundice—all the elaborate machinery of the nursery provides a stark contrast to its tiny patients. Next to each incubator stands a nurse who, from time to time, may reach into the porthole to administer medications or take vital signs. At least twice a day, an entourage of physicians stops by each incubator as they make their daily rounds. A group of doctors and nurses may enter the nursery, moving rapidly to bring in a new patient who may have been transported by plane from the hinterland.

The newborn intensive-care unit stands as a monument to science and technology, a living testament to the vast resources that our society has committed to saving life at its beginning. There are, however, times in the social life of the intensive-care nursery when neonatal intensive care may seem less a symbol of progress than a confrontation with the problematic. These moments occur when parents and health professionals, faced with an infant who is terminally ill or who may survive with serious disabilities, must decide whether the infant will live or die. These life-and-death decisions are the subject of this book.

NEONATAL INTENSIVE CARE

Until very recently, this subject would not have been studied at all, for newborn intensive-care units did not always exist. Neonatal intensive

1

care is a nascent specialization in medicine and nursing that has developed rapidly over the past three decades. The ever-widening knowledge base of perinatal research, coupled with a sophisticated technology, has dramatically advanced the care of seriously ill newborn infants. In 1976, it was estimated that there were twenty newborn intensive-care units in California alone. In 1980, the number of hospitals in the United States having neonatal intensive-care units was estimated to be about six hundred. Each year, approximately two hundred thousand infants, or about 6 percent of all live births, are sufficiently ill to require intensive care.[1]

Neonatal intensive care has been directed toward infants with an array of problems. Conditions associated with prematurity, such as respiratory distress syndrome (also called hyaline membrane disease), are the most common reason for hospitalization in an intensive-care nursery. The second largest group of patients is those with congenital anomalies (e.g., congenital heart disease) that require immediate treatment.[2] However, infants having a number of other serious problems find their way into the newborn intensive-care unit—including, for example, infants born to diabetic or drug-addicted mothers, those born to Rh-negative mothers with increasing quantities of Rh antibodies in their blood, and those suffering from gastrointestinal disorders or generalized infections.[3]

Since their inception, the technologies of neonatal intensive care have increased in both scope and sophistication. Some of the innovations that have been introduced include devices for monitoring blood gases and blood chemistry as well as techniques for continuously monitoring heart rate and rhythm, breathing rate, and blood pressure. Some diagnostic techniques used for adults, such as CAT scans (brain scans) and cardiac catheterization, are now used for newborn infants as well. Therapeutic technologies include respirators and positive pressure ventilators to treat respiratory problems, phototherapy and exchange blood transfusions to treat jaundice, and intravenous hyperalimentation, a technique for providing nutrition to very sick infants.[4] Although it is difficult to evaluate the precise contribution of advances in neonatal intensive care to changes in mortality and morbidity,[5] available data suggest they have played a major role in reducing mortality among critically ill newborn infants.[6] The long-term outlook for very small, very premature infants, however, is still being evaluated and is the subject of considerable debate.[7]

Although neonatal intensive care is a recent phenomenon, some technologies for the treatment of sick newborn infants have been in existence for some time. A historical perspective illustrates the radical reorientation that has occurred in the treatment of sick newborns. At the turn of the century, most premature infants died during the first hours of life.[8] The first incubator, or "warming chamber," was developed by Dr. E. S. Tarnier in 1878. Dr. Pierre-Constant Budin, who was later to write the first textbook on neonatology, displayed his "child hatchery," consisting of six premature babies in incubators, at the 1896 Berlin Exposition, in order to attract attention to the techniques that he and Tarnier had developed. This type of equipment was publicized in the United States by Dr. Martin Couney, who exhibited premature "incubator babies" at international fairs and ultimately reared five thousand infants on Coney Island. Eventually, the incubator became a standard feature in the care of critically ill premature infants.[9]

By 1923, when the first American hospital for sick newborns was established, childbirth had already been transformed from a natural, family event to a medical and hospital-centered event.[10] Care of the sick newborn infant became the province of the obstetrician or the family doctor. The approach to newborn infants remained largely noninterventionist. Throughout the first half of the twentieth century, those infants who were considered too young or too sick to benefit from existing therapies were not seen as viable and were simply not treated. In the early and middle 1960s, as intensive-care techniques were developed and as a number of pediatricians began to specialize in the care of high-risk infants, the number of infants who could be treated increased significantly, and the horizons of viability expanded. The development of neonatal intensive care, then, signaled a dramatic transformation to a treatment philosophy of active, aggressive intervention.

LIFE-AND-DEATH DECISIONS

Neonatal intensive care represents a triumph of sophisticated medical technology. At the same time, however, a number of difficult ethical dilemmas have appeared in its wake. Improved medical management and surgical techniques have made it possible to save the lives of many infants who previously would not have survived. Among them are infants who may survive with serious physical or mental disabilities and who may require numerous medical and surgical treatments.

Consequently, many physicians, bioethicists, and parents have asked whether it is always appropriate to try to sustain the lives of these infants.

Consider, for example, three of the better-known dilemmas. Among the most controversial life-and-death decisions are those concerning infants with Down syndrome, a genetic defect accompanied by mild to moderate mental retardation. Thirty years ago, infants with Down syndrome who also had intestinal defects died in infancy, but pediatric surgery to correct these defects has now become routine. Is it right to withhold life-saving surgery from an infant who will be mentally retarded?

Spina bifida (incomplete development of the spinal column) is among the more serious of birth defects. It is often accompanied by hydrocephalus, or an abnormal accumulation of fluid in the brain. The development of the shunt in 1958 made it possible to control hydrocephalus, and refined surgical techniques made it possible to close the spinal lesion. While some children with spina bifida may have normal intelligence, those who are most severely affected are likely to be paralyzed and incontinent and to require numerous surgeries. Is it right to withhold surgery from these infants?

A third example concerns infants who are on the frontiers of viability. Neonatology has made it possible to resuscitate infants who weigh as little as one pound and who are born three months prematurely. Many of these infants die, and those who live risk damage to major organ systems, including brain damage. While these smallest of infants constitute only a tiny fraction of babies in the neonatal intensive-care unit, their costly care consumes a disproportionate share of the nursery's economic resources.[11] Is it right to resuscitate infants who may have only a slight chance for normal survival? Is it right to decide, as has been done in other countries, that treatment of some infants is too costly?[12]

Each of these dilemmas poses the hard question of whether what *can* be done *should* be done and calls into question the basic principle on which neonatal intensive care is premised: that of active, aggressive intervention. Each case raises serious questions about the price of medical progress and illustrates how medical decision making has been expanded to embrace judgments about the kind of life that is desirable. Among other issues, the first case raises the question of whether a decision to withhold therapy should be made on the basis of mental retardation. The second dilemma is sometimes character-

ized as a conflict between the principles of preserving life and preventing suffering.*The third case raises an additional question that typifies
neonatal intensive care: what to do in the absence of sound information concerning the future of an infant whose life is in question.

Life-and-death decisions may arise at any point during an infant's
stay in an intensive-care nursery. They include decisions to resuscitate
an infant at the moment of birth, decisions to undertake medical or
surgical procedures, decisions to terminate life support (e.g., to "disconnect" respirators), and decisions to resuscitate an infant whose
heart has stopped beating or who has stopped breathing ("code/no-
code" decisions). These decisions are not merely objects of theoretical
concern but are actual dilemmas frequently faced by parents and
health professionals. The accounts of physicians, journalists, ethicists,
and social scientists suggest that these life-and-death decisions are
being made in intensive-care nurseries throughout the country.[13]

✗ The question of which infants should receive aggressive treatment
raises an array of difficult issues of policy and morality. What criteria
should be used to determine when to resuscitate or provide life support for infants who may be terminally ill or severely damaged? Who
should be the final arbitrator of such decisions? Can these infants be
said to possess a "right to life" or a "right to die"? How can one
impute rights to or determine what is in the best interests of those
unable to speak for themselves? These decisions involve what Guido
Calabresi and Philip Bobbitt call "tragic choices," or decisions made
in the face of conflicting values.[14] Inevitably, life-and-death decisions
involve judgments about the kinds of lives that are worth saving—
and, by implication, the kinds of lives that are not worth saving.

WHY STUDY THIS SUBJECT?

A very rough measure of the importance that our society attaches to
life-and-death decisions in the nursery is the sheer number of publications about this subject. Yet a quick glance at the vast literature that
has appeared in the past two decades reveals a glaring paradox. It is
hard to imagine a topic about which so much has been written, yet so
little is actually known. In the past decade, at least seven books by
legal scholars, journalists, and social scientists have been published.
At least two books and more than a hundred articles have been
written about the ethics of newborn intensive care. Because the law
has failed to provide clear guidelines for life-and-death decisions, legal

scholars have debated whether these decisions are permissible, and their opinions differ dramatically.[15] If, on the one hand, we are to believe legal scholar John Robertson, those who make some life-and-death decisions face potential charges of homicide by omission. If, on the other hand, we are to believe Elizabeth MacMillan, decisions not to treat infants with the severest mental disabilities, who are unable to survive infancy, can be made with impunity.[16]

Ethical and legal discussions of neonatal intensive care are often prescriptive—that is, they tell us how decisions should or should not be made. Yet we know surprisingly little about how life-and-death decisions actually *are* made. Joel Frader, a physician who has written about decisions in the nursery, commented that after more than two decades of research on this subject, we still do not know the dimensions of the problem, or, as physicians say, its incidence or prevalence.[17] Much of the information we do have about life-and-death decisions is indirect and comes from three sources: surveys of physician attitudes, reports of individual nurseries, and well-publicized legal cases.

One source of information about how physicians *think* about life-and-death decisions comes from attitude surveys, in which pediatricians are asked how actively they would treat infants with a number of physical or mental disabilities. Although these surveys ask different questions, a common pattern can be discerned. The vast majority of physicians say they would not treat infants with the severest defects, who could not survive infancy and would be seriously retarded. Responses in the 1970s were divided on the question of treating infants who would survive with physical and mental disabilities—that is, babies with Down syndrome or spina bifida. Most pediatricians surveyed in the 1980s, however, seem reluctant to let these babies die.[18] While highly informative about the beliefs and values of physicians, these attitude surveys do not tell us what physicians *do* in actual practice.

Another piece of evidence comes from a few published reports of the practices of individual nurseries. During the early 1970s, several physicians began to report their policies for making life-and-death decisions in professional journals. One of the first published reports appeared in 1973 in the *New England Journal of Medicine*. In this article, pediatricians Raymond Duff and A. G. M. Campbell reported that they had withheld life-saving treatment from 14 percent of the 299 infants who had died in the Yale–New Haven Nursery. In a companion article in the same issue, pediatric surgeon Anthony Shaw described actual cases in which he and the parents had decided not to treat several infants with physical or mental disabilities. Dramatically different from the practices of the Yale–New Haven Nursery is the reported policy of Children's Hospital in Philadelphia, under the leadership of former Surgeon General C. Everett Koop, in which all infants—including those with very serious mental and physical disabilities—are treated very actively.[19] These isolated reports, however, can hardly be taken as representative of decisions made in nurseries throughout the country.

A third source of information is the body of legal cases that have been publicized in the media. The inconsistent rulings in these cases suggest that our society is deeply divided about decisions in the nursery. For example, a 1974 decision, *Maine Medical Center v. Houle,* involved an infant who was born blind and had some brain damage and multiple physical malformations, including one defect that could be repaired surgically, a tracheoesophageal fistula. Unless the defect was repaired, the infant would not survive. Although both the parents and the physicians argued against performing the surgery, the court held that the surgery should be performed because it was medically feasible. The Mueller case in Danville, Illinois, involved Siamese twins who were joined with a single trunk and had three legs. Nurses were told not to feed the twins. An investigation began when an anonymous caller informed the Illinois Department of Children and Family Services that the twins were being neglected. The district attorney filed criminal charges against the parents and the physician, which were ultimately dropped for lack of evidence when the nurses refused to testify against the parents and physician.[20]

Nowhere are the deep divisions and ambivalence in our society more apparent than in the well-known Baby Doe cases, which have been discussed extensively by ethicists and legal scholars.[21] In 1983, in Bloomington, Indiana, an infant was born with Down syndrome and an obstruction of the throat. Although the parents decided against performing surgery—that is, to let the baby die—some hospital physicians took the case to court. The Indiana Supreme Court ruled in favor of the parents, but the case came to the attention of the Reagan administration. Baby John Doe died before action could be taken. On October 11, 1982, the infant known as Baby Jane Doe was born with spina bifida, hydrocephalus, and microcephaly (an abnormally small head). Although the parents decided against surgery, a pro-life attorney mounted a challenge to this decision in the courts. New York's Court of Appeals upheld a lower court's ruling that the parents had a right to make the decision.

In the Baby Doe cases, for the first time, decisions in the nursery became a public issue. Pro-life activists, disability rights groups, the medical profession, and the Reagan administration became embroiled in a national debate. The cases also signify a growing trend toward state involvement in medical decisions.[22] President Reagan directed Secretary of Health and Human Services Richard Schweiker to draft a series of regulations forbidding nurseries from withholding food, water, or medical treatment from disabled infants. Outraged by these regulations, the American Hospital Association, the American Medical Association, and the American Academy of Pediatrics mounted legal challenges to the policies of the Reagan administration. The Baby Doe rules were finally struck down in the U.S. Supreme Court.

In 1985, three years after the death of Baby John Doe, Congress passed Public Law 98-457, which requires state child-welfare agencies to investigate cases of "medical neglect," defined as withholding medically indicated treatment from critically ill infants. Carefully crafted in response to the competing demands of disability rights organizations, the American Academy of Pediatrics, and pro-life groups, the Child Abuse Amendments and the Department of Health and Human Services rules to implement them were viewed by some as a compromise. Nevertheless, the amendments and the rules continued to mandate aggressive intervention for almost all infants.[23]

However dramatic these cases may be and however great their impact on public policy, it is difficult to view them as typical of life-and-death decisions in nurseries throughout the country. In fact, there is reason to believe that these cases are *atypical*. Despite the widespread attention given these cases, most life-and-death decisions do not concern infants with Down syndrome or spina bifida. Rather, they concern low-birthweight infants who pose dilemmas that are not well publicized. Moreover, despite the Reagan administration's concern about the medical neglect of disabled infants, one study of actual life-and-death decisions suggests that many infants are in fact over-treated rather than undertreated.[24]

In short, pediatricians have openly acknowledged that life-and-death decisions *are* being made; bioethicists have discussed the ways they *should* be made; jurists have discussed the ways they should *not* be made; physicians and sociologists have surveyed the array of physician attitudes toward them; and social scientists have discussed how life-and-death decisions are made in some settings.[25] Yet there remains a curious imbalance in the literature: we still know far more about how people think life-and-death decisions *should* be made than how they actually are made. We also know more about the decisions of physicians than those of nurses, and we know still less about the role of parents in life-and-death decisions.

THE STUDY AND RESEARCH DESIGN: AN OVERVIEW

Much remains to be learned about how physicians, nurses, and parents actually make life-and-death decisions in the nursery. For this reason, this research had three major objectives: first, to identify the major *criteria* parents and professionals use in making life-and-death decisions; second, to examine the decision-making *process,* or how participants communicate to arrive at life-and-death decisions; and third, to explore the influence of the hospital setting and the wider social and historical *context* on life-and-death decisions. Communication and context can best be studied by observing decisions directly, spending time in the nursery, and discovering the concerns of those who work in it. Because they allow the researcher to observe decisions as they are made, field research methods (participant-observation and interviewing) are ideally suited to studying the decision-making process and its social context.

This book is based on data collected in the course of sixteen months of field research in the intensive-care nurseries of two hospitals. I spent twelve months in the setting I call Randolph Hospital. Located in a demographically heterogeneous section of a large urban area, the Henry Maynard Randolph Hospital is part of a major medical school, is closely affiliated with a major university, and is commonly recognized as an elite institution.

The reputation of Randolph Hospital seems to permeate the entire institution. If neonatology may be characterized as medicine on the frontier, the Randolph Intensive-Care Nursery may be said to be on the frontier of that frontier. Several of its attending physicians are pioneers in the field, and discoveries made at the Randolph Nursery have become standard features in the armamentarium of contemporary neonatology.

The prestige of the nursery is apparent throughout its organizational hierarchy. At the top of this hierarchy are the nursery's five attending physicians, all of whom hold full-time university faculty appointments. Scientists as well as clinicians, the attending physicians alternate their clinical responsibilities in the nursery with research and teaching. During the months they are in charge of the nursery, the attendings (as they are called for short) are formally and legally responsible for all decisions concerning medical management, including life-and-death decisions.

Next in line are the five neonatology fellows, who have completed pediatric residencies and are training to become subspecialists in neonatology. During their rotations in the nursery, fellows perform a teaching and administrative role and are responsible for the nursery in the attendings' absence.

Routine clinical decisions and most diagnostic and therapeutic procedures are the responsibility of the pediatric residents and interns who rotate through the nursery. Admission to the pediatric residency program at Randolph is highly competitive, and most residents have trained at prestigious medical schools. Rotations in the intensive-care nursery are considered an important part of the clinical training of pediatric residents, who are required to complete at least four nursery rotations. The nursery rotations at Randolph are also considered to be among the most demanding, with the heaviest night-call schedules. Although staffing patterns vary considerably, the usual complement of physicians includes the attending physician, three residents, three interns, and, on occasion, one or two medical students.

The Randolph Nursery also employs one full-time and one part-time social worker, who help parents apply for insurance coverage and are formally charged with meeting the various "socio-emotional needs" of the families. The social workers conduct support groups with the parents, arrange for conferences with parents whose babies have died, and lead weekly social service rounds in which the nursery staff exchange information about the families.

Among the most important staff members are the forty-five to fifty intensive-care nurses (including two head nurses and a senior staff nurse). The nurses perform the critical functions of monitoring changes in infants' medical conditions and assisting in resuscitations. Randolph nurses actually perform some procedures usually done by interns, such as changing respirator settings. Like social workers, nurses maintain close contact with the families. Intensive-care nursing demands a high level of knowledge and technical skill and, for this reason, is often viewed as the vanguard of nursing specializations.

Even by the standards of intensive-care nurseries, the Randolph nurses are a highly educated group: all but one are registered nurses (R.N.s), and more than two-thirds hold baccalaureate (B.S.N.) nursing degrees.

The Randolph Nursery occupies one wing of a floor shared with the obstetrical delivery service. The domain of the nursery actually reaches to the "set-up room," located adjacent to the delivery room, which is equipped with sophisticated machinery designed to facilitate the immediate resuscitation of infants distressed at birth. The nursery itself, which has a bed capacity of twenty-two, is divided into three areas, each corresponding to a different intensity of care. The "high-intensive" room accommodates up to six of the most critically ill infants. Most of the babies are on respirators, in incubators, and require frequent biochemical tests to monitor changes in their precarious respiratory function. In the "low-intensive" room, some of the infants require some form of respiratory assistance but need less intensive monitoring. In the "intermediate-care" room, one can already begin to witness some perceptible signs of recovery: many of the infants are able to breathe with minimal or no assistance, and many have begun to feed on their own. Those patients who are no longer critically ill are sent to the "admit-recovery" area of the well baby nursery, where the nursery's physicians continue to follow them.

As one proceeds from room to room, the level of monitoring decreases, and the nurse-patient ratio decreases accordingly. For example, the nurse-patient ratio decreases from 1:1 in the high-intensive room to 1:6 in the intermediate-care room. In addition, the nursery includes a small isolation area for babies with infectious diseases, an office used by the head nurse, a tiny breast-feeding room, and a conference room. Ironically, the prestige of the Randolph Nursery is not reflected in its physical plant, for the nursery is plagued by the problems that attend a chronic lack of space. Physicians frequently find it difficult to locate an area in which they can confer privately with parents.

In 1968, following statewide regionalization of services for the newborn, the Randolph Nursery became a major referral center for a geographic area that spans half the state. Thus, the approximately 480 infants admitted annually to Randolph enter the nursery via two paths. About half are "inborn admissions," delivered in the hospital's obstetrical service, whose medical conditions range from the most routine to the most complex. The others are "outborn admissions," some born in nearby hospitals, others transported by ambulance or plane from outlying areas.

The patients who are outborn admissions fall into three major categories. First are those referred to the Randolph Nursery for critical care by secondary-care facilities that lack the requisite support technologies to treat these infants. The conditions of these infants range from "simple" respiratory distress syndrome to birth asphyxia or congenital anomalies. Second are infants referred for diagnostic procedures (e.g., cardiac catheterization) or evaluation by pediatric subspecialists. Third are those referred for pediatric surgical procedures that cannot be performed elsewhere. Many of these infants have congenital anomalies (e.g., intestinal malformations and heart defects) that require surgical repair.

In the past few years, with the proliferation of nurseries that are able to provide critical care (tertiary-care facilities), the Randolph Nursery no longer enjoys undisputed hegemony over referrals, and competition for patients among tertiary-care nurseries in the region has become rather intense. Consequently, the nursery's attending neonatologists have developed a complex web of delicate diplomatic ties with the hospital's pediatric surgeons (who perform procedures that can be done in few other hospitals) and pediatricians in the nurseries located in outlying areas (on whom the Randolph Nursery depends for referrals). It is also significant that there are considerable fluctuations in the Randolph Nursery census. In the winter months, the nursery depends largely on referrals from other hospitals, whereas in the summer months, the rate of inborn admissions rises, and some infants from other hospitals must be turned away.

Because the Randolph Nursery serves a wide-ranging geographic area, parents of sick newborns are an ethnically, economically, and occupationally diverse group: migrant farmworkers from rural areas, farmers and carpenters from the mountainous woodlands, physicians, psychologists, and other professionals, and parents from the urban ghettos. This diverse distribution creates a checkered pattern of financing. In the Randolph Nursery, services are financed through a combination of private insurance, Crippled Children's Services, and Medicaid. Owing to the state's rather ample financing of neonatal care through Crippled Children's Services at the time this study was conducted, most parents found that their babies' care in the nursery was financed by one or more of these third parties, although occasional—and very unfortunate—lapses did occur.

To provide a comparison, I conducted four months of fieldwork in the Special Care Nursery of General Hospital, a setting that contrasts sharply with Randolph in terms of its size and the social class composition of its patients. Located in another region of the same state, General Hospital is a large (over a thousand beds) acute-care hospital for the indigent, financed by a combination of federal, state, and local funds. Like Randolph, General Hospital is closely affiliated with a large medical school and serves as a teaching institution for medical students, residents, and nurses. It is situated in a poor area (although by no means the poorest) of a large metropolis. Like other public hospitals for the indigent, General Hospital's adult services suffer from overcrowding and an almost chronic lack of funds caused by the capricious vagaries of government financing. Residents who had completed their medical training at General related bleak anecdotes of adult patients overflowing into the halls of the wards.

The Special Care Nursery at General provides a striking contrast to the conditions that often obtain elsewhere in the hospital. It is located in one of the newer wings, which it shares with the obstetrical and gynecology service. It is equipped with the most up-to-date technology, and its parent conference room is spacious and well furnished. The nursery's attending neonatologists are actively engaged in research, some have national reputations, and all are closely involved in direct supervision and teaching. Perhaps the reputation of the head of the nursery, the sheer size of the nursery's patient population, and the steady influx of third-party payments spare the nursery from many of the pervasive problems that plague the adult services. However, even the Special Care Nursery is not impervious to the problems created by the formidable task of caring for large blocs of patients who are separated from the staff by the barriers of language and social class.

The obstetrical service at General Hospital is one of the nation's largest, having a delivery rate of approximately fifty live births each day (eighteen thousand annually). Presumably because of the association between high-risk pregnancies and poverty, many of these infants find their way into the Special Care Nursery, which is extremely large (forty to fifty beds). In contrast to the Randolph Nursery, virtually all the infants who enter the General Nursery are inborn admissions, delivered in the hospital's own obstetrical service. Faced with a volume of patients that already strains its bed capacity to the limits, the nursery cannot accept infants referred from other hospitals. This leads to one of the more fundamental and recurrent dilemmas that confront the General Nursery staff. Owing largely to a critical shortage of highly trained nurses in the area, the General Nursery can accommodate only five infants who require intensive care (i.e., who must be placed on respirators). So while the total bed capacity of the General Nursery is nearly twice that of the Randolph Nursery, the General Nursery has fewer than half the number of intensive-care beds. Faced with an unremitting pressure upon a limited number of intensive-care beds, the staff must make frequent triage decisions to transfer critically ill babies to other tertiary-care facilities in the region. Thus, the General Nursery is not a referral center, and the admission patterns and triage dilemmas that confront its staff differ dramatically from those at Randolph Hospital.

Babies are delivered in General's third-floor obstetrical service, and if they are deemed sufficiently ill to require additional care, they are admitted to one of three nurseries. The Newborn Intensive Care Unit (known as the NICU) has a bed capacity of five, maintains a 1:1 nurse-patient ratio, and is designed to accommodate those infants who are most critically ill. In the same large room is the Acute Care Nursery, designed for the care of twelve infants who no longer require ventilatory assistance (respirators). Separated by a hallway and a conference room is the Convalescent Care Nursery, which accommodates twenty-four infants who require the least intensive monitoring and care. As in the Randolph Nursery, the nurse-patient ratio decreases in each of the nurseries with the decreased intensity of the care provided. However, in contrast to the Randolph Nursery, each of the General nurseries constitutes an administratively separate unit. Although all are under the authority of the head of the nursery, each maintains a separate nursing staff with its own head nurse. In any given month, the medical staff of the NICU includes one full-time faculty member, one fellow, and two residents (interns do not rotate through the NICU). The Acute Care and Convalescent Care nurseries are managed by two large medical teams, each of which includes an attending, a fellow, three residents, and four to six interns (usually including two obstetrical interns). Because the nurseries are divided administratively, the continuity of care is sometimes compromised; as the babies recover, their parents are confronted with not only a changing cast of physicians, but an entirely new group of nurses as well.

Although the formal occupational hierarchies are identical in both nurseries, the staffing patterns in the General Nursery are somewhat more complex. In addition to the neonatologist who is the head of the nursery, the medical staff includes seven neonatologists who are members of the faculty. Five full-time faculty members head the NICU. However, because of the sheer volume of the patient population, the Acute Care and Convalescent Care nurseries are sometimes staffed by "outside attendings," neonatologists in the community who serve the nursery on a part-time basis. In addition to the residents who rotate through the nursery, there are five neonatology fellows, who tend to be quite closely involved in patient care. The nursery also maintains a program for training respiratory therapists, who are considered members of the "health care team." They participate actively in rounds and occasionally in life-and-death decisions.

The full-time nursing staff includes seventy-four nurses and three head nurses. All of the nurses who work in the NICU and all but one of the nurses in the Acute Care Nursery are registered nurses, many of whom have completed their training in the hospital's three-year diplomate nursing program. The NICU nurses have also completed a special program for critical-care nursing. However, of the thirty-two nurses who work in the Convalescent Care Nursery, more than half are licensed vocational nurses, and three are nursing assistants.

The staff of the nursery also includes one full-time social worker, a part-time social worker, and a full-time discharge planning nurse, who communicate and work with the families. Like the Randolph Nursery, the General Nursery has developed a set of procedures to mitigate some of the potentially disruptive consequences of neonatal intensive care for the families of critically ill infants. While the Randolph Nursery conducts parent support groups and conferences for parents whose babies have died, the General Nursery has developed the concept of discharge planning. A discharge planning team, consisting of a neonatologist, the social workers, the head nurses, and the discharge planning nurse holds weekly meetings and helps families plan for the future care of their babies.

Perhaps the most significant distinction between the two nurseries is to be found in the social class and ethnic composition of their patient populations. All the parents in the General Nursery are poor, and approximately 90 percent are Hispanic. Consequently, care in the General Nursery is financed almost exclusively through Medicaid and Crippled Children's Services. However, some of the parents are undocumented workers, who are occasionally reluctant to apply for funds that may in their view jeopardize their chances for attaining permanent residency and lead to detection by immigration authorities. One of the major dilemmas of the General Nursery is the communication barrier between the many parents who do not speak English and the many attendings, residents, and nurses who are conversant only with the rudiments of "hospital Spanish." Thus, members of the nursery staff rely heavily on the social worker, who also serves as an interpreter and participates in most of the conferences between staff and parents, including those in which life-and-death decisions are made.

I intentionally selected the Randolph and General nurseries to provide maximum contrast along the dimensions of size, referral patterns, and clientele. Each of these characteristics has a discernible effect on the life-and-death decisions made in both nurseries. I selected more than one setting to approximate a natural experiment that could illuminate the influence of specific features of each organization upon life-and-death decisions. Undertaking fieldwork in more than one setting enabled me to distinguish aspects of decision making that are unique in each nursery from those that are common to both and, in so doing, enhanced the generality of my conclusions.

The reader may ask—and with considerable justification—whether the nurseries that were studied are typical or representative of other newborn intensive-care units. Both the Randolph and General nurseries are variants of one type of newborn intensive-care unit: tertiary-care centers in teaching hospitals located in urban areas. It is reasonable to assume that the life-and-death decisions made in these nurseries would differ from, for example, those made in certain religious hospitals or in small secondary-care facilities located in rural areas. For example, secondary-care facilities characteristically do not face the dilemma of whether to remove infants from respirators (since their patients usually are not receiving ventilatory assistance). Instead, they confront the dilemmas of whether infants should be resuscitated, certain forms of care should be initiated, or patients should be transported to larger referral centers.

The professionals who work in the nurseries I studied probably exhibit more "permissive" attitudes toward nontreatment decisions than those in hospitals subject to close scrutiny or tight controls by religious groups or local communities. By the same token, smaller community hospitals might allow more latitude for negotiation between parents and family physicians than might obtain in teaching hospitals, in which the relationship between parents and physicians is apt to be more impersonal. However, it is significant that most newborn intensive care is delivered in tertiary or critical-care facilities. More important, by studying large nurseries, in which many patients are critically ill and in which patients exhibit a variety of medical conditions, it is possible to observe not only a greater number but a wider variety of life-and-death decisions than can be observed in smaller nurseries. Although it is impossible to generalize beyond the boundaries of the particular nurseries I studied, the types of decisions and dilemmas I encountered in the Randolph and General nurseries may be suggestive of those that take place in other similar intensive-care nurseries.

There is one sense, however, in which the Randolph and General nurseries may *not* be typical of newborn intensive-care units—a feature that was not unrelated to my entree into these settings. The staff of both nurseries attached considerable importance to ethical issues, and each nursery had developed a set of procedures for reaching life-and-death decisions, some of which may have been unique. For example, the Randolph Nursery had for some time been using a bioethicist to help the staff reach life-and-death decisions. Each month, the ethicist conducted regular "ethics rounds," in which the social workers, nurses, and physicians participated in a group discussion of a particular case that was considered problematic. Although ethics rounds were designed primarily for didactic purposes, they often became an arena in which life-and-death decisions were made when the attendings were present. In certain decisions (usually those considered to be highly significant or problematic), a formal conference was scheduled, and the ethicist was asked to serve as a consultant. In point of fact, however, most decisions were made in rounds at the patient's bedside or in less formal, impromptu conferences. (There were, of course, many variants of the process—as, for example, when decisions needed to be made at night, in urgency, or by specialists.) If the staff reached a decision to discontinue life support or not to perform a surgical procedure, a conference was held with the parents.

The General Nursery had introduced its own innovations into the decision-making process. Under the leadership of the head of the nursery and one of its neonatologists, the nursery was in the process of developing a written "protocol" that delineated the specific procedures to be followed when life-and-death decisions were reached. Briefly, these included: (1) obtaining complete diagnostic information before reaching a decision; (2) keeping the family and all staff informed of recent changes in a baby's condition; (3) holding a conference among members of the nursery staff to discuss an impending decision; (4) holding a conference with the parents to elicit their opinions; (5) placing a note by two attendings in the infant's chart if treatment was withdrawn or withheld; and (6) providing the infant with food, warmth, and social stimulation if life support was discontinued. When I was conducting this research, the protocol had not been adopted formally but was under consideration by the hospital's administration and was being discussed with some other neonatologists in the community. However, for some time, the staff had attempted to implement features of the plan on an informal basis. In fact, as part of my entree into the nursery, the head of the nursery asked me to ascertain whether the protocol was being carried out in actual practice.

The decision-making process in both nurseries shared some common features. When a decision not to resuscitate an infant or to discontinue life support was made, it was considered appropriate for the attending to place a note in the patient's chart. Both nurseries acknowledged that the attending physician bore the formal and legal responsibility for making life-and-death decisions and for this reason was the ultimate authority in deciding what was to be done. By the same token, life-and-death decisions were also considered "group decisions." Conferences were held whenever possible, at which residents and nurses could voice their opinions in an effort to negotiate a consensus. When a decision to terminate life support was made, parents were consulted and were encouraged to be with their babies when they died. These efforts to make the life-and-death decisions at least partly a collective enterprise are not confined to the two nurseries I studied. There is reason to believe that these features of the decision-making process have become part of the accepted practice of many other newborn intensive-care units following the Baby Doe controversies.[26]

What may have distinguished the two nurseries that were studied from many others were, first, the somewhat heightened "ethics consciousness" on the part of members of the nursery staff; second, the use of an expert in making life-and-death decisions (Randolph); and third, the attempt to formalize the process by constructing a protocol (General). However, these developments reflect larger trends within newborn intensive care (as well as other fields of medicine) to develop normative guidelines for reaching life-and-death decisions—that is, to

rationalize the process, in the sociological sense of the term. For this reason, by examining life-and-death decisions in the Randolph and General nurseries, I witnessed developments that would come to prevail in other newborn intensive-care units throughout the country.

My research activities in both nurseries proceeded along similar lines. Because life-and-death decisions are made infrequently and without advance notice, it was necessary to spend considerable time in the nurseries to be present when decisions were made. Each day I accompanied physicians on their daily rounds, not only observing many life-and-death decisions but also acquiring background information concerning patients who might later become the subjects of these decisions. I also spent considerable time in informal conversation with physicians and nurses, many of whom became my informants. In addition, I regularly attended events that were relevant to life-and-death decisions—for example, weekly social service rounds and ethics rounds (at Randolph), mortality review conferences, and formal decision-making conferences.

The purpose of this participant observation was twofold. First, it provided the context of life-and-death decisions. By participating with members of the nursery staff in the daily round of their activities, I attempted to acquire a sense of the circumstances of their work and their routine concerns. Second, I hoped to become familiar with the array of formal and informal activities that constituted the decision-making process. Under optimal circumstances, I could follow a particular life-and-death decision as it was discussed informally in the conference room, presented on daily rounds, debated in a formal conference, presented to parents, and (in cases in which the patient died) reviewed in a morbidity and mortality conference. In the Randolph Nursery, I obtained permission to tape-record a total of eight ethics rounds and conferences in which life-and-death decisions were made or discussed. When recording other conferences, I tried to approximate a verbatim transcription of the participants' discussions.

In an effort to draw more representative conclusions about the perceptions of members of the nursery staff than could be obtained through informant interviews, I conducted fifty-nine semi-structured, focused interviews with residents, fellows, and nurses. These interviews, which averaged about an hour in length and were tape-recorded, contained a series of general questions about life-and-death decisions; most important, seven actual life-and-death decisions were included in the interview schedule. Two major goals of the interviews were, first, to explore in considerable detail the values, beliefs, and modes of reasoning used by participants in life-and-death decisions and, second, to pursue theoretical leads that had been suggested in the course of observations. The interviews also served as a validity check, letting me know if my observations and perceptions were consistent with those of respondents. Finally, I examined the case records of all the patients in the General Nursery who were the subjects of decisions.

In the course of this research, I collected information (in varying degrees of exhaustiveness) concerning a total of seventy-five infants who were the subjects of life-and-death decisions—fifty in the Randolph Nursery and twenty-five in the General Nursery. Particularly in the Randolph Nursery, I was able to collect information concerning the major types of decisions and dilemmas encountered in neonatal intensive care: decisions to resuscitate infants at delivery, decisions to initiate life support or to undertake surgical repair of congenital anomalies, decisions to resuscitate infants whose hearts had stopped beating or who had stopped breathing, and decisions to terminate life-sustaining treatments.

The information that already exists concerning life-and-death decisions in neonatal intensive care has generally been obtained through large-scale sample surveys that ask physicians to comment on hypothetical dilemmas.[27] Although my methods do not allow for the large samples that can be studied by survey methods, my research strategies do have several advantages (the limitations of this research are detailed in Appendix 1 and Appendix 2). First, I examined actual decisions rather than hypothetical dilemmas. Second, I studied more than one participant in life-and-death decisions. This is not a trivial point, for although the attendings are the final authorities in life-and-death decisions, residents and nurses often initiate decisions and, in the course of debate, may influence the ultimate decisions. Third, the only way to capture the processes by which members of the nursery staff discuss, debate, or exchange their views is to employ a research stratagem that examines decisions directly.

THEMES OF THE BOOK

This, then, is a sociological study of life-and-death decisions in two intensive-care nurseries. Just as philosopher William Frankena explicated what is meant by the "moral point of view," I believe that it is important to explain what I mean by writing from a "sociological point of view."[28] The meaning of this term is far from self-evident, and a few explanatory comments will help to clarify the arguments that unfold in subsequent chapters. I also believe that it is important to be explicit at the outset about the premises and themes of this book because they provide the logical scaffolding for the arguments that follow.

A first theme is that *decisions are collective acts, not individual acts*. This point, while axiomatic to the sociologist, is a radical departure from much of the professional and public discourse on this subject. Bioethics, for example—whether deontological, utilitarian, or contractarian—assumes that life-and-death decisions are the actions of individuals. To be sure, participants bring their personal values, beliefs, and principles to the life-and-death decision. But at the same time, they must also debate with colleagues, answer to superiors, and interpret the law. The process by which the decisions are reached and the context surrounding them, no less than the principles of individuals, combine to shape the ultimate decision that is made. To write from a sociological point of view, then, demands an interactive model that treats decisions not as individual undertakings but as interactions between individuals. This book also has a hidden agenda, for it seeks to demonstrate the relevance of sociology to understanding moral and medical choices.

A second theme is that *people's decisions arise out of their location in the social structure*. Throughout this book, I show how the decisions of participants are shaped by the practical circumstances of their work. As both Rosabeth Moss Kanter and Eliot Freidson have noted, the lion's share of our days is consumed by the work process.[29] Yet we all too frequently fail to notice its impact on our lives. In the case of life-and-death decisions, we are inclined to assume that they are a "personal" matter and to situate them in the private sphere. This book challenges that assumption. A major argument is that members of the nursery staff, because of their different work experiences, develop varying views of the "facts" and conflicting conceptions of the right thing to do. For example, an infant who is likely to be severely disabled has a different social meaning for a nurse who sits at the bedside than for a physician whose contact with the baby is confined to technical interventions. Parents are somewhat outside the social structure of the intensive-care nursery, but, as I will argue, this is part of the problem.

A third theme is that *decisions are shaped by the social context in which they are made.* At one level of analysis, I argue that the organization of the intensive-care nursery as a work environment structures the perspectives of those who work within it. At another level, I argue that decisions within the nursery are shaped by institutional forces outside it. This point is also not always self-evident to those who make life-and-death decisions and to some who write about them. At the end of the book, I show how life-and-death decisions within the nursery are affected, in ways that are far from self-evident, by the allocation of resources in the society at large. This approach is sociological because I argue throughout the book that matters of the heart and crises of conscience are social activities anchored in a social context.

A final theme is that *much of what is wrong with life-and-death decisions is not the fault of the individuals who make them, but rather rests with the broader social context.* This theme is a corollary of the first and third points. When decisions are made that adversely affect the lives of all concerned—staff, parents, and patients—the temptation is to locate the source of the problem in the individual. This book will resist that temptation. It follows quite logically from this premise that if we wish to improve the quality of decision making, we must do more than change the behavior of individuals who make decisions. Rather, we should direct our analysis and interventions upward and outward toward the way the intensive-care nursery is organized and resources are allocated.[30]

Having described the scope and purpose of this research, let me say a few words about what this study is *not.* First, it is not a "total ethnography" of the newborn intensive-care unit, but rather a portrait of only a small segment of its social life. (Readers who wish to learn more about the culture and social structure of neonatal intensive care should consult Fred Frohock's *Special Care* and Jeanne Guillemin and Lynda Holmstrom's *Mixed Blessings.*)[31] My intent was to study only those decisions that would result in the life or death of an infant and in which participants discussed this outcome. Despite the intensity of emotion that was attached to these decisions, those who worked in the intensive-care nursery devoted only a fraction of their time to discussing these issues—the majority of their days being consumed by the many other patients who made claims on their attention. These other patients and their families were not the focus of this research. To be included in this study, an infant's condition must have been sufficiently severe for staff members to consider whether the patient should be treated. Several infants ultimately died; many faced the prospect of significant mental or physical handicap. This necessarily narrow choice of patients to be included in this study may mislead the reader to believe that the often tragic and problematic outcomes are "typical" of those encountered in the newborn intensive-care unit. In fact, the infants who were the subjects of life-and-death decisions constitute an exceedingly small proportion of the total number of patients in the intensive-care nursery. Members of the nursery staff routinely balance the occasional tragic situation against the many healthy infants who have recovered and joined their families. Readers are urged to do the same.

Second, this research was not undertaken by a physician, an obvious fact that is not without its theoretical and practical consequences. Particularly at the beginning of the research, I expended considerable effort to understand discussions among medical personnel, conversing among themselves in a highly specialized, coded vocabulary that I could hardly expect them to "translate" for my benefit. However, although the more arcane details of infant pathophysiology eluded my grasp, I believe I was able to comprehend the criteria—both medical and moral—upon which life-and-death decisions were based. If parents are able to participate effectively in life-and-death decisions—as indeed they are—so, too, sociologists who spend months in a field setting ought to be able to negotiate even the most recondite of medical realms. There were, however, some questions that my lack of medical training prohibited me from answering. For example, physicians who study life-and-death decisions are able to question whether medical judgments about particular patients are "correct" or "incorrect"—an issue that I, as a sociologist, was unable to address. However, by the same token, my training as a sociologist may have enabled me to "see" certain social features of life-and-death decisions that may not have been apparent to the physicians who made them. This, of course, is the usual warrant for the continued ventures of sociologists into the medical world.

Finally, this is not a study in biomedical ethics, in the strict sense of the term. My primary concern is to understand how life-and-death decisions are *actually* made, rather than to determine how they *ought* to be made. This distinction is, of course, much too facile. Just as the ethicist must come face to face with the actual empirical context of life-and-death decisions, so, too, the values of any social researcher influence the definition of the problem and the findings that are produced. This research is by no means value-free. Rather, this is a study in commonsense ethics, for my concern is with the modes of moral reasoning of ordinary people in everyday life. How a study of commonsense ethics can contribute to more formal and disciplined bioethical inquiry is a subject that is addressed in Chapter 2, in which I introduce the central arguments of the book, acquaint the reader with major approaches to decision making, and situate this study in its broader intellectual context. The chapter is theoretical, and readers may wish to return to it after reading the empirical materials in Chapters 3, 4, and 5.

CHAPTER 2

Theorizing About Life-and-Death Decisions

A Critical Review

The debates about life-and-death decisions began in the 1970s, not in the courts but in the scholarly journals. Even before the case of Baby John Doe transformed private dilemmas into a public controversy, writers in several disciplines had begun to ponder the problems of the intensive-care nursery. The work of these scholars had consequences that reverberated far beyond academic circles; indeed, many writers were to play a key role in shaping the public policies that affect decisions in the nursery today.

Life-and-death decisions have been examined from three perspectives. A first approach, bioethics, locates decisions in the individual conscience. A second perspective attempts to identify the norms and values at stake in life-and-death decisions and locates decisions in the collective conscience. A third perspective, the situational, shows how the immediate social environment shapes decisions. Each perspective contains a set of broad assumptions about the nature of decision making and moral action.

THE INDIVIDUAL CONSCIENCE PERSPECTIVE

As physicians face dilemmas for which the canons of medical training provide few guidelines, they often look to experts for guidance. Bioethicists are one group of experts who have assumed an influential role in developing policies for making life-and-death decisions. When

I refer to *bioethics,* I am using the term quite broadly to mean any attempt—whether by a physician, philosopher, or theologian—to examine the ethical principles on which decisions in medicine or the biological sciences are or should be premised. In other words, I am using the term to refer to a characteristic discourse rather than to a particular discipline or disciplines.

Most bioethicists have had training in ethics or moral philosophy. The field of ethics has been divided traditionally into two types of inquiry, each of which addresses different issues. Metaethics asks basic questions about the nature of moral discourse: whether, for example, ethical discourse induces emotions or prescribes conduct. Most bioethical analysis of newborn intensive care, however, has been written from the standpoint of normative ethics, or that branch of moral philosophy that concerns the values and principles that characterize right and wrong conduct. Normative ethics is itself loosely divided into two major orientations. Consequentialist or teleological ethics assumes that the morality of an act can be judged by reference to its consequences. This type of moral reasoning includes the utilitarianism of Jeremy Bentham and John Stuart Mill. By contrast, deontological or formalist ethics holds that there are rules and acts that have a transcendent moral validity apart from their consequences. Regardless of their particular intellectual orientation, ethicists examine and develop guidelines for moral conduct: that is, they attempt to arrive at rules, procedures, and methodologies of reasoning that determine whether actions are right or wrong.[1] The goal of ethics is not to describe how decisions are actually made, but rather to determine how they *should* be made. For this reason, bioethics is a venture into the realm of the elusive "ought."

Bioethicists are not only divided in their views, but, in addition, they have diverse visions of their own projects and professional roles. The more academically oriented philosophers view bioethical analysis as a theoretical enterprise and use decisions in medicine or biology as vehicles for examining classical issues in moral philosophy. Others use philosophical skills to clarify the concepts, precepts, and principles implicit in medical decisions. Still others have a more "applied" vision of the enterprise; following quasi-consultant roles, they attempt to develop principles and policies that can assist clinicians in reaching life-and-death decisions.

Bioethical analysis of newborn intensive care addresses the ethical principles on which decisions to treat—or not to treat—seriously ill newborn infants are or should be based. However, bioethicists are deeply divided over questions of what should be decided, which babies should be treated, and who should have the authority to make life-and-death decisions.[2]

"Restrictive" Policies

At one end of the continuum of opinion are writers who argue that all infants should be treated actively, except those already dying. Believing in an unqualified sanctity of life that extends to infants likely to survive disabled, these authors hold that all life is sacred, even the life of an infant who, in the words of Orthodox Rabbi Immanuel Jakobovits, "has teeth and tail like an animal."[3] One of the first and most articulate advocates of this position is Christian ethicist Paul Ramsey. Ramsey proposes a "medical indications policy" that treats potentially disabled and "normal" infants equally, a policy that is designed to compare treatments rather than infants. Under this policy, an infant with Down syndrome would, like any other infant, be entitled to receive treatments that are medically indicated. Ramsey, then, advocates providing medically necessary treatments for all infants, regardless of the severity of their disability. Even a baby with Tay-Sachs disease, born "destined to die," is entitled to full medical care up to the point at which the dying process has begun. Physicians are not obligated to *treat* a dying patient aggressively, however. They are obligated only to *care for* a dying infant and need not prolong the dying process.[4]

Ethics based on the sanctity of life was highly influential in shaping the policies of the Reagan administration. Pediatric surgeon C. Everett Koop, formerly surgeon general of the United States and a major architect of the Reagan administration's Baby Doe rules, believes, like Ramsey, that all infants who are not already dying should be treated aggressively. Koop believes that many of his medical colleagues are unduly pessimistic about the quality of life of infants with physical or mental disabilities, noting that "disability and unhappiness do not go hand in hand."[5] He also notes that disabled children can bring deeper meaning to the lives of others. All too often, he argues, physicians discriminate against disabled infants by asking *whether* to treat rather than *how* to treat.

Koop, Ramsey, and other advocates of this position are deeply disturbed by proposals to withhold treatment from newborn infants

on the basis of their anticipated quality of life.[6] Quality-of-life arguments, according to this view, erode our society's most fundamental
values about the equality of all human lives and discriminate against
the disabled. Many view abortion, decisions to withdraw or withhold
treatment from potentially disabled infants (sometimes called "infanticide" or "benign neglect of defective infants"), and euthanasia ("the
chosen death of the old, the infirm, and the unwanted") as part of a
widespread and destructive secular trend ("humanism") in Western
societies. Appealing to what is known as the "slippery slope" argument, these writers cite a 1949 article by psychiatrist Leo Alexander,
who participated in the Nuremberg trials, that appeared in the *New
England Journal of Medicine*. Alexander noted that genocide in Nazi
Germany began with the extermination of those viewed as "defective." The process started with an attitude, echoed in the euthanasia
movement, that there is such a thing as a life not worthy to be lived.
According to this logic, physicians who withhold treatment from
potentially disabled infants have taken a step onto a slippery slope,
setting in motion a process that may culminate in the death of all those
deemed undesirable.[7]

"Permissive" Policies

At the other end of the spectrum are advocates of more permissive
policies that allow infants to die under a wide range of circumstances.
Consider, for example, Australian ethicist Peter Singer, a founder of
the animal liberation movement. Singer has little sympathy for sanctity-of-life arguments, which, he suggests, are really arguments about
the sanctity of *human* life. If it is in fact consciousness that we value,
Singer comments in a highly controversial article, we might find that
members of other species—such as chimpanzees, dogs, cats, dolphins,
and whales, along with human adults—more closely resemble conscious beings than do newborn human infants. We value human
infants, Singer argues, because they are cute and appealing, much like
baby seals. But to insist that only the lives of human infants are sacred
is to commit a presumptuous kind of species-ism that reveres our own
species while devaluing others.[8]

Like several other philosophers, Singer is drawing a distinction
between genetic or biological personhood and personhood as a moral
concept. These writers offer another justification for letting infants
die: that the newborn infant, much like the embryo, is not a person

in a moral sense and for this reason does not have a right to life. Only persons can have rights—the most significant of which is the right to continue living. According to this argument, it is not enough to be a member of the species *homo sapiens* to qualify as a person in the moral sense of the word, but one must have other qualities as well. These writers then go on to list the prerequisites of personhood. For Australian philosopher Michael Tooley, personhood requires self-consciousness and a desire to continue existing. For philosopher Mary Ann Warren, the necessary qualities include consciousness, the ability to reason and communicate, and self-awareness. Above all, she believes that sentience, or the capacity to experience pleasure and pain, is the fundamental basis of all rights. For physician and philosopher H. Tristram Engelhardt, the cardinal attributes are self-consciousness and rationality. For Peter Singer, they are rationality, self-consciousness, and sentience.[9] While these definitions do not tell us precisely where to draw the line between persons and nonpersons, they suggest that most human adults and perhaps some animals are persons in the moral sense, whereas newborn infants clearly are not. Following this logic, since human infants are not persons, they do not have a right to life and for this reason need not always be treated.

Although these writers assert that infants are not full-fledged persons, they stop short of advocating killing babies indiscriminately. The strongest moral argument against ending their lives at whim is the high social value that most people accord to human infants. According to Mary Ann Warren, it is wrong to kill infants much as it is wrong to destroy natural resources or objects of art that give pleasure to others. According to H. Tristram Engelhardt, because newborns are persons in a social sense—that is, we attribute personhood to them in daily interaction—a decision not to save their lives requires serious moral justification. This justification might include the effect of a disabled child on family members and society's ability or willingness to care for infants.[10] But however compelling the arguments against killing infants, the act does not constitute the murder of another person.

The idea that human infants are not persons with a right to life has been highly controversial. Some observers object that the personhood standard is far too inclusive and permissive, since it applies to all newborn infants as a class and not merely to those with physical or mental disabilities. In the words of ethicist Robert Weir, personhood arguments "open the door to the *unlimited, indiscriminate termina-*

tion of an indeterminate number of newborn lives." Others object to personhood arguments because these suggest logical possibilities that contradict our deepest moral intuitions—for example, that someone who kidnaps and kills a baby has not committed murder. The personhood argument was imported into the nursery from the abortion debate, but some writers object to the idea that abortion and infanticide are morally equivalent acts. Still others argue that newborn infants are potential persons, and it is wrong to prevent them from realizing this potential. According to Canadian philosopher Eike-Henner W. Kluge, because infants have "constitutive potential," they are persons in the ordinary use of the term. In short, however deftly philosophers may spin the web of concepts and definitions, infanticide is in fact "the murder of persons."[11]

So far, I have discussed two justifications for not treating newborn infants actively: that the dying process should not be prolonged and that the infant is not a full-fledged person with a right to life. Still another justification for withholding life-saving treatment from newborns with serious physical or mental disabilities is based on their future quality of life—as well as the hardships they may create for their families and society. Several physicians who developed and publicized their decisions to withhold treatment have justified these policies on quality-of-life grounds. For example, pediatric surgeon John Lorber has developed one of the first selective nontreatment policies for babies with spina bifida to receive widespread publicity. Once an advocate of aggressively treating all babies with spina bifida, Lorber became convinced that "the pendulum has now swung too far . . . , [and] there are now many [infants] with dreadful handicaps who a short time ago would have died." On the basis of his clinical experience with 524 spina bifida patients in Sheffield, England, Lorber developed several prognostic criteria designed to identify infants who, if treated, would survive with serious physical handicaps. Lorber does not operate on infants who meet these criteria, but instead gives them analgesics and normal nursing care.[12]

Lorber's policy has been the subject of a heated debate in the British and American medical communities. Pediatric surgeon John Freeman, for example, is concerned about the fate of babies who go untreated. These infants, he argues, do not die quickly, but are likely to survive even more seriously disabled than they would have been if treated. Lorber's colleague at Sheffield, R. B. Zachary, suggests that, despite

Lorber's opposition to euthanasia, infants selected for nontreatment actually die of starvation because they are ostensibly fed on demand but are too heavily sedated to demand food. Ethicist Robert Veatch criticizes Lorber for committing the "technical criteria fallacy"—that is, for disguising value judgments about the kinds of lives worth saving beneath technical and medical criteria. While Lorber sometimes does treat his decisions as though they were based upon purely medical judgments, he occasionally provides ethical justifications, such as the suffering of severely disabled infants and "the disastrous effects on family life."[13]

Pediatrician Raymond Duff, whose open discussion of life-and-death decisions set the debate into motion, has published widely on the ethics of newborn intensive care, often in collaboration with his former colleague, A.G.M. Campbell. Duff and Campbell have advocated policies that would permit parents and "their professional advisers" to withhold life-saving treatment from infants with a wide variety of physical and mental defects—ranging in severity from acute brain damage and inability to survive infancy to spina bifida and Down syndrome. The last two conditions are moral gray areas, in which the family's willingness to care for the infant should be the deciding factor. Duff and Campbell believe that the most significant criterion is "damage to the central nervous system, especially the brain," and a level of brain function "insufficient to allow a personal life of meaning."[14]

Like Duff and Campbell, pediatric surgeon Anthony Shaw believes that parents should be allowed to make decisions on quality-of-life grounds. Shaw presents a rule of thumb that roughly describes how he makes life-and-death decisions: $QL = NE \times (H + S)$. That is, quality of life is a product of the infant's natural endowment and the contributions of home and society. Thus, lacking a natural endowment, an infant born without a brain would have no future quality of life, whereas the quality of life of infants with Down syndrome would depend partly on the contributions of their families and society.[15]

The policies of these physicians have been seriously criticized—and not only by pro-life advocates such as Paul Ramsey, who would "rather be charged with morally justifying first degree murder . . . than to add a feather's weight on the balance in favor of quality-of-life judgments." Some writers have disputed Shaw's and Duff and Campbell's broad definition of an unacceptable quality of life—a standard that would allow parents to end the lives of, for example, infants with Down syndrome, who have the ability to give and receive love. Still others point to a fundamental ambiguity in quality-of-life arguments: it is not clear whose quality of life is at stake and whose interests are being served. At times, quality-of-life advocates refer to the interests of the infant, but at other times, they also consider the interests of family members and society. The danger, these critics note, is that the former (the well-being of the infant) may become a thinly veiled rationalization for the latter (the well-being of others).[16]

"Moderate" Policies

For the reasons I have just mentioned, some ethicists have developed criteria that steer a middle course between highly restrictive policies that insist on the sanctity of all newborn lives and permissive policies that would allow parents wide latitude for discretion. Writers in this group would allow quality-of-life judgments to be made in very limited circumstances. Father Richard McCormick, for example, advocates a quality-of-life standard based on the infant's relational potential. Life, he suggests, is not an absolute value to be preserved in and for itself, but rather should be balanced against other values. McCormick argues that the physician is not obligated to preserve the life of an infant who lacks the potential for human relationships or whose capacity for relating to others is submerged in the very struggle for survival. This standard would apply to the anencephalic infant, but not to the infant with Down syndrome.[17]

Other writers propose standards based on the infant's pain and suffering. Basing his arguments on the medical maxim "Do no harm," physician and philosopher H. Tristram Engelhardt suggests that the physician should not prolong the life of an infant likely to have a short, painful, or seriously compromised existence. In such a case, continued existence would be harmful to the child, and the physician actually has a duty to withhold treatment. Developing this idea, bioethicists Albert Jonsen and Michael Garland suggest that intensive care does harm to infants who (1) are unable to survive infancy; (2) are unable to live without constant, severe, or intractable pain; and (3) are unable to "participate minimally in human experience," to respond to human attention, or to communicate with others.[18] These criteria, like the ones suggested by McCormick, would most likely draw the line between Baby John Doe, who had the ability to communicate, and Baby Jane Doe, who would probably have suffered considerably and been unable to relate to others.

"Do no harm," or the principle of nonmalificence, as it is called in ethics, appeals to many writers because it draws our attention to the well-being of the infant. Physician Norman Fost, ethicist Robert Weir, and the President's Commission for the Study of Ethical Problems in Medicine and Biomedical and Behavioral Research, in its 1983 report *Deciding to Forego Life-Sustaining Treatment,* have used this principle to develop an infant-centered standard that justifies nontreatment only when it is in the *infant's best interest.* To apply the best-interest standard is to weigh the benefits and burdens from the standpoint of the infant, while excluding from consideration the interests of family members or society.

Proposed as a compromise between pro-life and quality-of-life forces, the best-interest standard has many advocates. Because, I believe, it allows physicians to play a central role in determining the infant's best interest, this standard has gained the endorsement of the medical profession.[19] The best-interest standard also has its critics. Some feel that the standard is hopelessly vague and difficult to apply in practice. Others argue that trying to imagine the best interest of those unable to speak for themselves is a misguided project. Still others criticize this standard for excluding what they see as the legitimate interests of family members and society.[20]

To summarize, while most bioethicists agree that the dying infant should not be treated aggressively, some offer two other justifications for not sustaining an infant's life: (1) that the infant has not attained "personhood" (usually defined as self-consciousness) and (2) that the infant's future quality of life will be impaired. However, ethical opinion is sharply divided over where to place the hypothetical line of demarcation between an acceptable and unacceptable quality of life. Many criteria have been suggested, including multiple physical handicaps (Lorber), mental retardation (Duff and Campbell), intractable pain (Engelhardt; Jonsen and Garland), a short life span (Engelhardt; Jonsen and Garland), or the inability to participate in human relationships (Jonsen and Garland; McCormick). Writers also disagree about what should be done with infants who are not treated. For some authors (Singer; Tooley; Weir), "personhood" or "quality-of-life" considerations may be invoked to justify active euthanasia; for many other authors (Kluge; McCormick; Zachary), these grounds may be used only in a decision to withdraw or withhold life-saving treatment.

Who Should Decide?

The arguments I have just summarized are about the *substance* of life-and-death decisions—*what* should be decided. An equally controversial question is *procedural*—*who* should have the authority to make life-and-death decisions? Many physicians, such as Zachary, Lorber, Freeman, and Fost, believe that physicians, because of their superior knowledge, should have the authority in decision making. They argue that life-and-death decisions should be placed in the hands of physicians because parents are too emotionally involved, are incapable of comprehending the medical facts, are compromised by their own self-interest, or are likely to experience guilt after allowing a baby to die.[21]

For Raymond Duff, however, those who would place decisions in the hands of physicians are guilty of the worst kind of "medical paternalism." Like Shaw, Singer, Tooley, and Engelhardt, Duff believes that parents should have wide latitude for discretion in decision making because they must bear the ultimate consequences for life-and-death decisions. Ethicist Earl Shelp provides another argument for placing decisions in the hands of parents. Given the lack of consensus around life-and-death decisions in our morally pluralistic society, Shelp suggests, parents are the appropriate decision makers—provided that their decisions are reasonable.[22]

Many advocates of the best-interest standard would give hospital ethics committees a central role in determining whether treatment is in the infant's best interest, mediating conflicts between parents and physicians and conducting retrospective case reviews. This is the view of the members of the President's Commission in *Deciding to Forego Life-Sustaining Treatment*—a view echoed by the American Academy of Pediatrics and the Institute for the Study of Law and Medicine.[23] Still another view is that the state ("society") should regulate decisions to terminate care through legislation or governmental regulations—a position implicitly endorsed by the Reagan administration. In its Baby Doe rules and its final regulations implementing the Child Abuse Amendments, the Department of Health and Human Services did not permit either parents *or* professionals to make decisions contrary to governmental policy. In a gesture of compromise with the American Academy of Pediatrics, the Reagan administration provided guidelines for establishing committees. However, it insisted on calling them Infant Care Review Committees, rather than Ethics Committees—charging them with enforcing government regulations rather than debating ethical issues.[24]

Some believe that the state should have the final authority for decision making, since it would presumably bear a significant proportion of the financial burden, can represent the interests of the infant, and, unlike parents, is not compromised by possible conflicts of interest. Ethicist Daniel Callahan, however, has argued against casting the state in the role of "ideal observer," since emotional distance and detachment from the problem do not necessarily improve the quality of decision making.[25]

A SOCIOLOGICAL VIEW OF BIOETHICS

Despite dramatic differences in their views of life-and-death decisions, bioethicists share fundamental assumptions about the nature of ethical decision making and a common model of moral action. In brief, bioethics is dominated by an image of an individual autonomous moral agent who reaches decisions apart from social constraints. This model portrays physicians as able to contemplate complex problems free from competing demands on their time, untroubled by patients with perplexing prognoses, and unconcerned with the threat of medical malpractice suits, legal reprisals, and consequences to their own careers. For the sociologist, however, these problems are not mere obstacles to moral choices but the very stuff of which life-and-death decisions are actually made.

A first issue that eludes bioethicists is the many uncertainties that attend decisions in the nursery. Because their major concern is with ethical dilemmas, most bioethicists have emphasized those medical conditions in which these dilemmas are posed with crystalline clarity. For example, Down syndrome has received much attention in bioethics because it poses an important ethical dilemma with particular acuity: whether life-saving treatment may be withheld from infants whose major defect is subnormal intelligence. Other frequently discussed but statistically rare conditions are spina bifida, Tay-Sachs disease, and anencephaly. Although these abnormalities have posed problems legally, they are rarely encountered clinically. In this study, only one discussion concerned a baby with Down syndrome, a discussion that would not have taken place after the Baby Doe controversies. Only one decision involved a baby with spina bifida, and none concerned babies with Tay-Sachs disease or anencephaly. These conditions are congenital defects for which the prognosis is predictable within a certain range. But as Albert Jonsen and George Lister first remarked in 1978, many newborns treated in intensive-care units have a prognosis that is uncertain.[26] Among the subjects of this research, more than one-third of life-and-death decisions involved babies whose medical futures were considered uncertain or were debated by health professionals. These cases included premature infants thought to be on the frontiers of viability, infants having atypical clinical courses, infants with birth asphyxia or brain hemorrhages whose future potential was difficult to predict, and infants who had received innovative or experimental medical or surgical treatments.

Cases such as these raise an issue that ethical discussions have only begun to address: uncertainty in medical decision making.[27] Perplexing prognoses introduce other dilemmas into the decision-making process, for they demand that physicians consider what level of certitude is required to reach a life-and-death decision and by what standards certainty should be established. Bioethicists, then, have focused on cases that are ethically complex but prognostically simple. However, most decisions that clinicians must make are both ethically and prognostically complex.

Second, bioethicists have directed their attention to the *principles* at stake in life-and-death decisions rather than to the *process* by which decisions are reached. Consider, for example, ethical discussions that advocate informed consent. In order to achieve a truly informed consent, the physician must present medical information and treatment options clearly, and the patient must understand that information. However, research over a period of more than two decades on the sociology of doctor-patient communication has discovered a number of difficulties that may complicate the consent process. Professionals often unintentionally control the structure of the conversation to restrict the flow of information to the patient (in this case, the parents), often deflecting patient concerns. Studies of terminally ill patients, breast cancer patients, polio patients, and parents of mentally retarded children indicate that health professionals are sometimes reluctant to communicate openly in the face of tragic outcomes. When confronted with the parents of a disabled infant, professionals may use what Jeanne Quint has called "institutionalized practices of information control," such as speaking in generalities, using euphemisms, and allowing parents to take the lead in asking questions. Even without intending to do so, professionals may influence parents' decisions by presenting their own interpretation of the facts in the light of their own values and ethical philosophies. Parents may also selectively attend to and interpret what professionals say in the light of their own beliefs.[28]

Additional issues may complicate the communication process. For example, low birthweight is known to be associated with poverty, so parents and professionals must often communicate across the barriers of culture and social class.[29] Interpreters may compound these problems by reframing what has been said. Many ethical discussions treat "the parents" as a uniform category. However, research concerning abortion gives us reason to believe that parents in different socioeconomic situations may differ dramatically in their views of the social, economic, and psychic costs of having disabled children.[30] Gender as well as social-class differences may introduce complexities into the consent process: a baby's mother and father may each bring different values and interests to the life-and-death decision. If parents disagree, whose wishes should prevail? Since the consequences of having a disabled child may vary according to the variety of social situations in which parents find themselves, it may be inappropriate to treat "the parents" as a single social and moral category, as is often the case in ethical discussions of life-and-death decisions.

In short, it may be difficult to achieve informed consent without also knowing something about the process by which parents are informed and their consent obtained. Until we know about the social dynamics of communication between parents and professionals, informed consent is likely to remain an elusive ideal rather than a practical reality.

Bioethicists, then, direct our attention to ethical principles but deflect our attention from the decision-making process. This limitation is due in part to the decision of some ethicists to focus on a single decision maker—usually the physician, less often the nurse.[31] This focus implies that the actor reaches decisions alone, apart from the influences of others. But the life-and-death decision is a complex social activity that embraces several participants—attending physicians, interns and residents, nurses, and parents—each of whom may have very different values, interests, beliefs, and ethical principles. Although senior physicians have the most authority in life-and-death decisions, they rarely act alone. Particularly in recent years, nurseries throughout the United States have tried to collectivize the decision-making process by incorporating other members of the health care team. For this reason, medical rounds, case conferences, ethics committee meetings, and conferences between parents and professionals are all arenas in which different, and often conflicting, points of view are negotiated in a process of reciprocal social influence. To this extent, decisions are not the exclusive prerogative of a single actor, but rather arise out of the interactions between participants.

This leads to my third and final point: many discussions of the ethics of neonatal intensive care individualize the decision-making process, obscuring not only the way decisions are made but also the social context in which they take place. A major feature of that social context is the organization of the intensive-care nursery as a work environment. Life-and-death decisions arise out of the negotiations of decision makers, but these participants do not bargain with equal resources. Hospitals are hierarchical settings that allocate different resources to health professionals with which to impose their views on others and influence the probabilities that some views may prevail. Nurses and house officers who disagree with the decisions of attending physicians may choose to defy them, but in so doing, they face possible repercussions on their careers. Attending physicians, too, contend with the possible consequences of reaching decisions that may be at odds with the views of influential colleagues, hospital policies, or the law—consequences that bioethicists rarely discuss. The fact that decisions are a matter of politics as well as principles does not mean that bioethics should abandon its traditional concerns in favor of purely pragmatic ones. Rather, new ethical issues emerge, such as obedience to authority, that can be incorporated into bioethical analysis.

While the set of power relations in medical organizations does not determine the way individuals will act, it does limit the options of decision makers.[32] It also structures the consequences of engaging in a particular course of action. To the extent that actors predict the consequences of their decisions and take these predictions into account, it is accurate to speak of organizational constraints upon decision making.

Encounters between parents and professionals are also influenced by the organizational context in which they take place.[33] Consider, for example, a nursery that delegates responsibility for communicating with parents to various staff members. Professionals may hold different opinions about a life-and-death decision, leaving parents confused by conflicting information.

In sum, many ethical discussions rely on what, from a sociological vantage point, appears to be an idealized vision of decision making in which both the medical and social dimensions have been simplified. Many writers assume that moral choice rests exclusively with the individual moral agent, who reaches decisions apart from institutional constraints. Life-and-death decisions, however, are not merely matters of individual conscience but take place in the context of organizations, institutions, and power relations. This fact challenges bioethicists to create new models that examine not only the principles in life-and-death decisions but the process by which they are reached and the social context in which they take place.

THE COLLECTIVE CONSCIENCE PERSPECTIVE

In contrast to bioethicists, sociologists examine how medical decisions are actually made rather than how they should be made. A major contribution of sociology to our understanding of the medical world is the discovery that medical decision making is a fundamentally social process. Sociological research has challenged what until recently was the conventional wisdom: that a physician's decision to diagnose and treat is based exclusively on a straightforward evaluation of a patient's medical signs and symptoms. Sociological studies call attention to the many social considerations brought to bear on medical decisions.

Sociologists who have approached medical decision making from the collective conscience perspective have emphasized that decisions are governed by social as well as medical norms. This approach takes as its point of departure Emile Durkheim's insight that occupations, like all social groups, develop shared beliefs, norms, and values—a collective conscience—that powerfully affect individuals.[34] This cultural perspective views decisions as the product of consensual norms and values, transmitted through a process of socialization. The collective conscience approach attempts to identify the norms governing medical decision making and to relate them to broadly based cultural values in the larger society—its collective conscience.

According to this view, the traditional norm governing medical decision making has been one of aggressive, active intervention. As the eminent sociologist Talcott Parsons pointed out, this activity bias of the physician is resonant with the cardinal American virtues of activism, worldliness, and instrumentalism.[35] Faced with a life-and-death decision, a physician would be expected to decide in favor of life and to summon the forces of scientific knowledge and technical skill in an unending battle with illness and death. Thomas Scheff's discussion of the rules of medical decision making provides a portrait of the active physician.[36] Drawing largely on observations of psychiatric screening and the results of X-rays of patients with tuberculosis, Scheff demonstrates that medical diagnosis and treatment decisions are premised on a decision rule to diagnose and treat illness in cases of doubt or ambiguity. Based on a presumption of innocence, this medical decision rule, "When in doubt, diagnose and treat," sharply contrasts with the legal decision rule, "Presumed innocent until proven guilty." Viewed from the collective conscience standpoint, medical decision making has been characterized by norms and decision rules that dictate active intervention.

Beginning in the 1970s, however, studies that explored decisions to use new medical technologies suggested that this activist ethic has been undergoing a critical reexamination by physicians. Renée Fox and Judith Swazey's *The Courage to Fail* examines the impact of new medical technologies on medical practice from the standpoint of the research physician. In this landmark study of heart transplants, kidney transplants, and dialysis, the authors show that these highly experimental technologies created new ethical dilemmas for research physicians, since there were no established norms and guidelines to help them make difficult moral choices.[37]

This problem was most apparent in the Seattle Kidney Center, a pioneering institution in the development of chronic dialysis. When dialysis was first developed, it was a costly and scarce resource that very few patients could receive. Besieged by desperate applicants who outnumbered the few available dialysis machines, physicians were forced to develop new criteria to decide who should live. The lifeboat problem, a classical conundrum in philosophy, had become a reality. The original committee of community representatives charged with selecting dialysis candidates displayed a "middle-class bias," favoring the married, those patients most compliant with professionals, and those seen as having the most social worth as measured by middle-class norms. Following this logic, a married, male corporate executive would be more likely to live than, for example, an unmarried mother on welfare. So biased was this screening process that it was ultimately turned over to professionals, who based their decisions on an individualized assessment of each patient's social, psychological, and clinical situation.

Fox and Swazey suggest that biomedical technologies create new dilemmas and types of decisions for which aggressive intervention may not be appropriate. Elsewhere, Fox argues that the popular and professional movement for "death with dignity" signifies that contemporary medicine is moving away from an ethic grounded in the unconditional sanctity of life to one based on the quality of life, and that this trend reflects major shifts in cultural assumptions about health and illness in American society.[38]

Among the most sophisticated studies of life-and-death decisions, Diana Crane's 1975 survey, *The Sanctity of Social Life,* attempts to identify some of the social norms that have emerged. Crane concludes that the criterion physicians use to make life-and-death decisions is the patient's social potential or ability to perform future social roles. Following an experimental-survey design, Crane examined life-and-death decisions in the medical specialties of general surgery, neurosurgery, pediatrics, and pediatric heart surgery. Physicians in these specialties completed questionnaires describing hypothetical patients and were asked whether they would employ supportive, diagnostic, or heroic measures. The cases were constructed to contrast along two dimensions: whether the patient could be saved and whether the patient would be physically or mentally damaged. Crane then compared responses to the questionnaires with information abstracted from case records, which she viewed as largely indicative of actual treatment decisions. Both the survey responses and the case records confirmed her central hypothesis: that physicians, including pediatricians, were more likely to treat a "salvageable" infant aggressively than an "unsalvageable" one. They were also more likely to save the life of an infant with a physical disability (spina bifida) than one with a mental disability (Down syndrome). Crane concludes that life is no longer defined biologically. Rather, she suggests, a new social definition of life, one based on the patient's capacity for social interaction, has emerged.[39]

During the late 1970s, several surveys of pediatricians and pediatric surgeons supported Crane's conclusions that new norms were emerging. A 1976 survey of San Francisco physicians by Helen McKilligan, a 1977 national survey of pediatricians and pediatric surgeons by Anthony Shaw and his colleagues, and a 1977 survey of Massachusetts pediatricians conducted by I. David Todres and his colleagues showed that physicians are generally willing to withhold life-saving treatment on quality-of-life grounds.[40] For example, when asked whether they would save the life of a baby with Down syndrome and an intestinal obstruction, between 50 and 65 percent of the pediatricians in these surveys said they would withhold life-saving surgery when parents did not want the baby to be treated.

However, surveys conducted by Betty Wolder Levin and Jeanne Guillemin and her colleagues in the midst of the Baby Doe controversies suggest that aggressive intervention once again became the norm in the 1980s.[41] In the study by Guillemin and her colleagues, 73 percent of physicians would operate on a baby with Down syndrome and an intestinal obstruction in spite of parental objections. In the study by Levin, 87 percent of the respondents (physicians, nurses, and other health professionals) would perform surgery for an intestinal defect on a similar patient. However, only 59 percent of her respondents would perform open-heart surgery on an infant with Down syndrome. This suggests that the quality-of-life ethic may still obtain when infants with Down syndrome require more complicated procedures. A third survey of neonatologists, conducted by Loretta Kopelman and her colleagues after the 1984 Child Abuse Amendments, found that many respondents felt constrained by government regulations, but they still were willing to make life-and-death decisions.[42]

We must be cautious in interpreting the findings of the attitude surveys I have just mentioned because they use largely indirect measures of treatment decisions—that is, physicians' responses to questionnaires. Such questionnaires, in which physicians are asked to comment on hypothetical dilemmas, evoke responses that are suggestive, but not indicative, of decisions in actual practice. Case records, the second source of data, are retrospective accounts of decisions, often written with an eye to the hospital administration and the law. Particularly in view of the highly charged legal climate surrounding life-and-death decisions, the relationship between resolving hypothetical dilemmas and making actual decisions is an open question.

Using both survey and ethnographic methods, Betty Wolder Levin attempts to identify the culturally specific models members of the nursery staff use in reaching life-and-death decisions. Unlike most studies of decision making, which address only the patient's prognosis, Levin proposes a more complex model in which physicians balance assessments of treatments against assessments of patients. Patients were categorized according to their quality of life, the degree of certainty about their prognosis, the nature of their critical condition, and their social value. Treatments were categorized according to their aggressiveness, their ordinary or extraordinary nature, whether they were withheld or withdrawn, and whether they involved active or passive euthanasia. Using this model, members of the nursery staff would, for example, withdraw treatments closer to the extraordinary end of the continuum when faced with an infant with an uncertain prognosis. Levin suggests that this two-dimensional schema, in which physicians balance treatments against patients, more accurately depicts the cultural categories used in life-and-death decisions.[43]

While useful in revealing the norms and values at stake in life-and-death decisions—norms and values that may not be apparent to those who make them—the collective conscience approach shares some of the limitations of bioethical analysis. With the exception of Levin's research, these studies emphasize those conditions in which the patient's prognosis is known or predictable. Usually, only one decision maker—the physician—is studied. And, as in bioethics, the focus is on the principles in life-and-death decisions (in this case, social norms and values) rather than the process and social context of decisions. The collective conscience perspective is useful in identifying the cultural norms and values in life-and-death decisions but less useful in examining the social relationships and organizational realities in which these decisions are embedded.

The collective conscience approach suggests that physicians began to question the norm of active intervention in the 1970s but that the sanctity-of-life ethic began to resurface in the 1980s. However, this perspective does not account sociologically for these transformations.

Moreover, in the course of my research, a number of events occurred that could not be easily explained in terms of either the individual conscience or the collective conscience approaches, leaving several questions unanswered. Why, for example, were babies with ostensibly similar prognoses perceived very differently by health professionals? Furthermore, since these babies were similar in their prognostic (and hence their ethical) parameters, why was the decision making in each case so very different? What could account for perceptible differences in the decisions of physicians and nurses? Why were the nurses so frequently the most willing to withdraw life support and the first to pressure the attending physician to hold a decision-making conference? The answers to these questions, to be discussed in later chapters, had little to do with either the norms or values underlying decisions, but rather concerned the politics and sociology of the intensive-care nursery. Neither the individual conscience approach nor the collective conscience approach, however, speaks to these issues.

THE SITUATIONAL PERSPECTIVE

A third approach—the situational—is closer to the one I use in this book. This perspective uses ethnographic data to examine directly the decision-making process and the social circumstances surrounding medical decisions. Those who write from a situational perspective draw upon a very different conception of behavior—and for this reason have a very different model of decision making—than do those who write from a collective conscience standpoint. Unlike the collective conscience approach, which views human action as resulting from a set of internalized norms and values, the situational perspective emphasizes that actors respond to the pressures of the immediate environment. In other words, its approach to decision making is situational rather than dispositional. Medical decision making emerges as a social process, influenced by such factors as the patient's social situation, the hospital setting, the treatment philosophies of physicians, and communication between patient and practitioner.

Several detailed ethnographic accounts of decision making place the social aspects of medical decisions in sharp relief. In a participant-observational study of a tuberculosis sanitarium, Julius Roth found that professional decisions to release patients were based not only on the patients' physical condition at the time of release, but also on their ability to bargain strategically with physicians.[44] This finding suggests that the relationship between patient and practitioner is a major factor in medical decision making.

Two seminal studies of terminally ill patients suggest that professionals base their life-and-death decisions on patients' perceived social worth. In an observational study of terminally ill patients, Barney Glaser and Anselm Strauss conclude that younger and more affluent patients—that is, those perceived as having more social value—received more aggressive intervention from staff and more vigorous efforts at resuscitation. The death of such patients is viewed as a significant "social loss" to their families and occupations. In an ethnographic study of private and public hospitals, Sudnow concurs that those patients the staff perceived as able to contribute to society were more likely to be treated actively. Conversely, those perceived as having less social worth—the old and the deviant (drug addicts, alcoholics, and prostitutes)—were less likely to be resuscitated.[45]

Social scientists have begun to examine newborn intensive-care units from a situational standpoint. Jeanne Guillemin and Lynda Holmstrom's work is the most comprehensive study of neonatal intensive care. Their *Mixed Blessings* is an ethnography of neonatal intensive-care units that examines how patients are referred to nurseries, how they are treated, and where they go when they are discharged. As is evident from the title, the authors view neonatal intensive care as a "mixed blessing," costly in both economic and social terms to society and to the families served by the units. Two important chapters analyze the organizational factors that lead to aggressive intervention and those that exclude parents from the nursery's social life. The authors also provide brief comparisons with neonatal units in Holland and England.[46]

Another study, by Anthony Rostain, provides a nuanced discussion of the negotiations between parents and staff in life-and-death decisions. Rostain also describes the complex influences on these negotiations, including the leadership style of attending physicians, the strains among team members, and the relationship that develops between staff and parents.[47]

By calling attention to the features of the social situation that influence diagnosis and treatment decisions, the situational approach presents a sophisticated view of decision making. This approach examines the views of a number of decision makers. Ethnographic methods provide more detailed, more direct, and richer descriptions of decision making than those provided by bioethical analysis and the large-scale survey. However, these ethnographic accounts would be enhanced by the use of transcribed conversations, which would capture treatment decisions "in flight," allowing readers to interpret the materials for themselves. Finally, the situational approach is often characterized by a lack of systematic theorizing. Moreover, with the exception of Guillemin and Holmstrom, the authors rarely combine microsocial analysis of everyday social interaction with analysis of larger social structures. How, for example, does the decision making of health professionals in hospitals, clinics, and tuberculosis sanitaria relate to the social organization of these institutions? What does the social organization of these settings tell us about the character of health care in contemporary America? Because of these unanswered questions, ethnographic studies ultimately leave the reader with accounts of practices in specific organizations and fall short of providing more general explanatory models of decision making.

APPROACHES TO DECISION MAKING:
AN ANALYTIC SUMMARY

Despite their diversity in discipline, theoretical goals, and methodological orientations, the three major approaches to medical decision making I have reviewed share several common features. At the risk of some oversimplification, it is possible to classify these approaches along two dimensions: (1) whether the perspective focuses on the principles underlying life-and-death decisions or on the processes by which they are reached and (2) whether the perspective describes and analyzes decisions in medical settings or seeks to provide more general explanations. By combining these two dimensions—the analytic focus and the goal of theorizing—it is possible to create a typology of approaches to decision making, as represented schematically in Figure 1.

Both the individual conscience and the collective conscience perspectives emphasize the principles underlying life-and-death decisions rather than the process by which they are reached or the context in which they take place. For the bioethicist, these principles are ethical ones ("do no harm," "humanhood"), whereas for the normative sociologist, these are the consensual norms and values on which decisions are based. Both approaches have common limitations: a

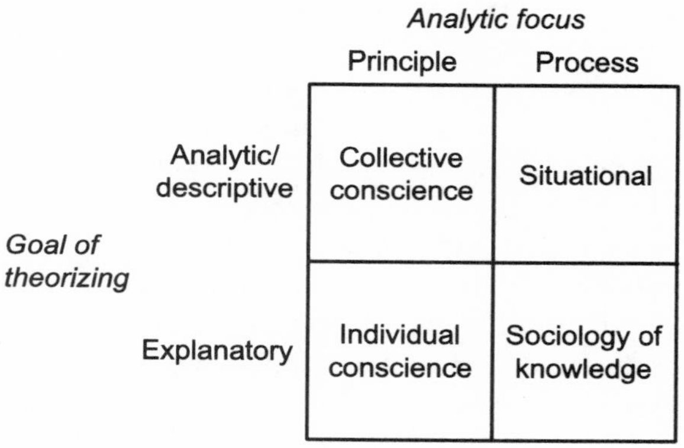

| | | *Analytic focus* | |
		Principle	Process
	Analytic/ descriptive	Collective conscience	Situational
Goal of theorizing			
	Explanatory	Individual conscience	Sociology of knowledge

Figure 1. Approaches to decision making

tendency to focus on cases in which the prognostic parameters have been simplified and a tendency to examine life-and-death decisions from the standpoint of a single participant.

As I have argued, this focus on principles—to the exclusion of process and context—creates a somewhat idealized image of decision making. In each case, significant information is omitted—information that concerns the interaction, the set of power relationships, and the organizational and institutional context in which life-and-death decisions are embedded.

There is, however, a major distinction between the individual conscience and the collective conscience perspectives. On the one hand, bioethicists seek to develop general explanatory models of decision making, such as deontological or teleological theories. On the other hand, sociologists writing from a collective conscience perspective emphasize "thick description" of norms and values and do not attempt a general explanation that accounts for how physicians come to adopt a particular stance, such as the "quality-of-life ethic," or how the norm of aggressive intervention comes to be transformed.[48]

The situational approach provides more detailed portraits of the decision-making process and examines the perspectives of more than one participant. This perspective's major contribution is its discovery of the many organizational factors brought to bear on life-and-death decisions, such as the negotiation between patient and practitioner and the patient's social worth. However, like sociologists who write from a collective conscience standpoint, many situational sociologists do not develop a theoretical framework that integrates their findings with more macrosocial explanations of medical organizations and institutions.

The fourth approach, which I use in this study, is that of the sociology of knowledge. In contrast to the individual conscience and collective conscience approaches, a sociology of knowledge approach assumes that life-and-death decisions are tied to the set of relationships in which they are embedded and the social circumstances that surround them. By examining the views and perceptions of several participants, this approach provides a more complex but less idealized model of decision making. Like situational studies, the sociology of knowledge approach focuses primarily on the process by which decisions are reached rather than on collectively held norms and values, but it relates situational and interpersonal factors to medical organizations and institutions—that is, it combines microsocial and macrosocial levels of analysis. In so doing, this approach attempts to go beyond analytic description and to provide more general explanations of decision making.

AN ALTERNATIVE PERSPECTIVE

This book approaches life-and-death decisions in newborn intensive care from the standpoint of the sociology of knowledge, an approach that relates these decisions to the social context in which they take place. The sociology of knowledge is part of a larger tradition in sociological inquiry. Sociologist Karl Mannheim may be credited with introducing the phrase into the sociological lexicon in *Ideology and Utopia*. However, the term has been used to embrace a highly diverse collection of classical and contemporary theories, ranging from Karl Marx's analysis of the Hegelians in *The German Ideology* to the more phenomenological approaches of Alfred Schutz, Peter Berger and Thomas Luckmann, and Dorothy Smith.[49]

The sociology of knowledge is not in itself a theory but rather an approach common to several theories. While writers in this tradition relate ideas and belief systems to a social context, they differ in the particular contexts they choose to examine, and hence in their units of analysis, which range from historical epochs to contemporaneous classes and economic strata, to occupational groups within organizations, to texts produced by bureaucracies.[50] What is common to the various "sociologies of knowledge" are three basic themes: (1) ideas about the world are relative to particular times, places, and social groups; (2) ideas are viewed as socially derived from the practical interests of these groups; and (3) the interests of a social group arise out of its position in a larger social structure.

While hardly new to sociology, this perspective has rarely been applied to the study of medical settings and has not been used in the study of medical decision making. A notable exception is Eliot Freidson's social construction of illness, developed in *Profession of Medicine*. Among this work's many contributions, one is most relevant to this book: Freidson shows that physicians' decisions are shaped by the practical circumstances of their work. For example, he distinguishes between first-line medical practitioners, who are selected by the patients themselves (client-dependent practices), and those specialties and settings in which physicians rely on their colleagues as a source of referral (colleague-dependent practices). In client-dependent practices, physicians are likely to provide treatments oriented to the preferences of their patients. In colleague-dependent practices, physicians are oriented to the approval of their colleagues rather than to the wishes of their patients. By making the work environment the centerpiece of his analysis, Freidson reveals that the social organization of medical practice profoundly affects medical decision making.[51]

I examine the ways that one set of ideas and belief systems—those brought to bear on life-and-death decisions—is shaped by a particular social context—the social structure of the intensive-care nursery. The sociology of knowledge approach, as used in this book, makes several assumptions about the nature of decision making.

Decisions as Multimeaning Transactions

A sociology of knowledge approach assumes that the participants in any decision do not have "objective," all-embracing views of reality, but rather perceive it largely from the vantage point of the specific social situations in which they find themselves. The social situations of participants influence not only their sense of the "right" course of action but the "facts" they select as relevant, and hence what they choose to designate as "data." The term *ideology* has often been used to refer to a self-justifying view of reality, cloaked in an ostensible objectivity. I use the term *treatment ideology* to denote any partial view of reality, hoping thereby to purge the term of its pejorative connotations. This book explores how physicians and parents apply these selective but sincere points of view in assessing the futures of critically ill infants and in assigning meaning to those prognoses.

Decisions as Interactional Emergents

More is implicated in decisions than multiple but static perceptions of reality. Perspectives are not merely the private property of participants. Rather, participants in decisions communicate with one another, debate their respective points of view, and attempt to influence one another. Informal discussions, formal case conferences, and conferences between parents and professionals are arenas in which this negotiation process takes place. I adopt an interactive model that views decisions not as individual undertakings but as the results of interactions among individuals. I also use a research strategy that examines these conversations directly.

Decisions as Organizational Products

Like many other decisions, life-and-death decisions take place within the context of organizations. My sociology of knowledge perspective assumes that the work environment—the social organization of the teaching hospital and the newborn intensive-care unit—creates particular pressures and problems for the professionals who work in them and shapes their decision making. Complex organizations in general, and medical organizations in particular, influence life-and-death decisions in several significant ways.

First, they allocate very different information to the participants that influences the knowledge each brings to the life-and-death decision. For example, experienced neonatologists can draw upon a vast reservoir of clinical experience, while nurses can draw on knowledge based on direct contact with infants and parents. This book examines how these different sources of knowledge shape the decision making of professionals.

Second, hospitals, as "advisory bureaucracies," allocate different resources to decision makers, thereby creating probabilities that the views of some will prevail. Medical knowledge is, of course, one such resource. Other resources include the relative authority and autonomy of occupational groups in the medical division of labor and the relative ability of groups to impose sanctions.[52]

Third, organizations structure the possible consequences that ensue from engaging in a given course of action. Because decisions take place within a framework of power relationships, health professionals who consider reaching decisions at variance with the wishes of influential colleagues and superiors must contend with the potential consequences of these decisions. While these consequences do not entirely determine how individuals will act, they do influence the probabilities that a certain line of action will be chosen.

Finally, organizations create commonalities of interest and occupational subcultures. Each group of workers confronts common problems posed by the work environment. It is the nurses, for example, who must contend with working in an understaffed nursery when its beds are full. Moreover, to the extent that members of each group communicate informally with one another, they may develop a common set of perceptions of a particular infant and a common perspective on decision making.

Decisions as Historical Products

Life-and-death decisions are influenced by developments outside the confines of the intensive-care nursery. Shifting legal rulings, changes in the focus of medical education, articles in the mass media, and public policy pressures toward cost containment—to name a few of the more obvious developments—combine to create a wider climate in which decisions must be reached. Less obvious, but no less significant, is the impact on life-and-death decisions of public policy decisions affecting resource allocation outside the nursery.

A sociology of knowledge perspective has several advantages over other approaches to decision making. First, it enables us to account for patterned variations in the decision making of occupational groups. By examining the work environments of doctors, nurses, and other health professionals and the dilemmas they confront, we can better understand the often conflicting points of view that each group brings to the life-and-death decision. Second, a sociology of knowledge perspective offers a view of decision making that is consummately sociological. It directs attention to features of the social context that shape decision making and eliminates the need for individual psychological explanations. Third, this perspective provides an analysis of decision making that is in many ways less personally judgmental than other perspectives. Because it calls our attention to the very real pressures parents and professionals face, we are less likely to account for unfortunate outcomes on the basis of the "unethical behavior" of individuals.

However, at this point it is important to raise a significant cautionary note. Some writers depict a sociology of knowledge approach as either a narrow, "debunking" tradition in sociology or one that is both reductionistic and structurally deterministic. The sociology of knowledge has on occasion assumed a "muckraking" tone in which the omniscient sociologist reveals the biases and group interests lurking beneath the actor's veneer of objectivity and altruism. Without plumbing the depths of this epistemological quagmire, suffice it to say that I try to avoid assuming a posture of omniscience, and I attempt, where relevant, to discuss how my own values, as actor and researcher, have structured my observations and conclusions. I also assume that the interests of professional groups and parents are more often than not legitimate attempts to come to grips with very real and pressing structural dilemmas.

The second criticism of the sociology of knowledge—that of structural determinism and reductionism—is at once more significant and more difficult to confront. It is said, not the least by students of moral philosophy, that a sociological approach promulgates a view of decision making that underestimates the role of the moral values that participants bring to decisions, thereby reducing conscious, free choice to social constraint and obscuring the moral responsibility of individuals. Some may also argue that a sociology of knowledge approach is deterministic, overemphasizing the role of social structure and underemphasizing individual action or agency.[53]

The point of this study is not to deny the importance of the values and ethical principles that actors bring to any decision—which may be acquired from the family, the media, professional training, or any other agency of socialization—but rather to call attention to the role of the social structure of the newborn intensive-care unit in shaping the decisions of participants. Ultimately, this book undoubtedly underestimates the significance of transcendent values and ethical principles. But an extensive literature that analyzes the ethical principles of individuals already exists. By proposing a more broad-based, sociologically informed model of decision making, I attempt to redress an imbalance in contemporary thinking on this subject.

The following chapters show how life-and-death decisions are shaped by the practical interests and realities of participants and are related to the social structure of the newborn intensive-care unit. I demonstrate that decisions reflect not only beliefs and values but a myriad of social, political, and management considerations, such as the relationship between staff, parents, and infants. This analysis focuses on the decision making of three participants. First are the attending physicians (neonatologists), who are both academicians and clinicians and frequently experience a conflict between their research and clinical roles. Second are the interns and residents (housestaff), who rotate through the nursery, are frequently overworked, and are rewarded for their mastery of technical knowledge. Their contact with families is infrequent and sporadic, and their interaction with babies is confined to technical interventions. Nurses, the third group, sustain a relatively continuous contact with both parents and infants and derive much of their work satisfaction from infants who are socially—and medically—responsive. Frequently they take a more pessimistic attitude than physicians toward infants who are unattractive, unresponsive, or require chronic care.

Each group has a set of interests that transcend patient care. Attending physicians have a research interest, interns and residents have an interest in learning, and nurses have an interest in the practicalities of patient management. Parents, who are somewhat outside the structure of the intensive-care nursery, also have other interests in alleviating the stresses that ensue from having an infant who is critically ill or in limiting the future social, psychic, and economic costs of rearing a disabled child. Each participant has an interest in getting by with a minimum of distress in what is often a difficult and stressful technological environment.

Throughout, my data illustrate how attending physicians, interns and residents, nurses, and parents differ systematically in how they view the life-and-death decision. These differences are in turn related to each participant's location in the nursery's social structure.

Chapter 3 discusses systematic differences in how health professionals and parents predict the futures of infants having an uncertain prognosis. A recurrent theme is the conflict between physicians, who make prognoses on the basis of "hard data" derived from sophisticated measurement instruments, and nurses, who make prognoses on the basis of subtle cues gleaned from their interactions with infants. Chapter 3 also addresses the impact of new medical technologies on medical practice. Following medical historians, I suggest that medical practice in the last hundred years has adopted what might be called a "post-clinical" mentality, characterized by a diminishing attention to patients' subjective symptoms, a waning confidence in clinical observations, and an increased reliance on sophisticated measurement instruments. While this development has improved the diagnostic capabilities of physicians, it has also augmented the social distance between patient and practitioner.

Chapters 4 and 5 consider the role of the parents in life-and-death decisions and their transactions with professionals. In Chapter 4, "Producing Assent," I argue that it is impossible to speak of "informed consent" without at the same time understanding the process by which parents are informed and their consent is obtained. As I also suggest in that chapter, staff do not actually obtain parents' informed consent, but rather elicit their assent or agreement to decisions professionals have already made. The goal of producing assent is to avoid conflicts with parents that could potentially enter the legal system and transform private dilemmas into public issues. However, as Chapter 5 suggests, two types of conflicts cannot always be prevented: those between the parents and those between the parents and staff. When conflicts between parents and professionals do occur, staff employ a set of strategies to diffuse dissent. By so doing, professionals attempt to maintain boundaries of professional jurisdiction and boundaries between the nursery and the outside world.

Chapter 6, the conclusion, discusses the policy implications of neonatal intensive care. I address our society's seemingly paradoxical investment in newborn intensive care rather than in other, less technological treatment modalities, such as preventive care and nutrition, which would reduce the incidence of prematurity. The chapter also shows how this and other seeming paradoxes in public policy complicate the process of reaching life-and-death decisions. Returning to one of the themes posed in this chapter—the limits of individual conscience—the conclusion calls for a broader, more sociologically informed model of organizational, institutional, and social morality, which might result in more just and equitable decision making.

CHAPTER 3

Predicting the Future

Why Physicians and Nurses Disagree

It was not an auspicious beginning. Robin Simpson's premature birth on May 13 was believed to be the result of a domestic tragedy. During a quarrel with her husband, Mrs. Simpson fell down the stairs, and nine days later she entered a small private hospital with the signs of impending labor. Five days after that, Robin, who weighed two pounds, five ounces, was delivered nine weeks prematurely by cesarean section. Months later physicians and nurses in the Randolph Nursery were to recall these unfortunate events in an effort to make sense of the unusual course of an illness that kept Robin in the nursery for seven months. During this time, Robin was never able to exist apart from the life-support equipment necessary to support her breathing. Robin's protracted stay in the nursery was also costly, culminating in hospital bills of over a quarter of a million dollars.

When Robin first arrived in the nursery, she appeared to be doing reasonably well. However, beginning one day after her birth, it became increasingly apparent that her case was unusual. Premature infants often begin to experience difficulties breathing (respiratory distress syndrome) in the first hours of life, and some require respirator support. As their lungs mature, they become less dependent on the respirator and ultimately are able to breathe on their own. Robin continually defied expectations of a "normal course" for a premature infant with lung disease. She was a day old before she developed lung disease, and, once placed on a respirator, she began to deteriorate rapidly. Moreover, in the days, weeks, and months that followed, Robin was unable to breathe without total respirator support, and attempts to wean her met with repeated failure. Faced with her lack of progress, the physicians and nurses began to wonder whether Robin's lung disease was incurable. By August, when Robin had been dependent on the respirator for three months, the staff held a conference to make the difficult decision about weaning her from the respirator, leaving her in an oxygen tent to support her breathing. The parents reportedly faced the news of this decision with a certain amount of relief. No one expected Robin to survive without the support of the respirator, but she began to breathe on her own, again defying expectations.

Three more months elapsed, but Robin's lung disease showed no signs of improvement. The nurses had become increasingly pessimistic about her chances for recovery and concerned about her mental development. Frustrated by the prospect of having to care for Robin indefinitely, they began to withdraw.

There were other problems as well. The Simpson's marriage was reported to be deteriorating. Mrs. Simpson, who at one time had visited regularly, was seen only rarely in the nursery. In November, after Robin had been in the nursery for six months, the head nurse discussed the case with Dr. Nelson, the attending neonatologist, and once again a conference was convened to decide Robin's fate.

The story of Robin Simpson's stay in the Randolph Nursery raises social and ethical issues encountered in intensive-care nurseries throughout the country. Protracted stays in a nursery are not only costly in economic terms; they also exact a less measurable price on the lives of patients, families, and those who provide care. Robin Simpson's case is not unlike the well-known case of Karen Ann Quinlan.[1] Both patients suffered from conditions that were not well understood and defied simple medical explanations. Both continued to live long after the equipment thought necessary to sustain their lives had been removed. In both cases, the central issue was prognostic. Both cases were clouded by the difficulty of concluding that these patients suffered from "incurable" and "irreversible" conditions and had no "reasonable" hope for survival. The case of Robin Simpson dramatically illustrates the subject of this chapter: how physicians and nurses predict the future of newborn infants and the difficulties that often attend their predictions.

Why should a sociological study of life-and-death decisions examine the process of prediction? At first glance, the issue of prognosis seems to be a purely factual, scientific question that lies beyond the pale of sociological inquiry. But predicting and prognosticating are integral features of the decision-making process that no study of life-and-death decisions can afford to ignore. At a deeper level, there is reason to believe that prognostic decisions are clearly within the realm of sociological analysis. In fact, a considerable body of socio-logical research suggests that practitioners' decisions to diagnose and treat illness are only partly based on an "objective" assessment of patients' signs and symptoms. As discussed in Chapter 2, studies undertaken from diverse theoretical perspectives and employing a number of research strategies have called attention to the many social considerations brought to bear on medical decision making.

A particularly promising direction in the sociology of medical deci-sion making has been the study of how organizations shape and structure diagnosis and treatment decisions. By relating a microsocial phenomenon—decision making—to its organizational context, this approach integrates micro and macro levels of analysis—a contempo-rary sociological concern.[2] It is also resonant with a classical premise in the sociology of knowledge: that ideas are shaped by the social settings in which they develop.

I examine the relationship of one type of decisions to their social setting: the relationship of life-and-death decisions to the setting of neonatal intensive-care units. This chapter considers only one kind of life-and-death decision: that in which the central issue is the prognosis of the infant whose life is in question. Perhaps the most difficult and controversial of life-and-death decisions, it raises a dilemma typical of neonatal intensive care as an enterprise: what to do in the absence of sound information concerning the future of the infant whose fate is being decided.

Briefly, I will suggest that life-and-death decisions may be ap-proached from the standpoint of the sociology of knowledge. This analysis will show how the organization of the intensive-care nursery as a work environment structures the perceptions of those who work within it. I will present data taken from interviews and case studies that suggest that members of the nursery staff, because of their differ-ing work experiences, may arrive at conflicting conclusions about the prognoses of infants whose lives are in question—differences that frequently result in conflicts concerning life-and-death decisions. This chapter, then, will be concerned with the relationship between one type of knowledge (knowledge involved in prognosticating and reaching life-and-death decisions) and one social context (the social organization of the newborn intensive-care unit).

In order to make any life-and-death decision, the participants must have some idea about the kind of future that awaits the patient. However, owing to the highly innovative, "experimental" nature of neonatal intensive care, these judgments often prove notoriously difficult. New drugs and surgical procedures are often not introduced in carefully designed protocols with randomized control groups. The infant is saved; the consequences are assessed later.[3] Applying techniques and therapies borrowed from adult intensive care may result in unforeseen iatrogenic consequences. Moreover, it is exceedingly difficult to determine the developmental potential of newborn infants who may have problems that will not become apparent for years. For example, it is now possible to resuscitate infants as small as 500g. (1.1 pounds) and as young as twenty-five weeks' gestational age. Many of these infants die, and the ones who do live risk damage to major organ systems, including serious brain damage.[4] Although many nurseries have undertaken follow-up studies to evaluate the degree of morbidity that occurs in their patients, these studies do little to clarify matters for professionals facing immediate life-and-death decisions. The very small number of survivors in follow-up studies, the fact that many disabilities make a delayed appearance, and the fact that many survivors have received what are by now outmoded treatments mean that it may be years before adequate data can be obtained.[5] These considerations suggest that it is often difficult to predict the viability or intellectual potential of many newborn infants and hence to make life-and-death decisions about them.

The analysis presented in this chapter grew out of several initial field observations. In both intensive-care nurseries I studied, a broad consensus around a *principle* had emerged. If practitioners were reasonably convinced an infant was unable to survive or would survive with serious neurological defects (e.g., severe mental retardation or cerebral palsy), then it was considered appropriate to withhold life-sustaining treatment from that infant. However, even when practitioners could agree on the principle involved in a life-and-death decision, they often could not agree on the *prognosis* of the infant whose fate was in question.

In some of the decisions to which I have alluded (those in which the underlying dilemma was prognostic), participants merely acknowledged difficulties in making predictions. More often than not, how-ever, the prognoses of infants whose lives were in question became the subject of debate, disagreement, and even acrimonious conflict among attending physicians, residents, and nurses. It also became apparent that these conflicts followed recurrent patterns: most often the nurses—and less frequently the residents—were the first to conclude that the infant would not recover or would have severe mental disabilities.[6] This observation suggested the hypothesis that when prognostic ambiguity is due to a lack of precise "scientific" knowl-edge, nurses, residents, and attending physicians may have different methods for arriving at prognostic assessments. In fact, each group of participants may be approaching the life-and-death decision from the standpoint of a very different "data base." That conflicts surrounding prognosis seem to have a systematic and patterned nature alerts us to the fact that predicting and prognosticating, an ostensibly "scientific" activity, may actually have a social and organizational basis.

In the following pages, I discuss how the newborn intensive-care unit qua organization allocates different types of information to those who work within it and in so doing defines the character of the "data" that each group brings to the life-and-death decision. Each occupa-tional group has a different set of daily experiences that define the contours of the information used in making prognostic judgments and in reaching life-and-death decisions. I am concerned with the judg-ments of three kinds of participants.

First are the attending physicians (neonatologists). Academicians as well as clinicians, they alternate their rotations with research responsi-bilities. Although attendings spend the least amount of time in the nursery observing individual patients, they can draw on a reservoir of clinical experience and have unique access to information from the follow-up study. Second are the residents and fellows, who rotate through the nursery. During their monthlong rotations, they spend considerable time in the nursery. Much of that time is spent in a number of rounds (e.g., working rounds, didactic rounds, perinatal rounds, X-ray rounds, and sign-off rounds) in which information concerning infants' medical conditions is exchanged. The remainder of their day is devoted to managing infants' clinical problems—in-cluding, for example, resuscitating infants at delivery, performing diagnostic procedures, reviewing the results of biochemical studies, and writing orders. Outside the confines of the physical examination, the residents' daily work routine affords little opportunity to observe patients directly. Neonatology fellows function largely in a supervisory capacity and engage in even less direct patient care. Not only do residents and fellows have little opportunity to observe individual patients in the course of a single day, but their ability to observe patients over time is further curtailed by the rotation system in a teaching hospital. In short, their contact with infants is limited, episodic, and confined to technical interventions. Finally, there are the nurses. Unlike the other participants, the nurses sustain continuous, close, and long-term contact with the infants who are their patients. Even in the least intensive areas, the nurse-to-patient ratio is sufficiently high to provide considerable opportunity for contact with and observation of individual patients. Moreover, nurses frequently care for particular infants repeatedly and hence may acquire a less episodic, longer-term view of their patients' progression. Finally, the nurses' activities are not confined to feeding, administering medications, and monitoring. Nurses also engage in types of patient care (e.g., verbalization and infant stimulation) that transcend the technical, and there is considerable social interaction between nurses and patients.[7]

Given these widely varying sorts of experiences, one would expect to find that each occupational group comes to construe the "facts" in different ways and to have differing notions of what constitutes adequate data or "evidence" to be used in reaching life-and-death decisions. I am suggesting, then, that the organization serves as a sort of interpretive lens through which its members perceive their patients and predict their futures, and therefore it functions as an *ecology of knowledge*.

THE ORGANIZATIONAL BASIS
OF PROGNOSTIC JUDGMENT

Viewed sociologically, medical prediction is a process of inference or typification. To arrive at a "best guess" about a patient's future, the practitioner collects empirical data concerning this patient and places him or her in a larger class of patients known to have typical or "normal" clinical courses.[8] A number of sources of information can be used to make predictions in medical settings. Each of these differs in the degree of patient contact that is required. *Technological cues* refer to any information obtained by means of diagnostic technology. *Perceptual cues* refer to information gathered through direct perception of the patient, including palpation, percussion, and, most commonly, observation. *Interactive cues* refer to information that arises out of the social interaction between patient and practitioner. In adult medicine, the major mode of interaction is the clinical history. However, if one defines social interaction broadly to include nonverbal aspects of communication, it is evident that social interaction between infants and practitioners can take place.

In order to explore their methods of prognostication, I asked residents and nurses, "How can you tell if an infant is doing well or poorly?" Responses given in an interview situation obviously may not reflect actual practice, but, taken together with field observations, they do provide useful information. My hypothesis was that physicians, because of their limited contact with patients, would be more likely to rely on diagnostic technology, whereas nurses would be more likely to mention interactive cues in their responses.

I examined the frequencies with which technological, perceptual, and interactive cues were cited. All the occupational groups relied primarily on technological cues and secondarily on perceptual cues. This suggests that the information from diagnostic technology assumes a superior epistemological status in the intensive-care nursery. However, a substantially larger number of nurses than physicians mentioned interactive cues in their responses. This difference, while statistically significant in the Randolph Nursery, is not significant in the General Nursery, as Table 1 suggests.[9]

In order to understand the nature of the prognostic process, it is necessary to go beyond gross tabulations and examine the interviews themselves. Unless otherwise noted, my question was: "Can you tell me what you know about the case and how you feel about it?" Nearly all the residents and fellows cited information gleaned from a variety of measurement instruments. These technological cues included changes in weight, laboratory results, and measures of respiratory function. In fact, four residents relied exclusively on this measurable information. As one of them stated: "It depends somewhat on the baby. In [the Acute Care Nursery at General Hospital], we can tell [the baby's condition] by whether the baby is growing or gaining weight. In the NICU [where the most critically ill babies are found], you can tell mainly by whether they're coming off the respirator."

Technological cues, however, were rarely cited exclusively. Instead, the largest group of residents and fellows based their diagnostic judgments on a combination of technological and perceptual cues.

TABLE 1

DIFFERENCES IN USE OF INTERACTIVE CUES BY OCCUPATION

Number of Respondents Who:	Randolph Nursery Occupation			General Nursery Occupation			Both Nurseries Occupation		
	Physicians (Residents & Fellows)	Nurses	Total	Physicians (Residents & Fellows)	Nurses	Total	Physicians (Residents & Fellows)	Nurses	Total
Did not mention interactive cues[a]	15	6	21	10	5	15	25	11	36
Mentioned interactive cues[b]	2	12	14	1	4	5	3	16	19
Total	17	18	35	11	9	20	28	27	55
	$\chi^2 = 6.88$ df = 1 p < .01			Fisher's exact test[c] $P = .097$ n.a.			$\chi^2 = 12.259$ df = 1 p < .001		

[a]These respondents cited technological cues, perceptual cues, or "other" types of information only.
[b]These respondents mentioned interactive cues in conjunction with technological cues, perceptual cues, and "other" types of information.
[c]The Fisher's exact test was used because of the very small sample in the General Nursery. χ^2 distributions, even when corrected for continuity, are likely to produce distortions when applied to very small samples (Blalock, 1960:221–25).

The following two responses are typical of this modal tendency to rely on a combination of measurable and observable information:

RESIDENT 1:   Well, we have our numbers. If the electrolyte balance is okay and the baby is able to move one respirator setting a day, then you can say he's probably doing well. If the baby looks gray and isn't gaining weight and isn't moving, then you can say he probably isn't doing well.

RESIDENT 2:   The most important thing is the gestalt. In the NICU, you have central venous pressures, left atrial saturations, temperature stability, TC [transcutaneous] oxymeters, perfusion [oxygenation of the tissues]—all of this adds in. You get an idea, when the baby looks bad, of the baby's perfusion. The amount of activity is also important—a baby who's limp is doing worse than one who's active.

That these physicians cited only those perceptual cues that could be obtained in the course of a routine physical examination—for example, color, activity, or muscle tone—attests to the limited nature of contact between physicians and patients. One resident lamented that the reliance on diagnostic technology was at odds with the ideals of his medical training:

Well, you really get dramatic kinds of information. I mean, the baby's blood gases can improve or deteriorate markedly. I think that you can tell best in the nursery by your clinical exam unless something really gross supervenes, like congestive heart failure, and even more by how his laboratory parameters are doing. . . . Is the child gaining weight, are they having apneic spells [episodes in which the infant stops breathing]? You know, do his electrolytes, does his CBC [complete blood count], do his blood gases look good? And, in a way, that's frustrating, because when you are a physician, you like not to depend on the laboratory, but . . . *the bottom line is what are this kid's values?*

Like the other participants, nurses cited technological and perceptual cues, but they also frequently cited interactive cues, including facial feedback, eye contact, and other aspects of the infant's facial expression. These cues may be seen as indications of developmental changes (particularly when infants are observed for a period of time) or, alternatively, as indications of the infant's general alertness or "level of awareness":

[You can tell a lot] by how well the baby responds, in terms of the medical parameters. Are you able to lower the oxygen? Is the baby having apnea or bradycardia [episodes in which the baby stops breathing or the heart rate falls]? You can also tell by how the babies look psychosocially—are they alert, bright, able to follow you with their eyes, to respond to noises? In [the less intensive area of the General Nursery], you can start to see some developmental changes, like smiling socially. In the NICU, you have to consider the baby's age and illness, but you can get some sense for how they interact.

Those nurses who discussed interactive cues frequently mentioned responsiveness. The cues nurses viewed as indicating responsiveness include not only facial expression and eye contact but also the baby's response to visual, tactile, and auditory stimuli, as the following nurse suggests:

> [When an infant is] breathing on his own . . . , it becomes a little more subjective, and some of the signs I use to judge are level of awareness, how alert I think he is, how he responds to noises in the room, to my touching him, to my knocking against the isolette, any kind of tactile or auditory stimulation, how active he is when he's left alone, whether he moves on his own, or whether he doesn't respond unless stimulated. Mentation, level of awareness, means a lot to me.

Another frequently cited theme was the infant's ability to respond to the nurses' attention:

> NURSE: I think if they're doing well, they just respond to being human or being a baby. . . .
> INTERVIEWER: Can you give me examples of how babies interact?
> NURSE: Basically emotionally. If you pick them up, the baby should cuddle to you rather than being stiff and withdrawing. Do they quiet when held, or do they continue to cry when you hold them? Do they lay in bed or cry continuously, or do they quiet after they've been picked up and held and fed . . . ? Do they have a normal sleep pattern? Do they just lay awake all the time, really interacting with nothing, or do they interact with toys you put out, the mobile or things like that? Do they interact with the voice when you speak?

This respondent explicitly formulates the procedures she uses to identify "appropriate" emotional responses from the baby's reactions. What appears to organize her interpretations is an implicit criterion for the attribution of humanhood: to be considered "human," infants should be able to interact in such a fashion that their actions can be seen as *intentional*.[10] Consider also the following quotation, in which a nurse describes an infant to whom she had become attached and who died rather unexpectedly:

> NURSE: That was the kind of disappointment I felt when Larry died, because he was a good kid. Intellectually he was doing terrific, and he was a reactive child.

INTERVIEWER: What do you mean by "reactive"?

NURSE: Does the things that normal newborns are supposed to do at this time. You know, look at you, give you some sort of facial feedback just in their mannerisms . . . , just reacting to their environment, appropriate reactions. Like Larry gave you an inner feeling that if you were going to do something to him, he knew that you were going to do something, because this is something that had been conditioned in him, because if you came toward him with a pointed object or something, he knows what's going on. . . .

INTERVIEWER: How did he act?

NURSE: When Larry first came off the ventilator . . . , we tried to give him contact . . . , and he just went crazy, because all that he ever associated with these uniforms and these colors was that people were coming by to either suction him, give him a shot, poke and prod, or everything else, and he reacted in a very paranoid way. . . .

INTERVIEWER: So what did you think about that?

NURSE: Well, I thought that was very appropriate, considering everything he'd been through up to that point . . . , so it just gave you a feeling that he was able to put two and two and put together a solution.

This nurse's interpretations of Larry's behavior seem to suggest an implicit model of social action, which presupposes the ability to remember, to attribute intentions, to typify or recognize objects, events, and actions as similar, and, in sum, to engage in rather sophisticated types of information processing.

In short, once interactive cues are employed, an interpretive framework is called into play that transcends the medical notions of "signs," "symptoms," and "disease." Instead, these nurses' answers suggest that they assign meaning to their patients' actions by reference to underlying conceptions of "level of awareness," "mentation," or "humanhood." Thus, the subtle cues many nurses noted may be said to be "interactive" in two senses of the word: (1) they arise out of social interaction between patient and practitioner; and (2) they are interpreted according to assumptions about "appropriate" social interaction. There is another sense in which the nurses differed from other respondents: they often characterized their knowledge as tacit, taken for granted, intuitive, or a "gut feeling": "I think that with a lot of nurses that have been here for a while, the gut feeling has developed from a lot of observation that they have recorded subconsciously and never put on paper, and that no one's ever written about, and I think that those are a lot of those things. So when people say, 'I don't like that kid; there's something wrong with him,' the gut feeling's really based on a lot of informal study that they don't notice that they're doing."

"Gut feelings" appeal to a different legitimation of knowledge than that designated as "scientific" evidence. To portray one's own knowledge as a "gut feeling" is to introduce information that, on the one hand, is shielded from debate (it is not necessary to document or defend what is called a "gut feeling") but, on the other hand, carries little weight in scientific argument and is excluded from the realm of scientific discourse. To paraphrase Pascal, gut feelings are "reasons of the heart."

In short, the nurses relied on cues gleaned from their interactions with infants, which they interpreted within an interactive frame of reference and characterized as "gut feelings." There is, of course, an alternative explanation for these findings. It might be argued that the differences in the knowledge of physicians (residents and fellows) and nurses result from the prior sex-role socialization of men and women. For example, psychologist Carol Gilligan argues that women are more likely than men to base their moral reasoning on social relationships.[11] Because there were no male nurses in either NICU I studied, it is impossible to resolve this issue definitively. However, since there were no differences in the responses of female and male residents, there is reason to accept a simpler explanation: that the contrasting responses of physicians and nurses reflect their experiences in the organization rather than prior sex-role socialization. Like the nurses, attending neonatologists spoke of having "gut feelings" or clinical experiences that enabled them to make predictions at a glance. However, these gut feelings were entirely perceptually based: "Of course I have gut feelings, based on clinical experience. I can often walk into a nursery and tell you how any patient might turn out, based on the patient's diagnosis and appearance. I've seen it so many times before. But I've also been around long enough to know I can be wrong."

Unlike the nurses, attendings placed little confidence in their intuitive judgments. No attending ever reached a decision to withdraw life support until diagnostic tests had been performed. Even when attendings had strong negative gut feelings about a baby's prognosis, they would continue to support the baby until tests had been conducted, as the following example suggests:

The Sanderson baby had a serious heart defect [an interrupted arch and a ventriculo-septal defect] and progressive liver failure. When the infant was about one month old, a decision was made by the attending, Dr. Nelson, and the housestaff to refrain from giving further transfusions to correct the liver failure and to remove the baby from the respirator. I was present for the discussion at chief of service rounds, which took place after the decisions had been made. Dr. Nelson provided the following account of his decision. He stated that the decision to terminate life support was an "active decision, because we could have continued almost indefinitely." Dr. Nelson commented that the major problem was liver failure, and the bilirubin level [a measure of liver function] had reached 25, which had exceeded the content that would have meant kernicterus [brain damage due to jaundice]. He also provided other evidence of "progressive changes in the sensorium," such as unresponsiveness and depression, which is also a sign of kernicterus. At that point, "we felt that continued exchange transfusions were in the realm of extraordinary measures," and "it was not fair to the child to continue." Following this account, an attending from another service said, "When did you first come to this realization?" Dr. Nelson replied, "When I first saw the child." The attending asked, "No, I mean when was it obvious that the child wasn't salvageable?" And Dr. Nelson said, "My guess is that if you wait that long for surgery, the chances of success are close to zero." Then the attending asked, "What is the estimated cost?" And Dr. Nelson answered, "From the nineteenth [when the baby was ten days old], the cost was about thirty thousand dollars." I think the other attending implied that the decision could have been made sooner. Nevertheless, Dr. Nelson had continued to support the baby long after his clinical impressions indicated that this was not appropriate.

In this case, the insistence on "hard" data, as defined by measurable information, led the attending to continue to support the infant even after his clinical judgment dictated an alternative course of action. The legal demand for documentation, coupled with a belief in the superior scientific status of measurable information, may contribute to attendings' insistence on measurable data. It is also significant that this insistence may propel attendings into highly aggressive lines of action.

There is one additional source of clinical experience that *is* the exclusive province of the attending and that is used as admissible evidence in life-and-death decisions. This is data from the follow-up study that is conducted by the nursery attendings in which infants under 1500g. (3 pounds, 2 ounces) are given a battery of psychological and neurological tests at periodic intervals. It is important to note that residents and nurses rarely, if ever, are present in the weekly follow-up clinic. This organizational fact, coupled with the fact that much of the follow-up data are unpublished, means that *members of the nursery staff are dependent on the attendings to provide them with reports from the study*. Often these reports take the following form: a resident will question why a particular patient is being kept alive, and the attending will describe a single patient or group of patients in the follow-up study who are normal neurologically. Because of the very small number in the follow-up study of survivors with certain conditions (e.g., very small, very premature infants), this information was the only available data. Although all parties view the presentation of particular cases as "anecdotal" information, the use of this information often assumes particularly persuasive power in refuting the pessimistic views of the residents, as can be seen in the following conference described in my Randolph field notes:

> This decision concerned one of a set of twins, who was very premature, weighing 800g. [1 pound, 12 ounces] and born fourteen weeks prematurely. One of the twins suffered a rather large brain hemorrhage. During the month, this twin also developed meningitis. The residents strongly suggested that a recommendation be made to the parents that the baby should be taken off the respirator. The attending then said, "You'd be surprised to see how many of these are normal or lead close to normal lives." The intern then asked, "How many end up in an institution?" The attending answered, "I'd say less than half a dozen out of five hundred—that's just a guess. Maybe we'll find out that more will end up institutionalized. We had one who came in [to the follow-up clinic] on the sixth. He was an 850g. twin [a very low birthweight] who had horrible lung disease. He looks weird, but his I.Q. is 120, and he's going to start college—I mean high school—next year. You'd be surprised, and that's why I say every one of you should visit the follow-up clinic. But you're right, there are those who turn out badly damaged. . . . So I'm hesitant to make the kind of decision you're requesting. I'm not prepared to do nothing—I'm prepared to work in making them self-sufficient." Another resident then asked, "Well, how many of those who pulled through are just better protoplasm?" And the attending answered, "Twelve years ago, the ones who lived weren't as sick but had more insults—we'd hope that management has improved, and we're more skilled at preventing insults. But it's hard to evaluate—there's really no good, firm evidence."

The fact that attendings have a virtual monopoly on highly valued information from the follow-up study has the effect of enhancing their authority in life-and-death decisions.

I have emphasized that the different daily work experiences of occupational groups in the intensive-care nursery may provide them with access to different types of knowledge to be used in predicting the futures of infants whose lives are in question. The following case shows how this may result in conflicts concerning how life-and-death decisions should be made.

THE CONFRONTATION BETWEEN MODES OF KNOWING: AN ILLUSTRATIVE CASE

Robin Simpson, the infant with severe, chronic lung disease who was hospitalized in the Randolph Nursery for a seven-month period and whom I introduced at the beginning of this chapter, is not necessarily representative of the medical conditions commonly encountered in neonatology. Quite the contrary: members of the nursery staff frequently alluded to features of Robin's clinical course that were unusual and frustrated their attempts at prognostication. Nevertheless, this particular case merits detailed discussion, since it represents a type of case encountered frequently in both of the neonatal intensive-care units I studied: it was extremely difficult to conclude that the baby would die or would be severely impaired neurologically. While most of the physicians and nurses agreed to the principle that these were grounds for terminating life support, it was on the issue of Robin's prognosis that they were divided, and the social basis of their judgments was laid bare.

What follows are highlights from the transcript of the final conference, which was more widely attended than usual. In addition to the regular participants—Dr. Nelson (the attending), Dr. Brandon (the ethicist), the fellow, four residents, the social worker, and a head nurse—four other nurses gathered inside the crowded room. Before the resident began his presentation, Dr. Nelson handed two adult-sized X-rays to Dr. Brandon. As the ethicist held the X-rays up to the light and shook his head, Dr. Nelson said, "These are distorted in size but give a more dramatic view of the lungs." The conference began with a presentation of Robin's history:

RESIDENT 1:   The problem is that this is a premature baby who, shortly after birth, showed signs of severe lung disease, which appeared in the chronic phase. There was no acute episode of RDS [respiratory distress syndrome]. One day after birth, the X-ray showed signs associated with chronic lung disease.

ATTENDING: You should note that the baby appeared fine within the first twenty-four hours.

RESIDENT 1:   Well, let's go in order.

ATTENDING: Well, this is relevant to the decision, since this is a situation unfamiliar to us.

RESIDENT 1:   This is a baby of 1044g. [2 pounds, 5 ounces] and twenty-seven weeks gestational age. The mother has three other children and was hospitalized after five days of prolonged ruptured membranes. The baby was delivered by elective C-section in St. Mary's Hospital. The initial Apgars [measures of the infant's physical status] were 4 and 8, and there was no immediate respiratory distress. The baby was transferred here for prematurity.

                                        . . .

RESIDENT 1:   There were several courses of antibiotics. Briefly, I want to summarize some considerations. She's had no obvious neurological deficits. The two brain scans were normal. She's had no biopsy of the lungs, although questions have been raised————. We continued her for three months on the ventilator, and when we decided to wean her, she was put in 100 percent oxygen to see how she did. She did surprisingly well after she was extubated. Since then, she's been on 100 percent oxygen or high levels and high doses of diuretics. Her pulmonary status has not improved, and she has severe chronic lung disease. She depends on 100 percent oxygen and large doses of diuretics and would not survive without them.

ATTENDING: There are other medical problems which are relevant. Her nutrition has only been sufficient to keep her alive and not to grow, and she's failed to keep up with the lowest level of growth on the charts. Equally alarming is the head size—it hasn't grown. Though she's received 100 calories per kilo, they've all gone into breathing and not into brain growth. This is the most disturbing neurological feature. Severe malnutrition doesn't have a good prognosis, and sometimes the brain is permanently affected, but the studies are not clear, and it seems that social factors go into this. I was here when the child was admitted, and since then she's been going slowly downhill. By May she was still here and getting 100 percent oxygen or 80 percent oxygen. By mid-August, when I was the attending again, she was still getting 78 percent oxygen and being ventilated at a rate of 25. The lungs, according to the X-rays and physical findings, indicated more severe lung disease. The lungs appeared to be irreparably damaged, and we were continuing to support her, and it became clear that this was not appropriate. This was discussed with the parents, and we suggested that she be weaned from the respirator and allowed to breathe on 100 percent oxygen. She was not to be reintubated if she went into respiratory failure. I was sure that this would happen and she would die. The parents agreed to this with some relief.

. . .

ATTENDING: At the end of this period, she's been watched closely and has made no progress and has in fact been getting worse since August. She hasn't gained weight, and her general appearance indicates she's not responding. I don't know what to do next. The lung damage is too extensive and probably won't heal. On the other hand, we can't be sure—we've had no one with that severe lung disease ————. The one other child who is at all similar is the famous Bobby Hauser, who's ————. After six months, the parents were told he would die. He was not to be reintubated when his CO_2 went up to 120. Also, he was given more Lasix [a diuretic], and he got better. The predictions are based on soft evidence. On the other hand, Bobby had gained weight and his head had grown—he was a different sort of child.

While presenting Robin's history, the attending and the resident establish parameters of a perplexing prognosis: the late onset of her symptoms, her failure to improve, and her surprising recovery when weaned from the respirator. Note that the evidence both physicians cited was obtained from diagnostic technology and the physical examination; nothing is said about Robin's ability to interact. The attending is concerned about Robin's neurological status. But examining evidence from Robin's normal brain scans and "unclear" epidemiological studies of malnutrition, he cannot conclude with any "certainty" that Robin is neurologically impaired. Although he suspects that Robin's illness might be irreversible, her remarkable recovery in the past and the miraculous recovery of another patient with chronic lung disease, Bobby Hauser, give him reason to doubt his own judgment. Unable to find "hard" evidence of neurological damage and unable to establish with "certainty" that Robin's lung disease is irreversible, the attending is at a loss to know how to proceed.

The nurses' comments, however, appear to inhabit an altogether different realm. They express "desperation" at having to care for an infant who "cries and screams" and is described alternatively as "unsocialized," "unrewarding," possibly "autistic," and "damaged":

ETHICIST: What is the nurses' perspective?
NURSE 1: Close to desperation.
(The other nurses seem to mumble in the background.)
NURSE 2: Desperation. . . . Everyone just feels sorry for her.
NURSE 1: She's unsocialized, and that's because no one tries to socialize her. Trying to socialize her is terribly unpleasant and unrewarding . . .

NURSE 2:   Bobby was socialized in the negative sense—he threw tantrums and he responded. Robin doesn't.

ETHICIST: Does she cry?

NURSE 3:   All the time, and she has been known to smile. But usually all she does is cry and scream. Part of the problem is that she's in that tent. You can't do anything for her.

NURSE 1:   The only thing she likes to do is eat. She doesn't get hypertonic when she eats.

ATTENDING: All children in 100 percent oxygen are stiff, and they stiffen up when held.

ETHICIST: What's Bobby like since he's been home? What kind of care is required?

ATTENDING: He went home in oxygen and now takes it on demand. He gets along with his sister. The mother worries, and they never do anything without asking me. They call me every time they want to take Bobby on a trip—which is actually quite reasonable because they are usually going up to 8000 feet. He's extraordinary in the social sense—we would have thought he'd be an emotional wreck. When he walked, he began to be independent—he was in oxygen and began to move around the room.

HEAD NURSE: Yes, he's very social. When he comes here, he talks to all the nurses.

NURSE 1:   He's a cute kid now.

ATTENDING: From that we learned that we don't necessarily bug up their psyches.

NURSE 3:   We can quiet Robin, she's not totally autistic, but I do think she's damaged.

ATTENDING: There are no autistics in the follow-up group. There are a couple of autistics who are also retarded. (Pauses and then says to the ethicist:) Is this research on children?

ETHICIST: It is innovative treatment.

The attending does not speak to the desperation of the nurses, but rather challenges the scientific status of their comments as prognostic signs. When the nurses express their frustrations with Robin's stiffness, the attending portrays this condition as a usual response to a medical affliction. When a nurse notes that Robin "likes" to eat, an attribution of emotion, the attending provides an alternative medical explanation. When a third nurse suggests that Robin might be psychologically damaged or autistic, the attending debates this with information from the follow-up study.[12]

In the dialogue between the attending and the nurses, one can witness the confrontation between two very different types of knowledge. The attending makes a set of claims concerning Robin's uncertain neurological status, and he summons technological and physical findings, the follow-up study, and the "extraordinary" social behavior of Bobby Hauser to support his conclusions. The nurses' comments, however, inhabit an altogether different realm of explanation. They organize their interpretations of Robin's behavior according to notions of "appropriate" responsiveness, most of which Robin has violated. The nurses support this portrait of an "unsocialized," "damaged," or "autistic" infant with interactive cues. Not surprisingly, it is the attending who has the last word in the discussion.

Dr. Nelson's query about whether Robin is being treated for research purposes reveals the depths of his distress about this case. So perplexed is the attending that he is unclear about his own motivation and is asking the ethicist to resolve the issue. Dr. Nelson begins to bring the conference to closure by posing three options: to continue the present course of treatment, which he later rules out; to increase the intensity of treatment; or to withdraw the oxygen necessary to support Robin's breathing:

ATTENDING: Well, the options are to continue what we are doing, to up the intensity of our approach, to set up the ventilator and juice up the caloric intake. The third option is to withdraw the oxygen— without question that would be fatal.

NURSE 1: And withdraw the Lasix?

ATTENDING: I'd say in this case that would be an extraordinary measure. The first option is not tenable—so we're left with either upping or stopping.

ETHICIST: I would stand by the position that what is going on is extraordinary and not obligatory. The extraordinary character comes from the dismal prognosis in the requisite organ systems, and secondly the long trial—you've made a long trial—and the third element is cost. We have to consider whether we can justify why we're putting so much effort in, and therefore to take the stopping course is justifiable. If we had more history, we could say keep going, because other cases turned out favorably. But we don't have this kind of information. So this constitutes extraordinary care, and there's no obligation to continue. The stop course is morally and legally justified. *(He pauses.)* However, to take the middle course and try an intensive effort for a short period of time—that might make everyone feel better, to make a last-ditch effort at changing the situation. It wouldn't draw more on our economic resources and our emotional resources, and we would be more certain that we've done everything.

ATTENDING: So the third option would be a little more intensive and demonstrate any reverses in her course—we could see if there's an increase in head size within ten days, and we could discontinue

ETHICIST: her if she should stay the same in ten days. So our options are to stop, to go all out, or to go all out for a short period of time.

ETHICIST: It makes psychological and emotional sense—it's easier to terminate if you're in the midst of a crisis than if things have evened out. An intensive effort would make a change in the baby, and it's sure to make a change in you. It's a leap on the side of life, and you need this.

ATTENDING: I'll be gone for two weeks, and then we can see if the time is up. When I'm back and there's no change, we can withdraw care.

The ethicist, whose comments up to this point have been confined largely to requests for information and opinions, now moves to his most "active" role in the conference, offering a set of moral assertions and justifications and making a recommendation. Continuing to treat Robin is "extraordinary and not obligatory"—"there's no [legal or moral] obligation to continue." He then offers three justifications: the long trial, the dismal prognosis, and cost. Pausing, the ethicist makes his recommendation: to try an intensive effort for a brief period of time. He then makes a number of assertions concerning the benefits of this option: it "might make everyone feel better," "it wouldn't draw more on our economic resources and our emotional resources," and "we would be more certain that we've done everything." Later he asserts that "it makes psychological and emotional sense . . . to terminate if you're in the midst of a crisis. . . . An intensive effort would make a change in the baby, and it's sure to make a change in you. It's a leap on the side of life, and you need this." It is interesting that the ethicist's major arguments in support of his recommendation concern the *beneficial psychological consequences for the staff* that would accrue from terminating life support in the midst of an intense effort. This consideration does not fall within the realm of what is commonly viewed as "ethical discourse." Rather, the ethicist's recommendation emanates from his assumptions about the social psychology of the intensive-care nursery and his inferences about the nurses' attitudes.

The ethicist's recommendation is presumably based on the "middle course" formulated by the attending. But the ethicist has also added a new feature to the original plan, the time limit. The attending then elaborates specific features of the plan: particular therapeutic maneuvers, a measurable criterion to assess Robin's improvement (an increase in head size), and a specific time limitation (ten days). The specific contours of the treatment plan emerge from this process of negotiation, and it is finally decided to make a brief effort to increase Robin's caloric intake and to postpone the final decision for a ten-day period.

The plan was carried out. During this time, however, Robin died— unexpectedly and without warning. At about 6 A.M. on December 9, shortly before Dr. Nelson was to return from his trip, Robin suffered an episode of bradycardia (her heart rate dropped). Those who were present characterized their attempts to resuscitate her as a "slow code." According to the intern, "the nurses called us in very late; we got there for essentially a last gasp." When I asked the resident who cared for Robin at the time what had happened that night, he said: "Robin . . . had been labeled a no-code. . . . I did do bag and mask respiration for a few minutes and stopped, knowing in my mind it was the last time I was going to do that. I placed a call to the fellow at that time . . . , asking for his support, which he gave to me. And at that time, I determined she was most likely dying and actually not to try to change that course." The head nurse, echoing the sentiments of other nurses I interviewed, said, "Robin surprised us all by dying. . . . I mean we were all in a state of shock, and I think that the interesting thing about it was that she finally made the decision, and we were not left with making another."

Robin Simpson's protracted stay in the Randolph Nursery raises significant social and ethical issues, for the task of caring for an infant who failed to improve had a negative impact on the lives of the parents, the staff, and, not least of all, Robin herself. But the central dilemma in this case was prognostic, for how one construes the "facts," "data," and "evidence" concerning a patient's neurological status and prospects for recovery, perhaps more than any other consideration, influences one's sense of the right thing to do. Recall, for example, some of the major decisions that were made: to wean Robin from the respirator, rather than to "disconnect" it; to support her in an oxygen tent for some time without monitoring her electrolytes; and finally, to make a brief "last-ditch" effort to increase her caloric intake. These decisions, in which the patients are left partly to their own devices, are the kind that sometimes ensue when attending physicians remain perplexed to the end.

The attending and the nurses who participated in the conference not only articulated contrasting conceptions of Robin as a patient, but had differing visions of the central dilemma. For the attending, the dilemma was one of profound prognostic perplexity. Torn between continuing to treat a patient who might be doomed and ending the life of a patient who might otherwise recover, he steered a middle course that spared him from confronting either alternative. For the nurses, the dilemma was one of continuing to care for an infant whose "unsocialized" behavior provided them with few rewards and who, in addition, may even have been damaged by their own neglect.

Interviews confirmed what the conference had suggested: that the physicians and nurses had radically different views of Robin's prognosis and, for this reason, different perspectives on the decisions that were made.[13] The largest group of residents agreed with the major decisions that were made; most of the nurses disagreed with them, stating that life support should have been discontinued much sooner. Citing the unusual features of Robin's case, most of the residents and fellows felt that Robin might have had a small chance for improvement, and for this reason a decision to terminate life support would not have been right. As one resident said when asked how he felt about the case: "It's a difficult bind that [the staff] were in because the chances of her surviving would seem small. But this is a case where very little was known, and I don't think they ever got a definite diagnosis of what was wrong with her lungs, and the case is very unusual, and it's therefore unpredictable. No one could know what her prognosis was, and I think it would have been wrong to withdraw support at any point in her course."[14]

By contrast, more than half the nurses said they had "long ago" reached the conclusion that Robin would never recover.[15] Moreover, all but two of the nurses (and none of the physicians) cited interactive cues, which led them to two conclusions. Some felt that Robin was neurologically impaired:

> NURSE: Oh! Robin Simpson. . . . In the end, I refused to look after that baby—I just couldn't stand her . . . , she just didn't act like a baby.
> INTERVIEWER: How did she act?
> NURSE: Well, she would be rigid, she was just like a board . . . , and she just had a real terrible cry. And I don't know, she just sounded to me like she didn't have a brain . . . , she never cried for a reason.

Other nurses viewed Robin as "unsocialized," "autistic," or "psychologically damaged" from months of life in an oxygen tent or from their own neglect. One of them told me:

I think they should have stopped on her a long, long time before they did. . . . And you can tell me, and they can come along and say, "This little life can amount to something great." That doesn't make the decision right. Because, sure, you don't know exactly what's going to happen, but you have a pretty good idea she's going to be damaged. . . . She was psychologically damaged by the time she died. No one loved Robin for her seven months of life. She was handled only when something had to be done to her. . . . When you handled her, she'd cry and she'd just arch her back. . . . She could pick up the frustration in your hands. . . . Finally, I just said, "Well, I'll just gavage you [feed with a tube] and then just tuck you under your blanket so I don't have to see you. . . ." So no one talked to her . . . , no one handled her, she never felt loved. After seven months here, I was sure that psychologically she was damaged for life.

Taken together, the conference and the interviews suggest that physicians and nurses, by virtue of their very different experiences in the nursery, develop different views of the "facts," "data," and "evidence" and that the socially distributed nature of that knowledge can lead to conflicting views of how life-and-death decisions should be made. How can one account for what appear to be different conclusions about Robin's prospects for recovery? The answer, I believe, is organizational, for the patient who fails to improve has a different social meaning for the nurse who sits at the bedside for days, weeks, and months than he or she does for the physician who has much less exposure to the patient during monthlong rotations. For the latter, the survival of another, similar chronic patient provides grounds for hope; for the former, a protracted clinical course provides sufficient grounds for desperation.

When a patient's course is chronic and resists typification and when, in addition, conventional diagnostic technology fails to provide "unequivocal" evidence of brain damage, conflicting prognostic interpretations are likely to proliferate. It is at this point that the social origins of these interpretations are revealed. What is at issue are two radically different perceptions of the same patient. One bases its conclusions on diagnostic technology, physical findings, and epidemiological studies; the other, the perspective of continuous contact, bases its inferences on social interaction. The two perspectives meet in the ethics conference; and in the confrontation between the two modes of knowing, not surprisingly, the former prevails.

In life-and-death decisions, facts, values, cognitions, and affects become inextricably intertwined. The Simpson case reveals a complex interplay between the perspectives of engagement and detachment. Just as the physicians' structural and emotional disengagement from the patient and from the consequences of their decisions (coupled with a possible investment in learning something from the case) may have led them to insist on absolute "certainty," so, too, the nurses' pessimism may have been colored by their frustrations in caring for an infant who posed behavioral problems and failed to improve.[16] Continuous contact has its shadow side, permitting emotions (including negative ones) to develop—emotions that may compromise the quality of an infant's care. This analysis implies that each group of participants may be approaching life-and-death decisions from the standpoint of a very partial knowledge base, selectively filtered through the lens of structural circumstances.

INTERACTIVE CUES, COMPUTERS, AND THE FUTURE OF LIFE-AND-DEATH DECISIONS

So far, I have emphasized how the organization of the intensive-care nursery allocates different types of information to those who work within it, giving rise to conflicts in life-and-death decisions. Moreover, the types of knowledge participants use in decisions are not valued equally—that is, the status of the various forms of knowledge closely parallels the stratification of the various occupational groups. The neonatologists' follow-up data on similar cases are valued most highly, followed in descending order by technological, perceptual, and interactive cues. Clearly, developments outside the walls of the intensive-care nursery influence the value placed on different forms of knowledge. For example, the high valuation of technological information reflects broader trends in the history of medicine.[17]

The newborn intensive-care unit provides a microcosm in which it is possible to observe some of these historical transformations in the value of prognostic knowledge as they are taking place, thereby joining the history of ideas to the sociology of knowledge. This is not a trivial issue, since, given recent policy trends favoring "ethics committees," prognostication will undoubtedly assume even greater importance in life-and-death decisions.[18] It is possible, for example, to examine how "micro" sources of information (technological, perceptual, and interactive cues) come to be transformed—or fail to be transformed—into larger prognostic indicators and how they acquire validity as prognostic signs.[19]

In several intensive-care nurseries throughout the country (including the Randolph Nursery), attempts are being made to refine prognostic indicators by using certain information recorded in the charts of patients who are later seen in follow-up clinics at periodic intervals. This is presumably one step toward resolving one of the mysteries in the art and science of prognostication: why some premature infants do well and others of the same size, gestational age, and diagnosis do poorly, and what seems to distinguish the former group from the latter. For example, oxygen deprivation (hypoxia) in the neonatal period, once thought to be an ominous prognostic sign, is no longer viewed as a necessary precursor of brain damage. Rather, the duration of hypoxia seems more predictive of subsequent neurological disabilities.[20]

In some nurseries, this refinement of prognostic indicators is being carried one step further. Many newborn intensive-care units have begun to employ computerized data banks in which detailed information (pertaining, for example, to infants' respiratory and metabolic status) is fed into a computer by residents and stored for future use. This information has the potential of serving as an adjunct to (if not a partial replacement for) the physician's progress notes and can facilitate the testing of research hypotheses. The very detailed information stored in the computer can then be retrieved, correlated with data from the follow-up study, and hence be used in refining prognostic indicators. Neonatologists frequently express the hope that the development of more precise prognostic indicators by means of these methods will help them reach life-and-death decisions that rest on a more solid empirical foundation.

But the developments I have just discussed, while improving the art and science of prognostication, may take place at a certain price and may result in the loss of certain potentially valuable sources of information, for *only the measurable features of infants' conditions are correlated with information from the follow-up study.* This is at least in part because this information is recorded most systematically in the charts. Should neonatologists be so inclined, they could theoretically examine the perceptual information recorded in the charts of infants who are seen in follow-up clinics to determine if any of these perceptual cues (e.g., subtle changes in activity level) are associated with neurological defects. This would, of course, require a massive investment of resources to extract from the case record information that has not been recorded systematically.

This type of analysis has, in fact, been undertaken with the Apgar score, a system designed to measure an infant's degree of vigor at birth.[21] Despite its ostensibly "subjective" nature, the Apgar score has survived the test of time. For example, a low Apgar score at five minutes has been associated with neonatal mortality and abnormal neurologic status at one year of age.[22] But precisely *because many of the interactive cues nurses note are rarely entered into patients' charts systematically, they cannot be validated as prognostic signs.* The use of computerized data banks may only exacerbate this tendency toward losing certain types of information, since only measurable information (which excludes, for example, the physician's clinical observations) can be entered into a computer.

I am not claiming that information based on the clinician's perceptions of and interactions with patients has a high rate of "interobserver reliability," let alone "predictive validity." What I am suggesting is that, given current trends within neonatal intensive care, these are questions that are unlikely to be answered. Under present circumstances, the interactive cues cited so frequently by the nurses interviewed in this study are unlikely to acquire predictive validity and will remain in the realm of "gut feelings."

This brief discussion of the refinement of prognostic indicators is only a footnote in the sociology of medicine, suggesting how the scientific status of certain types of knowledge is enhanced while others are excluded from the realm of scientific discourse. But at the same time, a contrary trend is taking place within the field of pediatrics, where a systematic interest in infant development is emerging. Pediatricians trained in "infant development" or "behavioral pediatrics," sometimes in collaboration with social scientists, are engaging in detailed videotaped observation and analysis of infant behavior in intensive-care nurseries and are also studying the interaction between infants and parents and nurses. (However, the resources invested in this "soft" wing of pediatrics are not commensurate with those invested in the acquisition of computerized data banks.) As pediatricians acquire more systematic knowledge of the social interactions of infants in the first months of life, perhaps at some point in the future some of the interactive cues nurses note will come to occupy a less humble place in the hierarchy of knowledge in the intensive-care nursery. If this scenario does indeed take place, and if the diagnostic and prognostic legitimacy of the nurse's knowledge can be established, the nurse's authority in life-and-death decisions may also increase.

SUMMARY AND CONCLUSIONS

This chapter has approached life-and-death decisions from the stand-point of the sociology of knowledge. Prognostic conflict in these decisions was used as a paradigmatic case to illuminate how the organization of the intensive-care unit as an ecology of knowledge may result in disagreements over how life-and-death decisions should be made. A major finding was that physicians and nurses, because of their differing work experiences, may come to develop conflicting conceptions of the future of infants whose lives are in question. For example, residents, whose contact with infants is limited and techni-cally focused, base their prognostic assessments largely on "hard" data acquired by means of sophisticated measurement instruments (technological cues) and only secondarily on perceptual information. My point is not that physicians as individuals assume an uncaring attitude toward their patients, but rather that, structurally and organi-zationally, they are disengaged from infants (as well as parents).

The contrast between physicians and nurses provides a natural experiment, since the social situation of the latter is, to a certain extent, unique. Nurses are sociologically significant insofar as they, unlike physicians, sustain continuous contact with infants and derive much of their work satisfaction from interaction with infants who are medically and socially responsive. For this reason, nurses have unique access to a type of information that emanates from interaction with infants who are their patients. I have also suggested that this type of knowledge (interactive cues) merits more detailed study. This is not to say, however, that nurses' decisions are necessarily "superior" to those of physicians. The case of Robin Simpson suggests that the continuous contact between nurses and patients may not, ironically, be without its shortcomings. Indeed, the very structural engagement of nurses and patients may lead nurses to assume a more pessimistic attitude toward infants who are unresponsive, pose behavioral prob-lems, or require chronic care—infants, in short, who pose manage-ment problems.

This analysis implies that each set of participants approaches life-and-death decisions from a very partial knowledge base. Moreover, the types of prognostic knowledge used in life-and-death decisions are not valued equally. As the data indicate, technological cues and in-teractive cues do not carry equal weight within the realm of medical discourse. Although nurses have access to certain aspects of an infant's behavior that are not available to the other participants, the interactive cues nurses note are *devalued data*. I have also suggested that this knowledge, which can be gleaned only through continuous contact, be treated as an open question, subject to further study, rather than peremptorily cast out of the realm of medical discourse. A culture that allows only certain types of knowledge to be used as the criteria of "certainty" may impel physicians to continue supporting an infant's life long after this is appropriate.

The differential value attached to various forms of knowledge reflects broader trends in the development of medical practice that have been discussed by historians of medicine. Of particular interest are the historical phenomenologies of medicine presented by Michel Foucault and Stanley Joel Reiser. Foucault documents changes in the structure of medical perception in the eighteenth and nineteenth centuries that accompanied the rise of clinical medicine.[23] He traces the shift from a "preclinical" mentality based on taxonomic classification to an anatomical or "clinical" mentality, in which tissues, organs, and diseases, once beyond the horizon of visibility, were laid bare. The rise of the clinical mentality signaled radical transformations in how physicians conceived of their subject matter and restructured their relationship to patients. This is because the development of the clinical mentality required a hospital-based medical practice in which autopsies could be performed and in which the patient could become at once the subject of therapeutic ministrations and the object of medical study. The term *clinic,* then, has a double meaning, for it denotes both an emerging institutional form and a nascent way of "seeing" disease, both of which laid the foundations for diagnostic science and technical intervention.

Reiser's history of diagnostic technology implies that the "clinical mentality" may have receded in favor of one that may be designated "post-clinical" or technological (what he terms the abandonment of the *art* of medicine in favor of the *science* of medicine).[24] His analysis traces the development of medical practice as it evolved from a reliance on the patient's subjective narrative toward clinical perceptions (e.g., observation, palpation, and percussion), which in turn gave way to an increased reliance on sophisticated diagnostic instruments. (I have termed these interactive, perceptual, and technological cues, respectively.) While acknowledging that these developments have enhanced the diagnostic capabilities of physicians, Reiser also suggests that each juncture in this epistemological transformation was accompanied by an increasing alienation in the doctor-patient relationship.

Reiser's analysis is not, as it may seem at first glance, entirely technologically deterministic, for he notes that the use of diagnostic technology was accompanied by certain forms of organization that augmented the social distance between patient and practitioner. The very use of instrumentation interposes a physical barrier between physician and patient. Once it became possible to speak of "asymptomatic illness" (disease detected by signs apparent only to the expert), a phenomenological realm apart from the patient's subjective experience was created. The new diagnostic armamentarium also entailed changes in the physician's role, wherein history taking and interaction assumed less importance in medical work. A hierarchy among medical practitioners developed in which those who could master and interpret esoteric techniques occupied a superior position to the first-line medical practitioners who dealt directly with patients. Finally, as the locale of diagnosis moved from the patient's home to the laboratory, new forms of social organization emerged in which physicians became increasingly disengaged from their patients.

These cultural and structural features of technology-intensive medical settings complicate the process of reaching life-and-death decisions. Newborn intensive care is grounded in a "post-clinical" culture that accords privileged status to certain types of knowledge, and it also has a social structure in which physicians are organizationally disengaged from patients and parents. Furthermore, the task of interaction with the patient is vested largely in those subordinate in the occupational hierarchy. We are left, then, with partial and selective visions of reality, in the sense that Mannheim intended the term *ideology,* and with differential resources with which participants are able to promulgate their respective points of view.[25] Physicians have the medical knowledge for reaching life-and-death decisions, but they may lack potentially valuable sources of information that can be acquired only through interaction with infants. Nurses have access to this more "subjective" source of information, but they may be unduly influenced by the practicalities of patient management. As parents become increasingly reliant on physicians to interpret an increasingly esoteric knowledge, they run the risk of becoming peripheral to life-and-death decisions; therefore, a truly informed consent may become difficult to attain.

The analysis presented here also suggests something about how the quality of life-and-death decisions may be improved. To the extent that decisions cannot be extricated from the social organization of the intensive-care nursery, broader changes in that organization may be necessary. A culture that permits the exploration of other modes of knowledge, and a social structure that facilitates greater interaction among physicians, patients, and parents, may contribute to more informed and equitable decision making.

CHAPTER 4

Producing Assent

Parents, Professionals,
and Life-and-Death Decisions

Having read the last chapter, the reader may ask with considerable justification, "But what about the parents? What role do *they* play in life-and-death decisions?" The next two chapters, which discuss the role of parents in decision making, speak to this issue.

My decision to discuss the parents last reflects the natural order of decisions in the two intensive-care nurseries I studied: only after the professionals have reached a decision are the parents consulted. This practice has the effect of placing parents on the periphery of life-and-death decisions.[1]

FROM PRINCIPLES TO PRACTICE

In discussing the role of parents in life-and-death decisions, I am revisiting a classical problem in a new context: the relationship of theory and practice, ideas and action. The ideas are those of bioethicists who write about informed consent; the practice is that of physicians and other clinicians; and the setting is intensive-care units for newborn infants. Without plumbing the depths of the is/ought controversy, I assume at the outset that the ideas of bioethicists can be made relevant to the realities of clinical practice. One purpose of this chapter is to suggest ways to bring theory and practice into better accord.

Ethicists are sharply divided over whether, and to what extent,

*1 side
apart from
parents*

parents should participate in the decision-making process. At one end
of the spectrum are those writers who believe that the newborn infant
has a right to life apart from the rights of the parents, and for this
reason decisions should be made by physicians in accordance with a
"medical indications" policy. Some have suggested that physicians,
with their superior knowledge, should be the principal decision makers. At the other end of the spectrum are those writers who argue that

*1 side
for parents*

parents should have the final authority to determine whether their
babies should live or die. These commentators advocate the principle
of informed consent because they believe that parents bear the ultimate consequences of life-and-death decisions.[2]

*mid
point*

Midway between these positions are those bioethicists who contend that parents should play an important but limited role in life-and-
death decisions. In contrast to those who argue that parents have an
implicit conflict of interest with their babies, these authors argue that
parents are optimally situated to determine the interests of their babies and to place those interests over their own.[3] However, when
parents reach decisions that professionals believe are contrary to the
best interests of the infants, the dispute should be adjudicated by an
ethics committee.

The arguments in this chapter are directed toward those who believe that parents should be incorporated into life-and-death decisions
and, in particular, to those who advocate informed consent. All too
often, such writers simplify the social dimensions of life-and-death
decisions and treat social dynamics as relatively unproblematic. In the
following pages, I consider two issues that bioethical discussions of
informed consent frequently fail to address: the process by which
parents are informed and the context in which their consent is obtained. These considerations, which often elude bioethical analysis of
life-and-death decisions, are fundamental concerns for those who
make them. In the first part of the chapter, I discuss the communication process, for simply to articulate the *principle* that parents should
be involved in decision making does not consider the highly complex
and delicate negotiation *process* that often takes place between parents and professionals. In short, how should the principle of informed
consent be enacted in practice? How do we bridge the gap between
principles and practice, ideals and action?

Next, I turn to the context of consent and examine how the organization of the intensive-care nursery shapes the decision-making process. Writers have recognized that the nursery can create barriers

barriers.

between parents and their babies.[4] I discuss how the organization of the intensive-care nursery creates barriers between parents and members of the nursery staff—barriers that are consequential for life-and-death decisions. Health professionals confront the task of communicating devastating information to relative strangers—to say nothing of communicating across the lines of education, culture, and class. Parents must make often irreversible decisions while facing the harsh realities of seeing their babies connected to life-support equipment, traveling long distances, and negotiating with an ever-shifting array of personnel. Transcending these barriers is what informed consent is all about.

THE DECISION-MAKING PROCESS

Two Models of Decision Making

Writers who advocate incorporating the parents into life-and-death decisions leave unanswered a basic question: namely, *how* parents are to participate in decision making. Consider, for example, an ostensibly simple issue: how should professionals inform parents, and how should parents' consent be obtained? How should diagnostic and prognostic information be presented to parents? Should parents be presented with a *range* of prognostic outcomes, or should prognostic information be weighted toward the low or the high end of the continuum? Next, consider the decision itself: should parents be presented with the *option* of discontinuing life support, or should they be presented with a recommendation from the staff?

Variety of questions

Each of these alternative presentation strategies presupposes a fundamentally different implicit model of the role that parents should play in life-and-death decisions. In the first model—that of *informed consent*—parents are treated as the principal participants in the life-and-death decision. In the second model, parents are viewed as giving *assent* to a decision members of the nursery staff have already made. (The two paradigms should be seen as ideal types, as poles on a continuum. Actual decision-making may combine features of both models.) The quotations in Table 2, taken from my interviews with physicians and my observations of staff conferences, illustrate the contrast between consent and assent models.

Medical sociologists since Parsons have argued that there is an

TABLE 2

MODELS OF DECISION MAKING

Assent Model	Consent Model
*Infant with Down syndrome**	*Infant with Down syndrome**
Children with Down's syndrome are mentally retarded, and some die early from heart disease. Many develop multiple medical problems. Even the educable ones that have a loving family (are) . . . still a trauma to the family and . . . what happens when the parents die and the children are left alone as adults?	I think that the surgeons would have to give the parents . . . some kind of realistic appraisal of what a Down's syndrome child might or might not be able to do, the variability within Down's syndrome. . . . [The future is] really variable. Some Down's babies are very retarded and . . . have a miserable life; I think that's a minority. Most Down's children by our standards are moderately retarded and learn to take care of themselves in a physical sense. I've seen families where [children with Down's syndrome] are an integral part of the family. They are accepted and loved by all concerned. They require prolonged supervision and can work in sheltered . . . workshops, but . . . have the potential . . . by their amiable nature to be rewarding and to have rewarding relationships and to have a positive influence on society, and have enough intelligence and awareness to enjoy life . . . and some Down's children . . . are very bright compared to the others and can go to school and lead happy, productive lives. Some parents find taking care of a child with Down's syndrome can be very rewarding; others find it more stressful.

TABLE 2 (CONTINUED)

Dying Infant†	Dying Infant†
. . . Then the blood pressure continued to decrease and the heart rate slowed down. . . . We have been giving the medicines for 48 hours and it's not working. He is dying and there is no sign of recovery. In the last 48 hours [he] has gotten worse. We have done everything we can and we feel there is nothing more we can do. For these reasons, we have decided to stop the medicines that are keeping the baby's heart going. Continuing the medicines will not do any good and will only prolong [the baby's] suffering.	. . . since that time, the baby has deteriorated. He did have a bleed in his head. Now, his blood pressure is dropping and he has stopped urinating. Yesterday we did a CAT scan to see if the baby had a bleed, and we found that he did have a bleed in the head. Before we finish, there are two things I want to mention. Sometimes the parents want to hold the baby before he dies to say goodbye. We encourage you to do this, but don't want to pressure you in any way. If not, we can call you when the baby dies. We are here to support you in any way and to respect your wishes. Another thing is since we want to honor your wishes, sometimes parents prefer that their baby not suffer for a long time, and we will turn off the ventilator that is keeping him alive. Other parents prefer for us to continue to support the baby until he dies. It's entirely up to you.

*These quotations are taken from interviews with physicians who were asked, "What should the surgeon tell the parents?" and "What kind of future do you see this baby as having?"

†These quotations are taken shorthand from conferences with the parents and are close to verbatim.

inevitable "competence gap" between doctor and patient, and for this reason physicians hold some degree of hegemony over decision making.[5] However, as the examples presented in the right-hand column of Table 2 suggest, even within this constraint, physicians may structure the conversation so as to allow considerable latitude for parent participation. If a model of informed consent is practiced, clinicians can facilitate greater parental involvement by presenting parents with a range of prognostic outcomes, as shown in Table 2. Equally important, to ensure that the parents exercise an informed choice, practitioners must pose treatment options in a nonjudgmental fashion. In the following example from the General Nursery, presented in brief form in Table 2, the physician poses options without attempting to persuade the parents to discontinue life support. She also encourages, but does not pressure, the parents to hold the baby when he dies:

ATTENDING: Before we finish, there are two things I want to mention. The first is that sometimes the parents want to hold the baby before he dies, to say goodbye. If you want to do this, we can let you be alone with the baby. We encourage you to do this, but we don't want to pressure you in any way. If not, we can call you when the baby dies. We are here to support you in any way and to respect your wishes. Another thing is, since we want to honor your wishes, sometimes parents prefer that their baby not suffer for a long time, and we will turn off the ventilator that is keeping him alive. Other parents prefer for us to continue to support the baby until he dies. It's entirely up to you.

sw/ empowerment

Naturally, empowering parents to be the primary decision makers entails a "risk" for the staff: namely, that parents may make a choice that does not accord with professionals' point of view. This is, in fact, what happened in the case just cited: the parents decided not to remain with the baby when he died and chose to continue life support.

Some parents assume at the outset that life-and-death decisions are to be made by the professionals, and these assumptions require an effort on the part of the staff to empower parents to be the principal decision makers. Consider, for example, the case of María Sandoval, a baby who had a chromosomal disorder, Rubinstein-Taybi syndrome, in which those affected are moderately to severely retarded and also have physical abnormalities. The mother, a sixteen-year-old daughter of migrant farmworkers who was receiving welfare, was asked to decide whether the baby should receive surgery to correct a minor heart abnormality. When I interviewed the mother, she understood the implications of the syndrome and the kind of care and special schooling that María would require. The following is an excerpt from the conference with María's mother, her maternal grandmother, and the pediatric dysmorphologist (a specialist in birth defects):

(The resident draws a diagram to explain the nature of the baby's heart defect.)

RESIDENT: Your baby has what is called a patent ductus arteriosus, or PDA. This means that there is an opening between the heart and the lungs. In most babies, this closes, but sometimes it stays open and the blood doesn't circulate properly. Too much blood accumulates in the lungs, and then the baby can't breathe well or grow properly. There is an operation for this in which we tie off the ductus, or ligate it. It's a relatively simple procedure. Now, if we don't do the surgery, the baby will continue the way she is and will die in time.

MOTHER: So are you going to do the surgery?

RESIDENT: That's what we wanted to ask you.

PEDIATRIC DYSMORPHOLOGIST: Yes, we wanted to let you know what your options are. . . .
(The mother explains the dilemma to the grandmother in Spanish.)

GRANDMOTHER *(in Spanish):* Only you can decide.

MOTHER: She said I'm the only one who can decide.

PEDIATRIC DYSMORPHOLOGIST: We've added a new set of problems. The problem with the heart and lungs is part of the syndrome that we talked about. At the time we talked before, there didn't seem to be a problem, but now it's apparent she will need surgery to correct the defect. Now, one option we have is not to do the surgery, and it's clear that the baby will die. We want to ask you whether you would like us to do the surgery.

MOTHER: I know she's not a completely normal baby, but I don't want her to go on like this.

RESIDENT: Yes, she won't live forever with the heart problem.

PEDIATRIC DYSMORPHOLOGIST: Another thing—you understand that the surgery won't correct the genetic defect, the Rubinstein-Taybi syndrome that we talked about?

MOTHER: I know. I want the surgery.

PEDIATRIC DYSMORPHOLOGIST: Do you have any other questions you would like to ask us?

MOTHER: What are the risks?

Because the Baby Doe controversies have changed the climate surrounding life-and-death decisions, it is possible that staff members of today's nurseries would not have given this mother the option of withholding relatively minor heart surgery from a baby with Rubinstein-Taybi syndrome. However, while historical circumstances may have changed the *criteria* used in this particular decision, they have not changed the general point I am making about the decision-making *process*. The previous excerpt dramatically demonstrates that even a parent who is very young and is separated from the nursery staff by invisible barriers of culture and social class can understand the implications of the choices she faces and provide an informed consent. As in the previous example, the physicians structure the conversation by providing options so that the mother is empowered to make an informed choice.

Producing Assent

Unfortunately, the cases cited previously were the exception rather than the rule. Although professionals in both intensive-care nurseries I studied acknowledged the importance of involving the parents in the decision-making process, an assent model, rather than an informed consent paradigm, was most frequently used. In most conferences with parents that I observed directly (as well as those informants recounted to me), providers employed a number of practices, whether intentionally or unwittingly, that framed or shaped parents' decisions.

First, the decision-making process itself is structured to limit and constrain parental participation. Generally, the staff conference and the conference with the parents take place in separate arenas. The staff confer first—either in rounds or in a formal conference—and parents are not present during these deliberations. Only *after* the staff have reached a consensual decision to terminate life support or withhold treatment are the parents consulted. Members of the nursery staff refer to this process as "presenting a united front." This practice is said to protect the parents from being confused by conflicting opinions. While the practice indeed has this effect, "presenting a united front" has other consequences as well: when the staff's decision is to continue treating the baby actively, the parents are not consulted at all. While a consensus among both staff and parents is required to *discontinue* active treatment, the parents' consent is not required to *continue* treating a baby. This process automatically excludes the parents from life-and-death decisions in which the staff have decided in favor of treating a baby, as well as from those decisions in which it is simply assumed that the baby will be treated—for example, decisions to resuscitate the very small, very premature infants described in Chapter 3. Because such infants run a high risk of death or major brain damage, resuscitating them is arguably experimental. However, since resuscitating the tiniest newborns is not explicitly defined as an experimental protocol, the parents are not consulted. The babies are simply resuscitated, and the parents are in effect excluded from resuscitation decisions:

INTERVIEWER: How do you feel about resuscitating the very small preemies?

NURSE: It's really sad that parents don't understand their rights—that they can put their foot down and say no. . . .

INTERVIEWER: So what should the parents be told?

NURSE: I think they should be told realistically . . . that they usually don't live, they usually don't do well, [and] they usually have brain damage. And I think they should also be told that there are occasionally babies . . . that do respond to treatment. . . .

INTERVIEWER: Are they given the choice?

NURSE: I don't think they are. I think that automatically [the babies are] resuscitated when they're born.

In short, in both nurseries I studied, the decision-making process was organized to limit the options available to parents and to eliminate parents from some decisions altogether.

"Presenting a united front" has another important consequence: when the parents are consulted, they are not exposed to a range of opinions. Even when a decision has been reached after intense controversy, the parents are brought into the process only after the staff have reached closure. As the following example suggests, "presenting a united front" obscures controversy in favor of consensus and narrows the options presented to the parents. Vicente Duarte, a seven-day-old premature infant who was hospitalized in the General Nursery, had suffered a pulmonary hemorrhage and a massive intraventricular hemorrhage (bleeding in the brain). Vicente had been given vasoactive drugs (to support the blood pressure and increase the heart rate) after his heart rate had fallen dramatically. During the conference, the staff reached a consensus that the dopamine and isuprel that the baby was receiving to support his heart rate and blood pressure should be discontinued. Only the fellow was reluctant to discontinue life support.

ATTENDING: Well, in my view of the results of the CT scan and the massive bleed, the chances of getting this baby back undamaged are very slim, and I think we are doing excessive medical management if we continue to treat him aggressively. I am going to discuss this with Dr. Juarez, and you can talk to the parents. If they decide not to continue, then we should discontinue.

. . .

ATTENDING: He's already had two episodes where he suffered insults to the brain for a period of two hours.

FELLOW: I've read reports of severe asphyxia and acidosis, and there were infants who survived with normal mental function.

ATTENDING: But with the combination of shock leading to low blood pressure for forty-eight hours—has anyone reported such a case which survived undamaged?

FELLOW: It is reported.

ATTENDING: I know of no patient that survived. Besides the hypoxic episodes, this patient has had a documented bleed in the brain. There are a lot of other things involved, and you have to put the whole thing together and look at the whole picture and see whether doing something heroic is justified. But none of us is God, and we can't say this with 100 percent certainty. That is why it has to be a group decision to see if everyone goes along with the decision. Do you think we should continue?

FELLOW: Half and half, I don't know. Just by looking at the baby, I'm not sure there is no hope. Are we positive about this?

RESIDENT: No one can ever be positive—we have to think of the likelihood for the baby. He got maximal care. If you go on, the odds are low that he will survive undamaged. Also, you have to think of the quality of life the baby will have. . . .

ATTENDING: Yes, every patient is entitled to 100 percent care until you have no reasonable doubt that the baby will not be able to survive undamaged.

SOCIAL WORKER: Damage isn't the point. The question is, are we prolonging the baby's death?

ATTENDING: There's a 90 percent chance the baby will die. If there's the slightest chance that the baby will survive undamaged, we should continue. . . . That's why it has to be a group decision. When I started back in '70, I never gave up.

FELLOW: I guess I'm still at that point.

ATTENDING: Then, I had to be 200 percent sure. There would be babies where . . . people would ask me what I was doing, and I would say, "You can't just stop." But in that case, you see only what you are doing at the moment, and you're not looking beyond that.

Despite the fellow's reluctance, the nursery staff decided to discuss with the parents the option of discontinuing the drugs. That conference was attended by the fellow, the social worker, who translated to and from Spanish, and Mr. and Mrs. Duarte.

FELLOW: Tell them that we are here to give them the test results, but first I would like to review the history. The first day, the baby was born prematurely, and he had sepsis [a massive infection]. Then we suspected a bleed in the brain, because he began to have seizures. . . . We found blood in the lungs, but we also strongly suspected that he may have bled elsewhere. We replaced the blood he lost. Then the blood pressure continued to decrease, and the heart rate slowed down. We have been giving medicines to try to raise his blood pressure and heart rate. We've been giving the medicines for forty-eight hours, and they're not working. Yesterday, we did a CAT scan to see if the baby had a bleed in the brain, and we found out he did have a bleed in the head. Because the medicines are not working, we feel there is nothing more we can do. Continuing the medicines will only prolong the baby's suffering, and for these reasons we have decided to stop the medicines that are keeping the baby's heart going.

The social worker then translated and asked the parents how they felt. Mrs. Duarte began to cry. Then, after several moments, she asked, "Is there nothing else that you can do?" There was a momentary, pregnant pause, because both the social worker and I knew that the fellow believed there *was* something that could be done. Then the fellow answered, "We can go on, but he will die within days, and this will only prolong the baby's suffering."

After the conference, the fellow continued to maintain that the bleed was not so bad and that there was hope for the baby. She felt that middle-class parents "know what they want and can express it," and she identified "much more with these parents—they belong to another culture, and we tell them what to do."

This case illustrates a major function of conducting the staff conference before consulting the parents. By the time the staff have reached their decision, all the ambiguities, hesitations, and disagreements that were expressed in the conference vanish in the face of the staff's illusory "united front." The additional ambiguity that was expressed in the staff conference—whether the decision to terminate treatment was a decision not to prolong the process of dying or was being made on quality-of-life grounds—also disappears from the conference with the parents.

In short, in both nurseries I studied, the decision-making process ✗

✳ was organized so as to limit parents' options—even to the extent of eliminating them from some decisions altogether. The actual, if sometimes unstated, aim of the conference with parents was to elicit their agreement to decisions staff had already made.

The example just presented illustrates another practice for producing assent: when there is a range of possible prognoses, it is not uncommon for professionals to "slant" the prognosis by presenting outcomes leaning toward the positive or negative end of the continuum, in accordance with their beliefs and values, as illustrated in interview materials on the left-hand side of Table 2. Thus, in the case just presented, the attending and the fellow allude to three possible prognostic outcomes: the baby will die; the baby will survive with brain damage; or the baby will have a very small chance of surviving without serious brain damage. The parents, however, are simply told that the baby will die.

✳ In a common scenario, professionals employ a set of strategies to persuade the parents to accept the staff's point of view. A pattern residents frequently use is the appeal to expert authority. In the course of informing the parents of a decision not to treat their baby actively, physicians assure the parents that the decision was reached only after consulting a number of highly respected specialists. Often this strategy is employed in the context of bearing the bad news of a very grim prognosis, as in the following excerpt from a phone conversation between a resident and the father of an infant with multiple heart defects:

> We talked to Dr. Walker [a world-renowned pediatric cardiac surgeon], and he says it's too dangerous to do the surgery now. Some babies do well with a temporary pacemaker. We've seen them left in for a month or so with no problems. I really respect his opinion, and this is the best way to go. We'll see how well she'll do, and we'll use a medicine to help pump the heart. *(He listens to the father's response.)* We won't feed her for a couple of days. Friday we'll try to feed her. *(He listens.)* That would be fine.

Or consider this dialogue from a conference between a resident and the mother of an infant with a kidney defect:

RESIDENT: So right now we'll correct any major complications that arise. And if his lungs improve, we can consider dialysis. But I really doubt if that will happen. He's already had two major complications today, and the next time that will happen, he may not pull through.

MOTHER: You think he won't make it?

RESIDENT: Yes, I think your son will die—maybe tonight, maybe in four days. That's also the opinion of Dr. Morris [the neonatologist] and the surgeons, who have gone over your son's situation in detail. The kidney specialists say there have been a few kids who have survived with very little kidney tissue, and their quality of life leaves much to be desired. But still, we'll do as much as we can. Dr. Morris is on rounds right now, and he wants to talk to you and your husband.

MOTHER (*crying*):   Thank you.

Appeals to expert authority are only one of a number of practices that staff employ to encourage parents to agree to decisions to terminate life support. Other devices commonly used in termination decisions include reviewing test results (thereby appealing to the authority of technology); noting that the baby has failed to improve; assuring the parents that the nursery has done everything in its power to try to help the baby; letting the parents know that the baby is being kept alive by artificial means; either informing the parents of the staff's decision or recommending termination of treatment, rather than presenting the parents with options; and finally, closing the discussion with a statement about the moral consequences of keeping the baby alive—that is, prolonging his or her suffering. So commonly used were these strategies in the General Nursery that conferences with the parents followed an almost canonical script. Consider the case of Ramon Martinez, a baby with severe liver disease, multiple skeletal deformities, and a possible brain dysfunction, who had failed to improve for a period of months:

RESIDENT: I want to talk in English—they know I speak Spanish. We want to tell you about the test results. We did a test, an electroencephalogram, and it showed a very slow brain wave. This means that the baby's brain is not functioning normally. In fact, the test results were very abnormal.
(*The pediatric dysmorphologist translates this into Spanish.*)

RESIDENT: We also have done several other tests and consulted several people, as I told you we would do a week ago. We did a CAT scan [translated as *rayos*], and it is very difficult to interpret these in very small babies. The CAT scan was read as normal, but there was something at the brain stem that could be a tumor. . . . The baby also has problems with his liver. In addition, he hasn't shown any improvement for a long time, although we have done everything possible. So we have talked this over with many experts and with

Dr. Cardenas, the head of the nursery. I want to assure you that we have done everything that we could do for the baby, and now there is really nothing more we can do. The respirator and the medicines are the only things that are keeping the baby alive, and we recommend not continuing the machines and the medicines. Keeping him alive would do him no good and would only prolong his suffering. *(The pediatric dysmorphologist translates this.)*

In this case, as in many others, the resident constructs the medical and ethical parameters to lead to the conclusion that nothing more can be done and that discontinuing life support is inevitable. He presents the test results that point to a conclusion of brain damage (the abnormal EEG), while discounting what might otherwise be viewed as countervailing evidence (he notes that the CAT scan was *read* as normal, but points out that the test is difficult to interpret in small infants). Supporting his medical claims with appeals to experts who have been consulted, the resident notes that the baby has shown no improvement although the staff have attempted to do everything possible. The resident also constructs a moral interpretation of the case, implying that the baby is being kept alive by artificial means. This construction suggests that continuing to support the baby would require an active decision, whereas terminating life support would only be allowing nature to take its course. Finally, he concludes the presentation with an appeal to the ethical principle of nonmalificence ("Keeping [the baby] alive would do him no good and would only prolong his suffering"). This is a moral precept with which most parents would find it hard to disagree. What parents would want to prolong their baby's suffering? In short, the resident has framed both the medical and ethical parameters of the case to lead to the conclusion that terminating life support is the only medically sound and morally correct alternative.

Given the persuasive practices that I have just described—framing the medical "facts" of the case, appealing to medical technology and expert authority, and formulating unequivocal moral precepts—it is hardly surprising that very few parents challenge physicians' interpretations or reject their recommendations. Although professional constructions shape parents' decisions, so powerful is the public acceptance of expert authority that few parents offer resistance. The production of assent, while managed and engineered by professionals, is in fact an interactional accomplishment in which parents are unwitting accomplices.

Which Model Will Be Used?—Differential Leverage
in Decision Making

Given the large number of parents and providers in both nurseries
who were involved in life-and-death decisions, there was considerable
variation in the extent to which parents were encouraged to participate actively in the decision-making process. The sociological question then becomes: under what social conditions can parents exercise
leverage in decision making?

The degree of latitude that parents exercised in decision making
varied according to a number of social contingencies, including: how
the staff viewed their own role in life-and-death decisions; how the
staff viewed the psychological consequences of incorporating parents
into life-and-death decisions; how certain the staff were about the
correctness of a particular decision; and how the professionals perceived parents' competency to participate in life-and-death decisions.

Professional Ideologies and Role Conceptions.   In both nurseries,
professionals differed in the degree to which they felt they should
manage the decision-making process. When interviewed, they revealed a range of communication philosophies and normative views
of the role that they and the parents should play in life-and-death
decisions. At one end of the continuum were those residents (decid-
edly in the minority) who felt strongly that they should not intervene
in parents' decisions. As one resident said, "It's the parents' decision;
we're only here to help. I don't believe this business about doctors
being God."

Professionals' views of the procedural question of *who* should
decide are sometimes related to their views of the substantive ethical
question of *what* should be decided. Those professionals who felt that
the infant's future quality of life and the family's interest should be
considered often viewed themselves as playing a limited role in life-
and-death decisions to be made by parents. At the other end of the
spectrum were those staff members who expressed the "child advocacy" ideology, which views quality-of-life decisions as a conflict
between the interests of parents and those of the infant, in which the
proper role of the pediatrician is to be an advocate for the child's right
to life.[6] Drawing on the rhetoric of child abuse, the child advocacy
ideology conceives the parent-child relationship in potentially adver-
sarial terms. Physicians who felt that they should advocate for the

child's right to life sometimes expressed the view that the courts should be consulted if parents refuse to have infants treated who are likely to survive with disabilities. When asked whether he felt that a child with Down syndrome and an intestinal obstruction should be treated, one resident responded: "In my experience [in another state], the courts went through that, and the child had surgery and was made a ward of the court because the parents decided not to [operate and] the physician disagreed. But I think that the child has rights beyond what the doctor and the parents decide. . . . If they can't agree to have surgery in the child's best interest . . . , that's when the parents should no longer be allowed to make the decision."

Perhaps most disturbing were the views of two nurses, whose responses indicated the conflict between the interests of parents and those of the staff. As members of the nursery staff, these nurses felt that they had an obligation to advocate for the child's right to life. However, they also identified with parents who could not care for a disabled infant. Torn between these two views, the nurses were profoundly ambivalent. When I asked one of them whether very small, very premature infants should be treated actively, she replied:

> See, I can't give answers to these things because . . . I always put myself in the place of these parents, and I always think that I wouldn't want to have one of these children. And on the other hand, I think exactly like all this thinking that goes on with these right-to-lifers. . . . The nurse's perspective is more like the right to life. I'm thinking of the child . . . , and this child has a right to life. The parents don't have the right to take a life away from this child. My other perspective is the way I feel and that I would not want this child, and that's it. You know, I put myself in the place of the parents.

In short, staff differed in their normative conceptions of their own roles and those of the parents. Those who argued that physicians should play a limited role in a parental decision were likely to advocate an informed consent model, whereas those who viewed themselves as child advocates were more likely to advocate an assent model.

Staff Commonsense Psychology.   Communication with the parents can be based on more than ethics, role conceptions, and ideology: staff also ground their communication strategies in what might be called "commonsense psychology." For example, in an ethics conference in the Randolph Nursery concerning an infant with spina bifida whose parents had been given conflicting information, Dr. Nelson expressed the commonly held view that physicians will inevitably influence the parents' decision, and for this reason physicians will *nolens volens* produce assent:

> Well, the only [legal problem] I can conceive of is the situation where the physician feels that the lesion is relatively minor and amenable to surgery, and the parents say no. And that is almost inconceivable, because the parents make their judgments largely on the basis of the information the physician gives them. So there I've always felt trapped, as is the case here, where [the parents] made one decision when they were given an optimistic point of view, and they made an opposite decision when they were given a pessimistic one. . . . So the physician has . . . the matter completely in his hands. I think having the parents well informed is always well informed on your grounds. . . . It's the way you see it. So ultimately the decision is made by whoever is calling the medical shots.

While correctly acknowledging the physician's power to influence parents' decisions, this belief in the inevitability of professional dominance ignores the fact that some physicians (as noted previously) can and do empower parents to provide informed consent.

Although most staff members who were interviewed felt that physicians are obliged to communicate openly with parents about their babies' diagnosis and prognosis, there were exceptions. For example, during a decision-making conference, a Randolph attending expressed reluctance to communicate a bleak prognosis to the mother of a baby with a serious congenital kidney defect that the staff had decided not to treat aggressively. His justification was that bearing bad news could damage the mother-child relationship. The mother was a seventeen-year-old unmarried black woman who was receiving public assistance, and the staff had found it difficult to communicate across the invisible lines of culture and social class.

RESIDENT 1:	We don't know what to tell Mom. We need to come up with a formula so we can tell her what to expect.
NEPHROLOGIST:	How old is she?
RESIDENT 2:	Seventeen. The other day, she came in and asked if we had any good news.
PEDIATRIC SURGEON:	It's been very difficult to deal with her. A week ago, I told her flat out the baby would probably die.
ATTENDING NEONATOLOGIST:	If that is the outlook, then can that be refuted? When you're not dealing with gross brain damage, I've always been hesitant to give a grim

picture. It's something I'm always hesitant to do, because it can damage a potentially good relationship between mother and child.

Other physicians based their decisions to use an assent rather than an informed consent model on a firmly held belief in the deleterious psychological consequences for the parents that might ensue from incorporating them fully into the decision-making process. A frequently cited "folk" psychological theory was that parents who are asked to play an active role in life-and-death decisions would later experience guilt. As the head of the General Nursery said, "I don't believe you should ask the parents outright, since that lays a guilt trip on the parents."[7] In the course of a staff conference in rounds about what to tell the parents of Vicente Duarte, the social worker and the resident in the General Nursery echoed this point of view, while arguing in favor of what I have called a policy of assent:

SOCIAL WORKER: I think we should present to the parents that we know the baby is dying. The father already doesn't have much hope. Yesterday, we told him that, depending on the scan, we should know if the baby would die or be seriously damaged. I think we should present our plan and let them know how we feel, but we shouldn't let the decision fall on them.

RESIDENT: I agree—it would produce a lot of guilt.

This belief that parents who are asked to make life-and-death decisions are likely to experience guilt is clearly paternalistic, insofar as it justifies reducing the power of parents on the basis of what is presumed to be in their best interest. This irony did not escape the head of the nursery, who noted in the context of a staff conference concerning a particular baby: "We usually end up making the decision for the family. We say it's not fair to them to ask them, 'What do you want them to do?' because they'll experience guilt, and then we end up maneuvering them into doing what we want." I refer to this viewpoint as a "folk psychological belief" because it has little support in social psychological research on decision making.

How Staff Perceive the Decision.   Professionals also varied their communications with parents according to the degree of moral certitude attached to a particular life-and-death decision. Although the observational evidence is indirect, staff were more likely to give

greater latitude to parents when the former were ambivalent or deeply
divided about a decision. In such cases, attendings shifted the locus of
decision making downward in the nursery's hierarchy, giving more
weight to the opinions of residents, nurses, and parents. As Guillemin
and Holmstrom also observe, those cases in which parents were repeatedly consulted were likely to be cases that the staff found highly
problematic (e.g., an infant with an unusual heart defect and possible
brain damage).[8] Conversely, when the staff felt certain or when there
was a high consensus (e.g., infants with the congenital abnormality
trisomy 18, all of whom were severely retarded and most of whom
would die in infancy), they were more likely to make recommendations to the parents.

The interviews provide further evidence that some staff members
varied their communication styles according to the degree of moral
certitude they attached to a decision, allowing more latitude for parental discretion in cases they viewed as morally ambiguous. Some
staff were reluctant to impose their views on parents in decisions that
they felt were ethically problematic and relative "gray areas," but they
were much more likely to impose their views on parents who wished
to treat an infant with trisomy 18. For example, one nurse had argued
forcefully for allowing parents to decide whether their very small, very
premature (twenty-five-week-old) infants should be treated. When
confronted, however, with the hypothetical case of an infant with
trisomy 18 whose parents wanted the baby to live, this nurse's commitment to the principle of informed consent faltered. Ultimately, she
suggested counseling the parents to "accept" the reality of their baby's
poor prognosis:

INTERVIEWER: What if the parents had wanted the baby [to live]?

NURSE: Yeah, it's definitely an inappropriate decision. God, that's really hard to say! I've never known parents who wanted a child
when you've explained to them that the baby usually has no
brain. You can't even offer minimal intelligence. I don't know;
that's a real hard one. I'd really have to think on that. The
parents' wishes have to be really considered, especially when
it's borderline. . . . I think you really have to delve in deeper and
find out why they want this baby . . . , because I don't think
anyone wants to take home a severely retarded, severely deformed child. I think there's something else going on when they
want to subject themselves to that.

INTERVIEWER: And if there's something else going on?

NURSE: I think you have to deal with that . . . , and continually work through that, and see if you can get them to accept the reality that the child is not going to live a normal life.

Perceptions of Parental "Sophistication."   On several occasions, staff varied their styles of communication according to their perceptions of particular parents' "sophistication." These attributions were, of course, based on the degree to which parents and professionals shared a common language and culture—which in turn reflected parents' social class, ethnicity, and educational attainment.

In both nurseries, staff consciously adjusted their vocabularies according to parents' perceived educational attainment, or what was called the parents' "medical sophistication." In the medical metaphor used by an attending at rounds, "Let's find out the level of the parents' education, and according to that we will titrate the information we give them." Judgments about parents' sophistication were often made at a moment's notice. For example, a resident calibrated her vocabulary "upward" in response to a mother's perceived medical sophistication as the resident explained the results of a cardiac catheterization:

RESIDENT: Well, he came through the catheterization well and doesn't have heart disease. What happened was that he was stressed by something. It was nothing you could have done anything about or prevented. Maybe the cord was wrapped around his neck and caused him to expel meconium.

MOTHER: Yes, we know what that is.

RESIDENT: Tell me if I'm being too simple. When the baby inhaled the meconium, this caused damage to his lungs. . . . The fact that the blood didn't have enough oxygen made it *look* like heart disease, but what he has is a problem with the lungs. The lungs aren't working properly and getting enough oxygen to the tissues, and we're worried that he won't get enough oxygen to the brain. The problem with the lungs is very serious.

Writing in the context of genetic counseling, anthropologist Rayna Rapp notes that the process of code-switching, or translating and simplifying medico-scientific discourse into the patient's vernacular, becomes even more complicated when practitioner and patient are divided by invisible barriers of language, culture, and social class.[9] Thus, "ventilators" and "drugs" become "machines" and "medicines" to the poor Hispanic parents of the General Nursery. The process of communicating prognostic information across class lines may introduce subtle transformations in connotative meanings. In explaining the consequences of her baby's brain hemorrhage to a twenty-year-old single black woman who was receiving welfare, an attending simplified his vocabulary and, in so doing, transformed the sterile, if stigmatizing, term *some damage* into the euphemistic *slow*. I reported this in my field notes as follows:

> I asked the attending about the Brown baby's brain hemorrhage, "How bad was the intracranial bleed?" He answered, "It's small, which means that there's a small chance that there'll be no permanent damage, a large chance that there will be some damage, and a small chance of severe damage." Later, I overheard him say to the mother, "Chances are the baby will be slow—that is, she won't learn as fast in school." She didn't respond. In rounds, the attending told the residents, "What I told [the mother] was that there was a small chance the baby would be normal, and there was also a chance the baby would be retarded. I said that the chances are that she would be—I used the word *slow*—she wouldn't learn to read and write as fast, and would have trouble with learning, and would require some special schooling. I don't know if she understood any of it."

In this encounter, the terms used with the mother are no more imprecise than is medical language. The term *some damage* has no clear empirical referent in terms of the baby's prognosis or future quality of life. (Does *some damage* mean mild mental retardation, learning disability, or temporary developmental delay?) However, by substituting the euphemism *slow* for *some damage*, the attending has removed the stigma and drastically transformed the connotative meanings. When interviewed afterward, Ms. Brown said that she had no objections to having a baby who was "slow," but she expressed serious concerns about having a baby who was retarded:

INTERVIEWER: What did the doctor tell you?

MOTHER: That the baby's small and premature, that there's a chance she'll be normal, she might be slow, and there's a chance she'll be retarded. If she's had another bleed, she'll be retarded, and they'll know by the end of the week.

INTERVIEWER: How do you feel about that?

MOTHER: I don't mind if the baby's slow or normal, but if she's retarded I can't keep her. I have to give her up for adoption. I can't have two kids and one is retarded—it's hard enough to have one. I want to go to work, too, when she's in school. I can't do that if the baby's retarded. It's just too much.

Thus, between the discourse of medicine and the vernacular lies the realm of connotative meaning. Just as staff may remove stigmatizing connotations in the process of code-switching, they may often unintentionally transform the routine into the stigmatizing. In communicating with lower-class parents, staff are sometimes not aware of the understandably ominous connotations of what seem to them to be routine bureaucratic procedures. Thus, Ms. Brown was understandably frightened when she was told that she should apply for Crippled Children's Services funds (to finance the baby's stay in the nursery), thinking that this meant a prognosis of disability. I asked her, "How does it feel to see the baby in the nursery?" She answered, "I was crying. It scared me that she wasn't breathing and to see all those machines. When the doctor talked about Crippled Children's, it scared me." The stigmatizing connotation attached to what staff view as a routine bureaucratic procedure may also account for the reluctance of some parents to apply for Crippled Children's Services funds.

Medical, technical, and bureaucratic language is only one discursive gap to be bridged in encounters between professionals and parents. There is also the language of the ethics of intensive care: "terminating" life support, "disconnecting" respirators, and "extraordinary" means are part of an arcane discourse that few parents can command. Thus, staff vary their styles of communication not only according to parents' perceived "medical sophistication" but also according to what might be called their "moral sophistication"—or how staff view parents' religious beliefs. In the Randolph Nursery, some staff were reluctant to discuss life-and-death decisions openly with Hispanic parents, who were presumed to be religious Catholics. These parents were believed "not to have a concept of" euthanasia. Here is an excerpt from my transcript of a tape-recorded conference concerning Roberta Zapata, an infant with an unusual brain defect, when the staff have decided to stop giving drugs to correct her heart failure:

FELLOW: The father definitely understands, I think he does, what's gonna happen. After they'd been here Sunday, it seems that the mother might have understood, but I'm still not sure, except I told them that the baby, there was nothing else that could be done for the baby, that they must understand that after these operations, there's nothing else that can treat the baby's heart, to get the baby's heart working, or to keep the heart working well, but that there was nothing else we could offer. It was just a matter of time before the baby was going to die, and then I told them, "We're going to try to get the baby off the ventilator," which for them to understand I had to use the word *oxygen* more than anything else. . . . We wanted to show them exactly, so that they could understand, and we wanted to talk to them about the medications, what we were going to do with that. And I can tell you that it's important, at least I think, for them to come in and see this, because . . . once you use the term *terminate oxygen*, they think you're killing the baby.

Consider also the following excerpt from my Randolph field notes:

When Larry Dominguez, a baby with a giant omphalocele [a protrusion of part of the intestine through a large defect in the abdominal wall at the umbilicus] and hypoplastic [underdeveloped] lungs, suffered a sudden cardiopulmonary arrest, I was told by the nurse that the staff had tried unsuccessfully to resuscitate him, that he was without oxygen for twenty minutes, and "his brain is just gone." The parents were called in, and the staff planned to turn off the ventilator. After the parents had come in, according to the nurse, "I talked to the sister who speaks some English. I told her, 'Larry died this morning, and we couldn't bring him back.' I said it that way because they don't understand things like resuscitation."

Another incident concerned Margarita Portes, a baby who had been referred to the nursery for multiple congenital abnormalities: an omphalocele, ambiguous genitalia, and defects of the bladder, vertebrae, ribs, and pelvic bones. She also developed a massive infection and serious respiratory complications (pulmonary hypertension). I overheard the surgeon, Dr. Smith, talking about the parents to the nurse and the chaplain, saying that it was hard for the parents to hear that there is anything wrong with the baby. Then I introduced myself to the surgeon, and we had the following conversation:

SURGEON: Well, this one is interesting for you—Portes.
INTERVIEWER: Are you deciding whether to do surgery?
SURGEON: Well, we can't do surgery until the baby's stable.
INTERVIEWER: So the main problem is the lungs?
SURGEON: Yes, the main problem is the lungs. But the other problem is interesting from a philosophical standpoint.
INTERVIEWER: Is it an omphalocele?
SURGEON: Yes, and the bladder is protruding. . . . You can make the baby survive, but you wonder what kind of life you're producing. . . .
INTERVIEWER: Are you going to continue supporting the baby?
SURGEON: Well, it's difficult to talk to the parents because of their background. They don't have a concept of euthanasia.[10]

In each of these cases, professionals voiced their discomfort about talking to Hispanic parents, presumed to be religious Catholics who lacked a concept of terminating life support. In the first two cases, this assumption led to code-switching and using a highly simplified vocabulary. In the third case, it led to the surgeon's decision not to broach the subject of alternatives to aggressive treatment—a decision that drastically limited the parents' participation in a life-and-death decision from the outset.

In the General Nursery, in which most of the parents were Hispanic, staff believed that parents were capable of understanding, in the social worker's words, "that all of [the baby's] systems are failing, and that he needs the medication to keep him alive, and we are only prolonging his suffering." However, in the Randolph Nursery, the staff's cultural assumptions about the parents' cultural assumptions drastically limited Hispanic parents' participation in life-and-death decisions. In fact, the only case in which a respirator was turned off without consulting the parents involved Hispanic migrant farmworkers.

At the other end of the socioeconomic continuum were those parents, usually professionals, who were perceived as knowledgeable, "sophisticated," and conversant with medical and ethical vocabularies. For example, a neonatology fellow accounted for a controversial decision to discontinue treating a baby with multiple genetic bone deformities (arthrogryposis multiplex congenita) by referring to a parent's moral sophistication. According to the fellow, the father's ability to articulate his wishes clearly and his mastery of ethical terminology figured into the fellow's decision to accede to the father's wishes.

FELLOW: This is a case of arthrogryposis multiplex congenita. The baby was born in ——— at thirty-two weeks with Apgars of 4 and 8. It was apparent to the physician and to the father, who was in the delivery room, that the baby had multiple deformities. The baby was put into oxygen, and an umbilical venous line was instituted. The nursery was called for consultation. After discussion with the family—and the family's wishes were for the baby not to survive—after discussion between himself and the family, it was decided to support the baby with oxygen but not to institute ventilatory therapy if it became necessary. We were called to find out, first, what was the situation with the arthrogryposis, and, second, would we care for the baby? When the baby arrived here, we found that the baby had severe arthrogryposis. Then the baby developed respiratory difficulties, grunting and retraction. The PO_2 [a measure of respiratory function] was 60—and 70 in 100 percent oxygen. We spoke with the physician, and we spoke with the father. He said that both he and his wife had discussed the situation and felt strongly that they didn't want the baby to survive, and asked that we not do anything regarding the ventilator.

DR. NELSON: Could you tell us something about the parents?

FELLOW: The father is an engineer, and I'm not sure what the mother does. Anyway, they were quite sophisticated. The father was conversant with the whole terminology of withdrawing support. He was adamant. We discussed the case with the attending at ———, and we decided to accede to the family's request. The baby had already developed metabolic acidosis, and it was decided not to ventilate the baby and not to use CPAP [a form of assisted ventilation]. The baby expired a few hours later. There are several questions this case raises: (1) the question of the extent of damage—whether the baby would be neurologically handicapped, and what would be the neurological outcome; (2) what kind of position do you take when the parents state their wishes clearly? They didn't use any euphemisms and stated very clearly that we should not continue to support the baby. This is very different from the usual case, where the parents are unclear and their feelings develop over a long period of time.

In the climate following the Baby Doe regulations, it is doubtful whether physicians would accede to parents' requests not to treat babies with physical deformities. The decision I have just discussed was highly controversial, and, as the ethicist's comments suggest, some viewed the decision as legally questionable:

ETHICIST: One issue is clear in this little debate. Victor [the fellow], the parents, and the referring physician are all liable to charges of manslaughter. There is an article by Robertson in the *Journal of Pediatrics*. . . . Robertson stresses that to make a decision that results in the death of a baby that has a chance for survival is to be liable to charges of homicide, and anyone who cooperates is an accomplice. . . . No longer do parents have absolute rights over their children in our culture.

Although the criteria used in this decision may have changed, the sociological point of this case remains true in today's climate: when staff are ambivalent about a decision, morally sophisticated parents exercise more leverage in decision making.

In the General Nursery, parents who were regarded as sophisticated were also likely to express their wishes clearly and in a vocabulary likely to be persuasive to staff. One example was Sonia Parducci, a college-educated mother of twins who gave birth while visiting this country from Italy. While not fluent in English, she was nevertheless able to assert herself in a decision to support one of the babies after he had suffered a brain hemorrhage.

INTERVIEWER: So then what happened after he had the bleed? What did Dr. Michaels tell you about that?

MRS. PARDUCCI: We stayed three or four days without knowing if they were going to stop the machine, so I stayed for a long time thinking about the death of the baby.

INTERVIEWER: Did they ask you about stopping the machine?

MRS. PARDUCCI: I told the doctor, if there is one hope, I want to keep trying, but if it's only for you for medical, and not for the baby, you know, for doctor school and not for the baby, stop.

Medical and moral sophistication—or, in more sociological parlance, socioeconomic status—has a double effect in the nursery that has been noted by other researchers. Working-class and lower-class parents receive information that is simplified and euphemistic, or they are excluded from decisions altogether, and, in addition, they are unlikely to express their wishes forcefully. Thus, they are doubly disadvantaged in their encounters with staff, and their leverage in life-and-death decisions is drastically diminished. Conversely, medically and morally sophisticated parents not only receive more sophisticated communications from staff but are more apt to assert their wishes and to articulate their points of view in a language likely to be persuasive to staff.

Medical sophistication, however, often proves to be a double-edged sword. Educated parents exercise more leverage in life-and-death decisions. At the same time, the ability of these parents to articulate and assert their wishes often brings them into overt conflict with the nursery staff—an issue pursued in Chapter 5.

THE CONTEXT OF CONSENT

The consent process is influenced by the *context* in which it takes place as well as the process of communication, and an equally important set of influences on parent-staff communication is the social organization of the intensive-care nursery. Several features of the organization of technology-intensive medical settings place barriers between parents and practitioners—barriers that complicate the process of reaching life-and-death decisions.

Technology, Critical Care, and Colleague Dependency

Perhaps the most visible and awesome feature of a nursery's landscape is its sophisticated machinery—the monitors, respirators, and incubators. The mere presence of this technology creates an atmosphere that is itself a barrier between parents, their babies, and the nursery staff.

As sociologists Diane Beeson and Barbara Katz-Rothman have observed that another medical technology, amniocentesis, can lead parents to suspend commitment to pregnancy, so having a critically ill child inside an "artificial womb," connected to tubes and wires, can lead some parents to suspend commitment to parenthood.[11] One parent noted that she had to place baby shoes on her bedstand at night to remind herself that she had a baby. Whether this behavior attests to the disruption of a biologically determined bonding process, as some would contend, or whether, as is more likely, it attests to the effect of the nursery's social organization on a socially constructed parent-child bond, suspending commitment to parenthood can affect the emotional context of life-and-death decisions.[12]

Moreover, the presence of sophisticated machinery, coupled with the tense atmosphere of critical care, said to contribute to burnout in professionals, can also lead parents to become profoundly alienated from both the nursery and those who work in it.[13] As one parent remarked to another in a waiting room, "Looking at all those tubes and wires is just creepy!" Along similar lines, an advice book written by parents for other parents of premature infants noted, "It is impossible to prepare yourself for the sight of your tiny baby. Your first look will leave you sick and stunned."[14]

In the General NICU and the high-intensive room of the Randolph Nursery, where the most critically ill babies were treated, parents found themselves in the midst of constant frenetic activity. At any moment, X-ray technicians, laboratory technicians, respiratory therapists, and physicians filed in and out of the nursery, remaining only to examine babies or perform procedures. Nurses took vital signs, made entries on charts, and administered medications. Periodically, an alarm sounded, indicating that a baby was in trouble. From time to time, a group of doctors clustered around a bed to resuscitate a baby. This atmosphere of constant crisis hardly motivated parents to initiate interactions with staff who were working with babies whose lives seemed to hang in the balance. As Sonia Parducci explained when her baby boy was hospitalized in the General NICU, she felt marginal, superfluous, and conscious of getting in the way:

INTERVIEWER: What was your overall impression of the staff?

MRS. PARDUCCI: Now that I know more things, I can understand a lot of things that, at the beginning . . . , I didn't understand. . . . At the beginning, I was so afraid for the babies that I [left] everything to the doctors. After the first week, I've seen that the doctors let me have a room, a time to be there. They told me, "Come there to visit your baby." But when I come there, I feel so extraneous—you know, a stranger to that place . . . , because of the machines, because of everything, because you cannot touch the baby in your arms. No mother has experience with incubators. You have to put your hand when you can into something, and you feel your presence is not good for the staff sometimes. They are in a hurry; they have to do something on your baby. A lot of times, they told me to go away because you're not used to seeing the blood. The last thing . . . was . . . the spinal tap. I wanted to see on Daniel. They don't let me stay to see. So it was very difficult in the beginning to stay. I understand how most . . . persons, that maybe they have other children at home, or other things to do, they don't go to visit the babies because it's too difficult to stay. . . . You only feel that your presence can disturb what the doctors do, and it's . . . like a defense for the person to go away. I had nothing to do, and in my mind there were only them, so I needed to stay there, and I begin to fight, to try to find my place there, and I told [myself] that it was my right to know everything.

While some parents withdrew, "coping through distance," others, like Mrs. Parducci, struggled to find a place for themselves in the nursery.[15] In either case, the technology-intensive and crisis-laden atmosphere alienated parents from both the nursery and its staff, placing them on the periphery of the nursery's social life—including the life-and-death decision.

The nursery also accentuates a phenomenon observed in other technology-intensive medical settings. As historian Stanley Joel Reiser argues, with the development of diagnostic technology, the patient's history and subjective experience of illness assumed less importance in the doctor-patient relationship.[16] However, in outpatient obstetrics or pediatric settings, practitioners continue to rely on patients to provide information about events that take place outside the interview, such as an obstetrical history or the development of a child's symptoms.

This information, uniquely accessible to patients and parents, becomes a resource in medical encounters. In the intensive-care nursery, however, the patient's history is compressed. Information about that history can be obtained from the chart or from the referring physicians, and the patient's true history begins at the moment of admission to the nursery. Once the baby is in the nursery, little information escapes monitors, laboratory technology, and the nurses' continuous observations. Since parents can tell staff little about their babies that staff do not already know, the parents' role as historians and their own observations become less relevant to staff. In short, the compression of history in the intensive-care nursery diminishes the parents' leverage in decision making.

According to historians, diagnostic technology was accompanied by dramatic transformations in the social organization of medical practice as physicians became reliant on hospitals and as medical specialties developed to interpret sophisticated machinery. With these developments, much medical care came to be delivered in what Eliot Freidson calls a colleague-dependent context.[17] In contrast to primary-care office practices, in which physicians depend on patients to refer themselves (client-dependent practices), in neonatology, as well as in other colleague-dependent practices, physicians are oriented to the opinions of their colleagues, on whom they depend for referrals. As in other colleague-dependent practices, attendings in the Randolph Nursery assiduously cultivated ties with referring nurseries and services. The colleague dependency of neonatal intensive care, then, empowers referring physicians and diminishes parents' leverage in medical decision making.

The Organization of Teaching Hospitals

Not only were the Randolph and General nurseries technology-intensive medical settings, but both nurseries were also part of university-run teaching hospitals—an organizational feature that shaped the contours of life-and-death decisions. In both nurseries, the staffing patterns of the teaching hospitals complicated the decision-making process. According to Eliot Freidson, the salient feature of teaching hospitals is the transiency of their housestaff.[18] At both hospitals, attendings, neonatology fellows, and consultants passed through the nurseries in staggered, monthlong rotations. Even the nurses, who were by comparison the stable residents of the nurseries and the

carriers of its culture, varied their assignments and shared patients
with nurses who worked other shifts. Each day, parents confronted a
large and changing cast of characters. The high turnover of personnel
in the nurseries, coupled with a system in which patients were
managed by teams of residents, compromised continuity of care and
prevented a stable doctor-patient relationship from developing, further alienating parents from the nurseries. As one group of researchers
wrote about parents of chronically ill children, "Rarely does anyone
teach the family about the structure of the hospital, the rotation of
interns who will care for the child."[19]

In the General NICU, the doctor-patient ratio is sufficiently high
for some parents to develop a relationship with a resident despite the
rotation system—only to encounter a new medical and nursing staff
as their baby improves and is transferred to the acute care and convalescent care nurseries. One parent explained how constant changes in
personnel frustrated her quest for information about her baby:
"Those last fifteen days, I wasn't able to have any news about the
baby, because he changed doctors three times. . . . He changed from
intensive care after Dr. Michaels, and he passed to the other side and
he had another doctor. Then he passed to the other side, into conva-
lescence, and he had another doctor. Then they changed doctors."

Large and fluctuating nursery staffs also make it difficult for some
parents to get consistent information in life-and-death decisions. In
the Randolph Nursery, parents had to deal with several professionals—attendings, residents, nurses, social workers, and consultants.
Since staff sometimes had conflicting opinions about a baby's condition—to say nothing of different ethical philosophies—parents sometimes received conflicting information or advice. As one mother complained, "Every day we run into a different person with a different
story." Perhaps the most serious instance of this problem occurred
when a baby with spina bifida was transferred to the Randolph Nursery from another hospital. Not only did neurologists at the referring
nursery speak with the parents after examining the baby, but, later, a
Randolph neurologist, neurosurgeon, and resident also spoke to the
parents after examining the baby. Several of the specialists had conflicting opinions about the baby's prognosis and whether the baby
should be treated. Receiving these conflicting opinions left the parents
feeling helpless and confused.

Another organizational feature of teaching hospitals complicated
the consent process: their commitment to the diverse and sometimes

conflicting goals of teaching and patient care.[20] Because both nurseries were part of university-run teaching hospitals, residents were implicitly rewarded for their mastery of medical knowledge. This knowledge, rather than communication skills, can be directly observed and tested in rounds and is the sine qua non of effective role performance. Because of excessive demands on a resident's time and a reward structure that provides few incentives for interacting with parents, residents implicitly rationed their time, giving contact with parents a low priority.

The rotation system, team management of patients, and the nursery's reward structure combined to place formidable barriers between residents and patients. Consequently, when asked, "How much contact do you have with families?" more than 70 percent of the residents in both nurseries lamented that they had "not much" or "very little" contact. In fact, one resident commented that "Eighty percent of the time, I don't recognize the parents." The residents offered several reasons, many of them organizational, for this lack of contact: language barriers (in the General Nursery); parents' fear of doctors; a team system that deprives parents of a primary physician; parents' reluctance to invest in transient residents who are "passersby"; and the need to set priorities in the face of intense job demands.

INTERVIEWER: How do you feel about working in the intensive-care nursery?

RESIDENT: What I didn't like about it was the incredible physical and emotional strains that it put on my life. I was fatigued, I was useless at home, I was uncommunicative and tired most of the time, and I was emotionally drained as well, because the very intensity that you tend to thrive on is also very draining.

· · ·

INTERVIEWER: How much contact do you have with families?

RESIDENT: Never enough—the demands of the place are so intense that when the family is there, the likelihood of your not doing something that needs to be done right now is small. . . . [It's] really sad that you don't have time to do the things you really would like to do, and seeing the families or calling 'em up on the phone are those kinds of things that always seem to get put into the background.

To summarize, the staffing patterns of the teaching hospitals and their implicit reward structure not only compromised continuity of

care and prevented stable doctor-patient relationships from developing, but also undermined one of the foundations of informed consent:
parents' needs for full and consistent information.

The "Steep Slope" of Neonatal Intensive Care

The ecology of professional work in intensive-care nurseries follows
an organizing principle found elsewhere in the medical world: as the
status of an occupation increases, the degree of patient contact decreases. In the medical division of labor, it is the lower-status occupations that have the most contact with patients, whereas the powerful
and prestigious professions are removed from direct patient care.[21] In
a curious—and gendered—organizational mirror of the Cartesian
mind-body dualism, "mental work" (diagnosing and curing) is the
province of physicians, while caring for patients' bodily needs is left
to nurses. According to Andrew Abbott, professions also become
internally stratified along the same lines: the highest-status professionals are specialists and consultants—"professionals' professionals,
who do not sully their work with nonprofessional matters"—whereas
the lowest-status professionals work directly with the public.[22] In
other words, neurosurgeons have less patient contact than do pediatricians, and registered nurses have less patient contact than do licensed
vocational nurses.

Less commonly recognized, however, is the fact that work settings
differ in the strength of this inverse relationship between occupational
status and patient contact; and to this extent, organizations may be
said to have metaphorical "slopes." When compared to a pediatric
clinic or a pediatric inpatient ward, the intensive-care nursery has a
particularly steep slope: there are few occupations in its division of
labor, and the core occupations in the hierarchy (attendings, residents,
and nurses) differ dramatically in the degree to which they engage in
direct patient contact.

Given the demands on their time, and given the nursery's reward
structure, residents are content to leave communication with parents
to subordinates in the occupational hierarchy (i.e., nurses).[23] In contrast to decisions about medical management, which can become
arenas for jurisdictional battles between nurses and beginning residents, interaction with parents is the nurses' distinctive organizational
niche.

The nursery's steep slope figures into life-and-death decisions in at least two ways. First, like the interactive cues noted by the nurses, which I discussed in Chapter 3, information about the parents and the "social situation" is lower-status information, identified with lower-status occupations. Second, although the nurses and social workers are likely to know the parents best because they interact with them routinely, they are least likely to participate in conferences with parents. Instead, the residents, fellows, neonatologists, and attendings from other services are most likely to communicate with the parents in the decision-making conference (see Figure 2). This pattern did not obtain in the General Nursery, in which the social worker, who knew the parents well, served as an interpreter, thereby providing a stable presence at many conferences. In the Randolph Nursery, however, the parents' most emotionally intense and significant encounter—the one concerning their baby's fate—was likely to be with a relative stranger.

Finally, because the lower-status occupations have the most direct patient contact, physicians are often forced to rely on information that has been preinterpreted by nurses and social workers, sometimes entered as cryptic notes in a patient's chart, devoid of behavioral referents ("mother appropriate and adequate," "has poor support system"). Secondhand information, divorced from its social context and behavioral referents and confusing statements of fact with subjective evaluations, becomes difficult to falsify. Moreover, as in the case of rumor generation and similar forms of collective behavior, information about the family can be transformed and even distorted as it filters up the nursery's occupational hierarchy and even further transformed as it is entered in the patient's case record.[24] The following incidents, taken from my field notes, illustrate some of the problems that can occur when information filters through the organizational hierarchy:

A baby was referred to the Randolph Nursery for diagnosis of a possible heart defect. His mother, a twenty-four-year-old single woman, was accompanied to the nursery by two friends. When I interviewed the mother, I learned her baby had been delivered by a lay midwife, and she had been involved in holistic health for several years. Reading her chart, one of the head nurses noted with some amusement that "the mother listed yoga and meditation as part of her prenatal care." During cardiac catheterization, it became apparent that the baby had a serious circulatory problem (pulmonary hypertension). The staff hand-ventilated the baby for almost an hour, but the baby died. After the neonatology resident had told the mother that her son died, the resident spoke to the cardiology fellow, obviously favorably impressed by the mother: "I've never seen anything like it. She was so calm and together. She was consoling

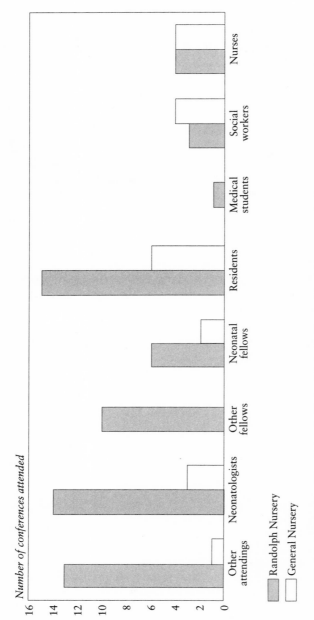

N = 65 at Randolph; N = 20 at General. Some of these data were obtained by means of informant accounts. In each case, I attempted to obtain at least two accounts of the conference.

Figure 2. Who communicates with parents in life-and-death decisions

me." The fellow then said, "That's interesting, because the social worker at Mount Sinai [the referring hospital] described her as not in touch and having a very poor support system." "Well, that's not what I observed," replied the resident. "She was very together and had great friends."

. . .

A twenty-six-year-old Mexican woman with three children gave birth to critically ill twins. A resident, who did not know the mother, told me that the mother had denied she was pregnant, that she didn't want the babies, and was going to give them up for adoption. A week later, I spoke to the social worker, who knew the mother quite well. She had not, according to the social worker, denied that she was pregnant, but rather had concealed the fact from her husband, fearful of what he would do if he learned that she had been raped by her employer's cousin.

Because of the nursery's "steep slope," some physicians received preinterpreted information that became distorted as it was filtered through the nursery's hierarchy. The "steep slope" of the nursery undermines one requisite of informed consent: the unrestricted flow of information between parents and practitioners. And, as the first example cited suggests, information about parents of babies who are outborn admissions may filter through the organizational hierarchies of more than one nursery. The "steep slope" of the nursery, then, interposes the barrier of hierarchy between parents and practitioners—a trend that is exacerbated when the nursery is also a regional referral center.

Regionalization

The Randolph Nursery serves as a referral center for a geographic area that spans half the state. For this reason, the complications in communication that I have discussed—staffing patterns that compromise continuity of care; colleague dependency that diminishes parents' leverage; diverse staff members who convey conflicting information; and information that is transformed as it filters though the hierarchy—are compounded. Originally implemented to contain costs and coordinate service delivery, regionalization exacerbates communication problems by interposing a barrier of geographic distance between parents and practitioners.[25]

Figure 3 presents the referral patterns of the Randolph Nursery. Most patients who were the subjects of life-and-death decisions were outborn admissions. Moreover, the largest single group of infants

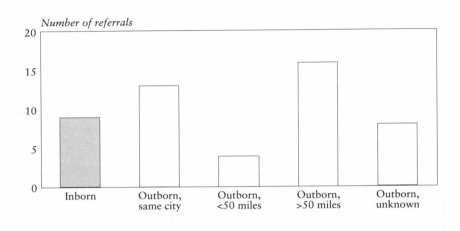

Figure 3. Where patients are from and how they are referred to Randolph

location

who were outborn admissions lived more than fifty miles from the nursery. Because of geographic barriers, visiting the nursery became an ordeal for many parents. Some had to travel long distances; some incurred significant expenses for transportation and lodging; some had to take time off from work; and some were unable to visit their babies at all, remaining separated from them during critical portions of the decision making.

Geographic barriers between parents and the nursery were exacerbated by another organizational feature: the nursery's acute-care orientation. Figure 4 presents referral patterns and the timing of decisions in the Randolph Nursery.

In Figure 4, almost half of the patients who were the subjects of life-and-death decisions were outborn admissions whose fates were decided less than one week after admission. Within this group, the largest single category was patients who lived more than fifty miles

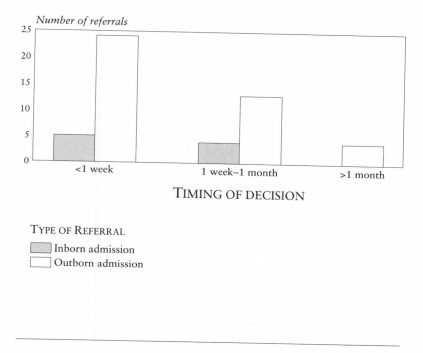

Figure 4. When decisions are made and how patients are referred to Randolph

from the nursery. The parents of these patients were the least likely to develop stable relations with members of the nursery staff, since geography combined with time constraints to create formidable barriers between parents and practitioners. These barriers were acknowledged by several residents when I asked them how much contact they had with families. One resident observed that he was "more likely to cross paths" with families of chronically ill infants who were in the nursery for more than a month.[26] Five residents indicated that they had more contact with the relatively few parents of patients who were born at Randolph and limited contact with the large number of parents who lived far from the nursery.

As Guillemin and Holmstrom have noted, the NICU referral system "weakens contact between parents and staff members while it reinforces communication between and among professionals and institutions."[27] Geographic barriers between parents and the intensive-care nursery also have significant consequences for the subject of this study, life-and-death decisions. First, because some parents from outlying areas found it difficult to travel to the Randolph Nursery, they remained at home, and consequently much of the communication between parents and professionals took place by phone. In the case of seven of the fifty infants who were the subjects of life-and-death decisions, the decisions were made exclusively by contacting the parents on the phone. In an additional five cases, major portions of the decision making took place on the phone. The telephone places serious constraints on the communication between parents and practitioners: participants do not have access to the nonverbal cues of the other conversationalists; and privacy is limited when physicians are forced to make calls in the presence of other staff members. Perhaps for these reasons, the mores of our society stipulate that the highly personal, significant, and emotionally charged communication that occurs in life-and-death decisions should take place in face-to-face interaction. While both of the parents and a number of staff members, including those who know the parents well, can participate in face-to-face conferences, usually only two conversationalists, a physician and one parent, can participate in decision-making conferences that take place by phone.

Second, when parents lived in outlying areas, often only one of them participated directly in decision making. Frequently, the mother remained hospitalized after delivery in the referring nursery, separated from her baby, while the father traveled to the Randolph Nursery and participated directly in fateful decisions, acting as an emissary between the mother and the staff. In these cases, an unintended consequence of regionalization was to increase the father's authority while diminishing the mother's leverage in life-and-death decisions.

Finally, many patients were referred to the Randolph Nursery for evaluation by surgeons, neurologists, cardiologists, and other specialists. Often these specialists had the responsibility of communicating with parents in life-and-death decisions. However, because of the nursery's "steep slope," exacerbated by barriers of geographic distance, the specialists usually had limited contact with and knowledge of the parents, and frequently were meeting them for the first time. Nevertheless, the specialists made sweeping inferences about the parents' background, competency, and intentions on the basis of very limited information.[28] In fact, on several occasions, specialists made attributions and inferences on the basis of demographic information gleaned from a quick glance at a patient's chart (e.g., age, ethnicity, marital status, and number of previous children).

Sometimes the specialists interpreted this demographic information against a background of cultural assumptions about parents' class, gender, and ethnicity. For example, a nephrologist incorrectly inferred that a single, black teenage mother was "ambivalent about the pregnancy." In another case, a neurosurgeon inferred that parents with a Spanish surname were "itinerants" (migrant farmworkers), when in fact they were permanent residents of an urban area. In the Margarita Portes case, discussed earlier in this chapter, the surgeon did not present the parents with the option of allowing the baby to die and not performing surgery because he assumed, largely on the basis of the parents' Spanish surname, that they were religious Catholics who did not have a "concept of euthanasia." The surgeon's inferences about the parents' cultural background did not consider their educational attainment. The father was a college-educated counselor in a community program, and the mother was a nurse; for these reasons they *were* likely to have a "concept of euthanasia."

All these demographic attributions resulted from organizational arrangements in which specialists, who were least likely to know the families, communicated with parents in life-and-death decisions. Unless contradicted by subsequent information, demographic attributions can, as in the last case, limit parents' participation in life-and-death decisions.

To summarize, several organizational features of the intensive-care nurseries complicated the consent process: the atmosphere of a high-technology medical setting; the rotations and rewards of teaching hospitals; the "steep slope" of the nurseries' hierarchy; and regionalization. Each feature placed a barrier between parents and members of the nursery staffs. Technology created spatial barriers; the rotation system introduced the barrier of time; the "steep slope" introduced the barrier of hierarchy; and regionalization placed the barrier of geographic distance between parents and professionals. The overwhelming effect of these organizational features, often additive and mutually reinforcing, was to place parents on the periphery of life-and-death decisions and to make the ideal of a truly informed consent elusive.

CONCLUDING REMARKS:
FROM PRACTICE TO PRINCIPLES

At the beginning of this chapter, I returned to a central theme of the book: the relationship between ethical principles and social practices. Next, I examined two issues that elude ethical discussions of informed consent—the process of communication between parents and practitioners and the context of consent—noting that process and context combine to place parents on the periphery of life-and-death decisions. Only by understanding social barriers to informed consent can participants transcend them. Only by understanding the social problematics of life-and-death decisions can they make the principle of informed consent relevant to actual practice.

When such decisions are examined, we find that staff usually do not employ an informed consent model but rather use practices designed to elicit parents' assent to decisions professionals have already made. The most common justification for producing assent is consequentialist ethics: assessing the rightness of an act on the basis of its consequences. Many staff members believe that parents who are asked to play an active role in deciding whether their babies should live or die will later experience guilt. Social science does not provide criteria to evaluate the ethics of this justification. However, to the extent that professionals make assumptions about the deleterious psychological consequences of informed consent, social science can assess the validity of these assumptions. In fact, the "folk" psychological belief that active participation in life-and-death decisions will produce guilt has little support in the social psychology of decision making.

There is evidence that participating in life-and-death decisions in the nursery is *not* psychologically harmful to parents. Moreover, psychologists Irving Janis and Leon Mann have noted that "postdecisional regret" (guilt) is less likely to ensue when decisions are made through what the authors call "vigilant information processing."[29] In order for vigilant information processing to occur, those who make consequential, emotionally charged decisions should participate actively in decision making and should be given time to weigh the alternatives carefully. Thus, clinicians can facilitate vigilant information processing by presenting parents with a range of prognostic outcomes, by introducing parents to others in similar situations, by presenting them with options, and by allowing sufficient time for careful deliberation. Conversely, post-decisional regret is more likely to ensue when parents are not provided with sufficient information or when they are not given enough time to weigh the alternatives.

It would seem, therefore, that members of the nursery staff systematically underestimate parents' competency to participate in life-and-death decisions, while overestimating the negative consequences of incorporating parents into these decisions. These considerations also suggest that a well-intentioned but paternalistic attempt to protect parents from guilt may, ironically, produce the very effect it is designed to minimize and may deter, rather than facilitate, vigilant information processing. In short, social science can contribute to the ethics of neonatal intensive care by identifying the consequences, often unintentional and unanticipated, of beliefs and practices in the intensive-care nursery.

By proceeding from principle to practice, I have addressed the relationship between the sociology and the ethics of neonatal intensive care, suggesting that the former can enhance the latter. But it is also possible to turn this argument on its head, proceeding from practice to principle. Having identified a set of social practices and their often unintended and unanticipated consequences, I can inquire about the ethical implications of these social practices and consequences. Two findings from this chapter illustrate this point. First, when a baby is transported to the Randolph Nursery from an outlying area, the mother often remains hospitalized while the father communicates with staff. This practice has an unanticipated consequence: although parenthood in our society remains largely the woman's responsibility, the parent who bears most of the long-term consequences of life-and-death decisions—the mother—has the least authority in decision making. There are other ironies as well: by producing assent, staff permit parental participation in life-and-death decisions without relinquishing their own power and authority. The actors who have the most at stake—the parents—have the least authority in life-and-death decisions.

Organizational practices that place parents on the periphery of decision making reflect a trend in the society at large that has been accelerated by the Infant Doe regulations and the amendments to the Child Abuse Prevention and Treatment Act. While Infant Care Review Committees have been praised by some as a practical innovation, others have criticized them for failing to provide parents with sufficient representation.[30] As growing state involvement has further eroded parents' discretion in life-and-death decisions, parenthood may become an involuntary institution.

In making life-and-death decisions, medical staff engage in social practices that have consequences that are unintended and unanticipated and ethical implications that are implicit and unexamined. A sociological study of life-and-death decisions, then, opens the door to further inquiry. Once we have identified social practices and their consequences, we can go on to ask the next question: are these practices right?

Diffusing Dissent

*Parents, Professionals,
and Conflict in Decisions*

On October 25, 1973, Drs. Raymond Duff and A. G. M. Campbell published a landmark article in the *New England Journal of Medicine* entitled "Moral and Ethical Dilemmas in the Special Care Nursery." Together with an article by surgeon Anthony Shaw that appeared in the same issue, the Duff and Campbell article represents the first time that physicians in the United States reported in a professional journal about their policies for making life-and-death decisions. Of 299 deaths that occurred consecutively in the Yale–New Haven Special Care Nursery, 43 (or 14 percent) of the infants died because parents and professionals had deliberately decided not to treat them actively.

News from the *New England Journal of Medicine* frequently finds its way into the popular press. For this reason, the authors' decision to publish their policy for making life-and-death decisions was at the same time a decision to subject that policy to public scrutiny. As the coauthor of *Sickness and Society,* a pioneering sociological critique of American hospitals, Duff had never been one to avoid controversy. Duff and Campbell were undoubtedly aware of the potential of their revelations to ignite a major public debate. In fact, the authors' explicit intent was to stimulate open discussion and debate, breaking the silence that had surrounded life-and-death decisions. Acutely aware that their decisions may have broken the law, Duff and Campbell concluded the article on a defiant note: "If working out these dilemmas in ways such as those we suggest is in violation of the law, we feel the law should be changed."[1]

Even more surprising than the bold decision to publish a potentially incendiary article in a major medical journal was the fact that the anticipated public outcry did not take place. To be sure, the article sparked a lively debate in the medical community. *Time* and *Newsweek* also reported favorably on the policy at the Yale–New Haven Special Care Nursery and received varied responses from readers, including some highly critical reactions from disability rights activists.[2] But the article failed to ignite a major public controversy.

Even more remarkable was another fact: despite repeated warnings from John Robertson, a conservative interpreter of the law, that parents and professionals who withhold life-saving treatment from infants with mental or physical disabilities risk criminal prosecution under homicide, manslaughter, child abuse, child neglect, or conspiracy statutes, no physician or parent has been successfully prosecuted for having made this type of decision. Although courts in several states have ordered infants to be treated under civil statutes, criminal investigations have been very rare. Undaunted by the risk of criminal liability, Drs. Duff, Campbell, and Shaw continued to publish reports of their policies with impunity.[3] In short, during the ten years following Duff and Campbell's revelations in 1973, life-and-death decisions did not assume the proportions of a public issue. It was almost a full decade later, on April 12, 1982, that the case of Infant John Doe became the center of a major national debate.

Sociologists who study social problems have been preoccupied with a central question: how do private moral problems become major public issues? But the case of neonatal intensive care raises an equally intriguing and relevant question: why did life-and-death decisions *fail* to become a public issue? Why did Duff and Campbell's article fail to ignite debate? What accounts for the decade of relative public silence between Duff and Campbell's initial revelations and the case of Infant John Doe?

Part of the answer lies outside the nursery, in the wider social and political climate. Both the rhetoric and substance of Duff and Campbell's article resonated with the dominant themes of the new social movements that mobilized around patients' rights in the early 1970s: the dangers of professional dominance and unfettered technological intervention; the need for greater consumer (in this case, parental) involvement in medical decisions; and the patient's right to die with dignity.[4] By the end of the decade, however, the political climate had shifted, the New Right gained ascendancy, and ultimately the anti-abortion movement, the disability rights movement, and the Reagan administration made Infant John Doe their cause célèbre.

But there are deeper and less obvious reasons for the decade of relative silence about life-and-death decisions—microsocial reasons rooted in the social practices of the nursery itself. Public issues originate inside the nursery when conflict around a decision cannot be resolved and a disputant takes the case out of the nursery and into the legal system. A decision can enter the legal system by several paths. First, professionals or parents can turn to the courts or the juvenile authorities when they disagree about a decision. Second, even when parents and staff reach a consensus, other staff may disagree with the decision and report the case to the government agencies. Third, a political group may learn of the decision and appeal to the authorities.[5] In fact, however, these avenues are traveled only rarely. For reasons I suggested in previous chapters, encounters with the legal system are very infrequent.

As in other nurseries, members of the Randolph and General nursery staffs attempted to negotiate a consensus among physicians, nurses, and other professionals, containing internal conflict by permitting subordinates to voice their opinions.[6] Once the staff decided not to treat a baby actively, the parents were consulted. Then, as I indicated in Chapter 4, professionals usually employed not an informed consent model but rather a set of practices designed to elicit parents' agreement to decisions already made by staff—such as presenting a united front, appealing to technology and expert authority, and moral suasion. Through these strategies, staff attempted to prevent dissent, which could disturb the flow of civil social discourse, undermine the premises of trust on which relations between parents and professionals are founded, and arouse painful emotions that disrupt the nursery's work routines.[7] In addition, conflicts with parents could bring a decision out of the nursery and into the legal system, threatening to transform a private disagreement into a public dispute. For these reasons, staff attempted to produce assent; and since they were usually successful, conflicts with parents were rare.

Nevertheless, two types of conflict could not be prevented: conflict between the parents and conflict between staff and parents. When conflicts with parents did arise, staff employed practices designed to diffuse dissent and contain its potentially disruptive consequences. In the remainder of this chapter, I discuss how conflicts arise and how staff manage conflicts with parents. By producing assent and diffusing dissent, staff are able to keep conflicts within the confines of the nursery, to prevent private decisions from becoming public issues, and to maintain the often fragile boundaries between the nursery and the outside world.

CONFLICT BETWEEN THE PARENTS

Ethical and legal discussions of decisions in neonatal intensive care typically treat the parents as a single moral unit having a single set of interests, rights, or duties vis-à-vis the newborn infant. However, because in our society parenthood is an institution that has different consequences for men and women, each parent may bring a different set of values and interests to the life-and-death decision. Moreover, since the responsibilities for parenthood in our society continue to rest largely with women, a decision to treat a seriously disabled infant actively may have different consequences for the mother and the father. In view of these facts, it is perhaps not surprising to find that conflict between the parents I studied was not unusual and occurred in at least five of the seventy-five life-and-death decisions observed in both nurseries.

In these five cases, conflicts between the parents followed a recurrent pattern. The father insisted that the baby be treated actively, and the mother, who was more acutely aware of the consequences of raising a disabled child, was more hesitant. The following case illustrates the tragic consequences that can ensue when parents disagree about a life-and-death decision and when the wishes of the father are allowed to prevail.

Case 1: Paul Gomez   Joan Gomez and Robert Smith gave birth to 800g. (1-pound, 12-ounce) twins, born fourteen weeks prematurely. The parents were unmarried, received welfare, and lived in a rural area more than fifty miles from the Randolph Nursery. One week after birth, one of the twins developed a very serious cerebral hemorrhage. The parents were called into a conference to discuss terminating life support. They were told that the baby had suffered a serious brain hemorrhage and would likely be severely retarded and probably unable to walk or talk. At one point in the conversation, Ms. Gomez said that she felt it would be better if the baby died. The father, however, dominated the interaction. He adamantly insisted that the staff continue to keep the baby alive because he had a nephew who had suffered a brain hemorrhage and nevertheless had become a perfectly normal child. In the ensuing months, the parents visited the babies only once. Ultimately, they abandoned the babies, who were placed in foster homes.

This case illustrates some serious ethical and social dilemmas that can arise from disagreement between the parents. When parents disagree about the fate of their child, whose wishes should prevail? Should staff have acceded to the wishes of the father, who seemed more vocal and adamant? Or should more weight have been given to the opinion of the mother, who in all likelihood would bear the social and economic consequences of caring for a severely disabled infant? In this case, the father's wishes prevailed.

For a number of reasons, the fathers' wishes were allowed to prevail in other cases of disagreement between the parents. First, parents may approach the life-and-death decision with dissimilar values and interests but may have different conversational resources with which to promulgate their respective points of view. A considerable body of research on gender and language suggests that men (in this case, the fathers) will be more likely to dominate the interaction, whether or not the staff are cognizant of this dominance.[8] Second, even when staff are aware that the father dominates the interaction, they may be reluctant to alter family dynamics. Thus, in one case, the father insisted on negotiating with the staff and asked that they not talk to the mother. When discussing the case in social service rounds, the staff were distressed by the father's dominance but were deeply reluctant to intervene in internal family dynamics. Third, in the nurseries I studied, as in other nurseries, consensus is required only for a decision *not* to treat an infant actively.[9] Given this bias in favor of active intervention, the father, who is more likely to insist on active treatment, is more likely to prevail. Finally, in a referral center such as the Randolph Nursery, in which parents are separated from the staff by significant geographical distance, the father may communicate with staff while the mother remains hospitalized in the referring nursery. For all these reasons, the outcome of disagreements between the parents contains an implicit irony: the parent who has the most at stake (the mother) is likely to have the least leverage in the life-and-death decision.

CONFLICT BETWEEN THE PARENTS AND STAFF

Given the power of practices for producing assent, overt conflict between parents and practitioners was rare. When parents who were poor disagreed with a decision to treat their baby actively, they rarely asserted their wishes, but rather withdrew from the nursery. Conflicting points of view compounded by conflicts of class, language, and culture culminated in a process of reciprocal alienation between the staff and parents. These parents usually responded to the situation by "coping through distance," disengaging from both the nursery and their infant, as happened with the Gomez twins and with Robin Simpson (see Chapter 3).[10] The following case illustrates this pattern of mutual disengagement.

Case 2: Ramon Martinez   Ramon Martinez was born four weeks prematurely, the seventh child of parents in their mid-twenties. Ramon required resuscitation at birth and was brought to the Randolph Nursery and placed on a respirator. When physicians examined him initially, Ramon seemed to be neurologically depressed, to have gross edema (fluid buildup) over his entire body surface, and to have multiple physical abnormalities. According to the geneticist who was consulted, the skeletal anomalies suggested a diagnosis of cleidocranial dysostosis (the absence of clavicles), but she was unable to determine the cause of the edema or the baby's neurological problems.

From September through November, Ramon had a complicated clinical course, characterized by inadequate nutrition, persistent hydrops (abnormal accumulation of fluid) of unknown origin, heart and lung complications due to respiratory dependency, and intermittent seizures. Although, according to the staff, Ramon was grossly malformed and had made little progress, they continued to treat him actively. For example, they made several unsuccessful attempts to treat his edema, and he finally responded to insulin/glucose infusions, a highly aggressive maneuver. Despite the staff's pessimism about Ramon's prognosis and their occasional comments about discontinuing therapy, a developmental assessment made in October suggested that he had intact central nervous processes and might have a "normal brain."

According to the social worker, Ramon's father was "repelled" by the baby and visited the nursery rarely, but his mother seemed concerned about him, was attentive, and was hopeful about his survival. However, when I interviewed the mother, this did not seem to be the case. During the interview, she expressed concern that the baby might be seriously disabled and severely deformed. Time and again, she asked, "What kind of life will he have?" She also seemed concerned about the effect of Ramon's stay in the newborn intensive-care unit on her six other children. When Mr. Martinez joined us, he expressed the same concern, only with more vehemence and apparent bitterness. It seemed to me that the staff, relying on their observations of the parents' nonverbal behavior, had misinterpreted the mother's wishes.

By November, both parents had withdrawn from the nursery and visited Ramon only infrequently. On November 19, the attending and the resident reevaluated the treatment plan. After staff members had conferred together and consulted specialists, they held a conference with the parents in which they unanimously decided to discontinue the life support that had sustained Ramon's breathing. The parents, physicians, and nurses made the decision with considerable relief—especially the nurses, who by that time viewed the baby quite pessimistically.

In the face of their earlier disagreement with members of the nursery staff about the kind of life Ramon would have, his parents had withdrawn from both him and the nursery. By contrast, when overt conflicts with parents occurred, they were likely to be with people whom the staff viewed as "medically sophisticated." Many were themselves health professionals.[11] These parents chose to be actively involved in treating their babies and were sufficiently knowledgeable to raise questions about the medical management and ethics of the case. Thus, the conflict between the staff and "middle-class," "medically sophisticated" parents resulted from the parents' tendency to assert themselves in all aspects of decisions concerning their babies.

Although one might think at first glance that "medically sophisticated" parents would be likely to share a common perspective with the staff, in fact there may be significant gaps between their perspectives because of the differing consequences of life-and-death decisions or the differing levels of emotional engagement. For example, parents may refuse to become emotionally committed to an infant whom the staff feel should be treated. One mother, a teacher of retarded children, questioned whether her 660g. (1-pound, 7-ounce) baby, born fourteen weeks prematurely, should be treated. Before the staff acceded to her request to discontinue treatment, the mother (according to the social worker) withdrew from the baby, talked about adoption, and delayed naming the baby, who ultimately received a county burial.

Conversely, conflicts may also arise out of the greater emotional engagement and attachment that may develop between parents and their babies. The different emotional contexts of the parent-child and staff-child relationships may result in conflicts in life-and-death decisions. For example, although babies with trisomy 13 (an extra thirteenth chromosome) and trisomy 18 (an extra eighteenth chromosome) have a similar prognosis—a short life span and severe mental retardation—these infants in fact appear very different. Whereas infants with trisomy 13 are often grossly malformed, infants with trisomy 18 have a more "normal" appearance. For this reason, parents of babies with trisomy 18 may become attached to them irrespective of the grim prognosis presented by staff. This attachment may lead parents to question the diagnosis and grim prognosis, as happened with a mother who was herself an NICU nurse—a case I discuss later in this chapter.

Finally, parents' greater attachment to their babies may lead them to challenge staff decisions to engage in what professionals view as routine procedures, which parents feel will cause their babies pain and suffering. Since the very definition of a routine or an invasive procedure may differ for parents and staff, ethical conflicts may arise around what staff view as a "standard operating procedure." One nurse whose baby had been hospitalized in the intensive-care nursery had this to say when I asked whether she had anything to add to the interview:

> NURSE: I think just the fact that a lot of things have changed my opinions . . . since I've become a parent.
>
> INTERVIEWER: In what way?
>
> NURSE: I guess I tend to look more at the parents' viewpoints on things than I used to. When you don't have any experience being a parent and knowing what those feelings are . . . , it's easier to say to somebody, "Oh, you can have more kids.". . . But you don't know how somebody feels about a newborn baby . . . , that nine months or six months or whatever you've had, being involved with that baby, you still have quite a feeling about him even though you've never seen [him]. . . . Just my baby being here, how it greatly upset me, even though he wasn't that sick.
>
> INTERVIEWER: What was wrong with him?
>
> NURSE: He had hyperbilirubinemia [jaundice], but he . . . just missed an exchange [a kind of transfusion] by half a point . . . , and I would come in and put signs all over the bed, "Do not put band-aids on me, and do not do this to me, and do not do that to my baby," because I knew all the things that went on, and I didn't want anybody doing it to him. . . . Coming in and

finding a band-aid on our baby's foot or a bruise on his head, what that must mean to a parent, we take for granted because we see it all the time. But when you come in, that may be the hugest thing a parent notices, this huge bruise on his head. It's routine for us, but not for a parent.

Consider also the example of Sonia Parducci, the college-educated Italian mother whose twins were hospitalized in the General Nursery. Mrs. Parducci began with the fundamental premise that she had the ultimate authority to make decisions concerning her babies ("Those were my babies, not their babies"). Here is how she described her struggle to find a place in the nursery and to make decisions concerning her babies' welfare, even to the extent of contesting what the staff viewed as "routine" medical procedures:

MRS. PARDUCCI: So I needed to stay there, and I begin to fight, to try to find my place there, and I told me that was my right to know everything. Those were my babies, not their babies, that I come to see sometimes. So I began to be insistent to stay, to look at everything they written, because they are *my* babies, not the hospital's babies. . . . I said to the doctor, "Don't do any more spinal taps on Daniel, because I feel that he don't need that." Because . . . they were going to do spinal taps and everything. For me it's terrible, because was terrible for routine, because, you know, I don't know if you have never seen. You have seen it?

INTERVIEWER: Yes.

MRS. PARDUCCI: You can understand, for your son you don't want them to do that, not for routine. I'm sorry, and if it wasn't routine, I had the right to know.

Parent-staff conflicts can take two forms, in both of which there are clear norms for conflict resolution. In the first type of conflict, the staff wish to terminate life support or not to treat the baby actively, while the parents insist on continuing active intervention. Given the bias in both nurseries toward aggressive treatment, a consensus is required for any decision *against* active intervention.[12] For this reason, the parents' wishes in this type of conflict should prevail, and ideally the child will be actively treated. In the second type of conflict, the parents feel that the baby should not be treated actively, while the staff favor active intervention—a type of conflict made famous by Robert and Peggy Stinson in *The Long Dying of Baby Andrew*.[13] In this case, the staff can theoretically ask a court to appoint a guardian *ad litem* and issue an order for active intervention.

Religion

However, in both types of conflict that I observed, the staff negotiated with the parents. With the exception of parents who refused ordinary treatments for religious reasons, the staff were notably reluctant to seek court orders. In fact, during the sixteen months of my observations in both nurseries, neither staff nor parents sought court intervention in a life-and-death decision. Rather than involve the legal system, the staff negotiated with the parents, employing a set of practices and strategies for managing, minimizing, or neutralizing dissent—that is, staff preempted and anticipated parental resistance, attempted to persuade parents to adopt their point of view, and, finally, employed a number of cognitive devices to neutralize parental disagreement or dissent when it did occur.

MANAGING DISSENT

Preemption

When staff anticipated that parents would disagree with or have difficulty accepting a decision to terminate life support, they often developed an explicit strategy to deflect parental resistance, as can be seen in the following case.

Case 3: Diana Jones   Diana Jones was a very small (700g. or 1-pound, 9-ounce), very premature (twenty-four- to twenty-five-week) infant who was born in a hospital bed before her mother could be taken to the delivery room. Her mother was a twenty-three-year-old African-American single woman with two other children. Although the baby was at the time considered to be on the margins of viability, she was nevertheless resuscitated and placed on a respirator in the slim hope that she could survive without serious disabilities.

Over the next four days, despite the staff's efforts to treat her actively, Diana developed multiple complications (serious lung disease, difficulties with ventilation and nutrition, and signs of kidney failure). In an ethics conference, the staff decided that it would be doing harm to the baby to continue treating her, since there was little hope of success. During the conference, the resident was concerned that, despite the grim picture conveyed to the mother, she had insisted that "her daughter was a fighter," she had developed a "significant emotional investment in the baby," and she was not prepared for the baby to die. During sign-off rounds that evening, the staff seemed reluctant to discuss terminating life support with Ms. Jones:

RESIDENT 1:   At the meeting, it was the consensus that we were prolonging the inevitable. I called the mother, and she was tearful. We felt it was unfair to present her with the decision when she got here.

ATTENDING: Then the decision should be made before the mother arrives.

SOCIAL WORKER: I think it's important that the mother be presented with a clear-cut decision, to make it real to her. Do you remember the Robbins baby? Bud [the fellow] had to go back over to redo the whole thing. They had to tell the mother that the baby had bleeds, and Bud still had to convince the parents that this was the only logical choice. They need time to absorb this. . . .

ATTENDING: The mother shouldn't be presented with any indecision. I feel the mother should not make the decision. The decision's already been made, and she'd have no option but to go along with it.

SOCIAL WORKER: But she doesn't know if the baby's gonna die because of the ventilator.

ATTENDING: We'd tell her the baby was terminal so we stopped, and the baby could be moved into another room.

RESIDENT 2:   In the times I've observed this in pediatrics, the family is always given the chance to take the baby and hold him.

ATTENDING: But this mother's had no physical contact with the baby.

RESIDENT 3:   This mother has not been appropriate. She's still hoping for the best. . . .

SOCIAL WORKER: What you're doing in a conference presents a reality to the parents. We don't know how she'll respond—whether she'll be overwhelmed or uncomprehending.

RESIDENT 4:   I think she can handle the baby's death, but not unplugging the machine.

FELLOW: That's really hard to get across.

NURSE: She kept saying, "Only this child's a fighter and will surprise us all."

SOCIAL WORKER: What is it about this mother that makes it so tough? Is there any anticipation that she won't accept the decision?

RESIDENT 4:   It's possible.

FELLOW: When I talked to her, she seemed to have an unrealistic attitude. She didn't seem to understand how serious the baby's age was, the chance of damage. Her reaction was, "I've had a premature before, and with God's help this one will do as well."

SOCIAL WORKER: But she's become more realistic.

RESIDENT 1:   Yes, she's more realistic now.

ATTENDING: So where do we stand?

FELLOW: She has to decide whether we should have the baby baptiz-
                 ed. . . .

ATTENDING: Well, if you're reluctant to discontinue care without discuss-
                 ing it with the mother first, we should. I personally would
                 not. But it should be put in terms that she has no option. The
                 baby will suffer terribly, and if we continue, it will be a fate
                 worse than death.

RESIDENT 4:   She'll accept that.

SOCIAL WORKER: It's close to the truth.

ATTENDING: It's important that we not be equivocal.

FELLOW: So we should wait until the mother comes before we discon-
                 nect the ventilator?

ATTENDING: Yes, we should wait until she arrives. We should say that if
                 we continue, the baby will suffer—that there is no possible
                 gain from continuing, and that the baby will die within one
                 or two days, but with terrible suffering.

The social worker commented to me later that Dr. Nelson, the
attending, found it difficult to speak with welfare mothers, but had no
trouble speaking with families with college educations. In fact, the
mother offered little resistance to the decision.

In this case, the mother's attachment and hope for Diana's recovery, most likely coupled with the professionals' difficulties communicating with poor clients, made the staff reluctant to broach this
decision directly. While Dr. Nelson's reluctance to discuss discontinuing active treatment was unusual, what is more typical is the strategy
that the staff used to anticipate and deflect the mother's potential
resistance: the plan to tell her that the baby would "suffer terribly."

Persuasion

Conflict with parents cannot always be so easily anticipated and
deflected, and parents sometimes offer overt resistance, actively questioning staff decisions. In these cases, usually involving educated parents, professionals redouble their efforts at persuasion, relying on
some of the strategies for producing assent already noted: appeals to
expert authority, appeals to technology, and moral suasion. Consider,
for example, the case of Silvia Lopez, in which relations between the
staff and parents became very strained.

Case 4: Silvia Lopez   Silvia Lopez was a small (1000g. or 2-pound,
3-ounce), premature (twenty-eight-week) baby who was born in late

August. She was the first child of Yolanda Garcia, a seventeen-year-old woman who lived with the family of the baby's father, Pedro Lopez, a college student. Ms. Garcia entered General Hospital when her membranes ruptured, and she gave birth to a baby girl two days later. The baby was asphyxiated at birth (her Apgar scores were 2 and 4), needed to be placed on a respirator immediately, and was treated for a possible infection. The lengthy list of problems in the case history, coupled with the use of the words *poor, remains unchanged,* and *no improvement,* suggest that Silvia's two months in the nursery represent what is known in the nursery vernacular as a chronic, complicated clinical course. Her problems included neonatal jaundice, a patent ductus (a heart defect common in premature infants), and several other serious complications. Seizures, which were noted in the chart on Silvia's third day of life, apparently became more frequent during October.

Although the physicians made some initial progress in weaning Silvia from the respirator, their success was short-lived. Soon thereafter, she deteriorated, remaining totally dependent on the respirator to sustain her breathing, developing bronchopulmonary dysplasia (a form of chronic lung disease caused by respirator dependency), and suffering several episodes in which major portions of her lungs collapsed. In late October, Silvia was believed to have developed congestive heart failure and shock resulting from a suspected infection of unknown origin.

During November, Silvia's condition did not improve and in fact worsened. She became increasingly lethargic and was described as looking "dead," "like a corpse." The staff began to treat her with infusions of dopamine (a drug that elevates the blood pressure, considered a measure of the last resort) after her heart rate and blood pressure had fallen and her urine output decreased, which the resident attributed to possible septicemia (blood poisoning due to a massive infection). Silvia failed to respond, developing serious jaundice, an electrolyte imbalance, and possible heart failure.

There were other problems as well, especially the staff's relationship with Mr. Lopez, which had become increasingly strained. The social worker described him as "young and immature," "not ready to cope with having a child," and "hostile." He upset the staff by raising questions about the medical management of the case, as the following discussion from rounds suggests.

NEONATOLOGY FELLOW:	As the nurses are frustrated, so the doctors are frustrated—she looks dead. . . . I feel funny about that family. The father has a lot of questions about what we're doing. He intellectualizes a lot. I'm not comfortable with that father. He's asking, "Why are you poking around here and there? What if? Why not?" He's asking repeated questions.
DISCHARGE PLANNING NURSE:	He's asking *inappropriate* questions.

The staff's relationship with the family reached a nadir after the physicians and nurses decided to discontinue the drugs that sustained Silvia's heart rate and to remove her from the respirator. According to the neonatology fellow, the attending had come in on Sunday and had written orders not to resuscitate Silvia. The resident had talked to the parents to "feel them out" about discontinuing treatment. During the conference, the father accused the staff of medical mismanagement, contending that the nurses had crimped the oxygen line and instead had given the baby carbon dioxide. According to the social worker, it hadn't registered on the father that Silvia might not make it, but the mother seemed more "realistic." I asked the fellow if they were going to have another conference with the parents. "Yes," she said, "but I don't want to be part of the discussion. There may be litigation."

On November 5, Dr. Martin (the attending who now had responsibility for Silvia's case), the resident, and the social worker conferred with the parents to try to convince them to discontinue treatment. If the parents refused, the presence of a terminal infant in the nursery would create serious morale problems for the staff.

DR. MARTIN:	Do you know what caused the baby's problems?
MR. LOPEZ:	Yes, being on the respirator.
DR. MARTIN:	But why was she put on the respirator?
MR. LOPEZ:	I know what you're going to say. Because of prematurity.
DR. MARTIN:	No. Let me give you the history.

Rather than beginning with an open-ended question such as "What kind of questions do you have?" which would empower the parents to initiate the topic of the exchange, Dr. Martin employs a didactic format—asking a set of "socratic" questions and evaluating Mr. Lopez's responses. This enables the attending to control both the form and the content of the encounter. Significantly, the father and Dr.

Martin imply different attributions of responsibility for Silvia's critical condition. When the father frames the history so as to suggest
iatrogenicity, Dr. Martin corrects him, indicating that the baby had
been put on the respirator because of her prematurity (for which, it
turned out, the father blamed himself).

Dr. Martin then recounts Silvia's history: The staff had been unable
to ventilate the baby, and recently the baby's heart had started to fail
because she had been dependent on the respirator for several months.
The baby had also been convulsing for weeks, which led Dr. Martin
to suspect that she may have had a bleed into the part of the brain that
controls respiration. Although the brain scan was negative, that type
of bleed does not show up on a CAT scan. Dr. Martin then presents
the conclusion:

DR. MARTIN: I and Dr. Singer [another attending] and a number of consultants
                have seen the baby, and it was their unanimous opinion that the
                baby was going to die. I believe in treating the baby as long as
                the treatment is effective, but now we have reached the point
                where the treatment was doing more harm than good. What do
                you think?

MR. LOPEZ: Are you a hundred percent sure that nothing can be done?

DR. MARTIN: No, one can never be 100 percent sure, but I can be 99.9 percent
                sure that nothing can be done. You can ask anyone around here.
                I am the last one around to fight for a baby. When everyone else
                has given up, I will still say there's something we haven't tried.
                But in this case we have tried everything, and while I am the first
                to say we should continue, here the treatment is not helping and
                is doing more harm than good.

MR. LOPEZ: I feel guilty enough about this already.

DR. MARTIN: That's another thing I can say with almost 100 percent cer-
                tainty—that there is nothing about this that was your fault. You
                are in no way responsible for this.

MR. LOPEZ: Are you asking us for a decision?

DR. MARTIN: No, this is not a decision for you to make. When I go to a
                mechanic, I don't know how the car works, and I must leave the
                basic decisions about how to fix the car to him. So here this is
                a medical decision that must be made by the medical staff.

wrong comparison

In this conference, the attending employed a number of persuasive
strategies, citing his own reputation for aggressive intervention,
claiming 99.9 percent certainty, appealing to the ethical principle of
nonmalificence, and, finally, asserting that the decision was a medical
one, thus removing the responsibility from the parents—a tactic that

succeeded, given the father's apparent feelings of guilt. After the conference, the doctors withdrew the drugs that had sustained Silvia's heart function and removed her from the respirator that had sustained her breathing. She died shortly thereafter. According to the pathologist who performed the autopsy, Silvia had an undetected, serious viral infection that was likely to have contributed to her deterioration.

Preemption and persuasion are strategies that professionals use to prevent and diffuse dissent. There are times, however, when staff are unable to contain conflict, and parents nevertheless reach decisions grossly at odds with the professionals' point of view. At such moments, another line of defense comes into play after the fact: staff invoke psychological explanations and attributions to account for the parents' perceivedly deviant decision making.

Psychologizing

Social scientists who have observed neonatal intensive-care units have commented on a recurrent pattern: the extent to which nursery professionals observe, interpret, and evaluate parents' behavior within a psychologistic framework. When evaluating parents, professionals draw on two distinct psychological frameworks. First is the framework of bonding, developed by Marshall Klaus and John Kennell. The separation of mother and child in the intensive-care nursery (fathers were not included until later formulations of bonding, and then only incidentally) is said to disrupt the "natural" attachment or "bond" that forms between mother and infant during a critical period. This disruption is said to impair the parent-infant relationship, even to the extent of leading to child abuse, although the evidence on the latter point has been disputed on methodological grounds. Concern with disruption of bonding has led neonatal units to liberalize visitation procedures and to develop social services to evaluate and encourage bonding between mothers and their babies.[14]

Second, the parents of critically ill infants are said to go through a grief reaction that is believed to proceed through a series of predictable stages, beginning with shock and disbelief or denial of their infant's illness, which then evolves into anger at the loss of a perfect child, which next develops into guilt for having a premature infant, which finally proceeds to acceptance of the child's illness or disability.[15] (Note that the highest stage is "acceptance" of disability, suggesting a commitment to an adjustment ethic.) Although some parents have questioned the utility of the stage model, it continues to

dominate the thinking of neonatal professionals. Perhaps the most
salient reaction is the feeling of guilt.[16] Staff believe that almost all
parents feel guilty—and, indeed, some parents I interviewed, like Mr.
Lopez, did express guilt. This is hardly surprising, given our society's
tendency to locate responsibility for prematurity in parents' health
behaviors. In the Randolph Nursery, social service rounds become
occasions in which residents, nurses, and social workers evaluate
parents' grief reactions and bonding behaviors.

The psychologizing that figures so prominently in the nursery's
social life has a number of consequences for parents and professionals
who participate in life-and-death decisions. First, it diminishes the
authority of parents in such decisions. As Guillemin and Holmstrom
forcefully point out, psychologizing transforms parents from "rational decision makers" into "second-order patients."[17] This tendency of
professionals to transform parents into secondary patients is also
characteristic of professionals who interact with parents of disabled
children in other settings. As John Gliedman and William Roth note:

> The problem of client-professional relationships touches upon some of the
> most troubling issues of our age. In a society that routinely creates or expands
> its publicly funded social service organizations in response to perceived social
> needs, the question of the proper relationship between the client and the
> professional is increasingly synonymous with the question of the proper rela-
> tionship between the citizen and the state. . . . It is striking to observe how often
> the structure of the professional's relationship to the parent automatically
> transforms the parent, in the expert's eyes, into a kind of patient.[18]

Second, just as psychologizing diminishes the authority of the parents in decision making, so too it enhances the status and authority of
the nursery's ancillary professionals: nurses and social workers. Concern about disruption of bonding has created a critical role for professionals, particularly nurses: namely, to evaluate parental visitation
behavior and to engage in interventions designed to encourage attachment between parents—particularly mothers—and their babies.
When babies are born, the social worker takes their photograph, to
make the babies seem "real" to the parents. Nurses encourage mothers to hold and touch their babies, to give them breast milk, and to
visit frequently. Combining the bonding and grief frameworks, nurses
and social workers believe that parental bonding or attachment to a
baby who subsequently dies will help parents resolve their grief.[19] To
this end, nurses and social workers believe that it is important for
parents to hold babies before they die.

In short, nurses (and to a lesser extent, social workers) have become *emotion managers*—a work force that functions to evaluate and manage parents' attachment to their babies. Sociologist Arlie Hochschild uses the term *emotion management* to describe the work that people do to change and manage their own emotions and notes that emotional labor is part of service work.[20] In the nursery, however, the nurses evaluate and manage the emotions of others—that is, the parents. Because nurses (and social workers) hold a near monopoly on information about the parents, their presentation of information about the parents' visitation behaviors, the kinds of questions parents ask, and parents' emotional attachment to their infants becomes the only area in which nurses can speak authoritatively and in which their opinions are solicited in decision conferences.

Consider, for example, this discussion of the parents in the conference concerning Robin Simpson, the baby with chronic lung disease discussed in Chapter 3. What follows is an exchange about the parents in which the attending, a social worker, and a nurse use a scheme of interpretation (the extent of the mother's contact and her behavior when she visits) to arrive at a "general impression . . . of withdrawal" and a "subconscious attitude," presumably of rejection:

ETHICIST: Are there any other perspectives?

SOCIAL WORKER: Since then, she called me on the anniversary of the SIDS [Sudden Infant Death Syndrome] death. She's gradually diminished calling Laura [the head nurse]. Laura was concerned with the diminished contact, as she said in her conference with you.

ATTENDING: They don't keep their appointments with me.

HEAD NURSE: She came in Friday and Saturday afternoon with the little girl, who asks about the baby—the four-year-old responds to Robin as if the baby's a real person.

ETHICIST: Is that the youngest?

SOCIAL WORKER: No, there's a two-year-old who's pretty attentive. It's now been six years since the SIDS death, and I haven't heard from the mother apart from the time she called me on the anniversary. The father hasn't come in for some time.

ETHICIST: So the general impression is one of withdrawal?

ATTENDING: Even though they have visited the baby.

NURSE: Last time, Mrs. Simpson brought in clothes for Robin. It seemed like someone had given them to her, and the clothes were really dirty. This made me ask, "What's going on here?" I think this may reflect a subconscious attitude.

ETHICIST: What's the family's socioeconomic status?

SOCIAL WORKER: The father works in a garage. He's an auto mechanic. The
                   mother's a cocktail waitress. She's the type of person who
                   seems to mother everyone. In fact, it was hard for her to let
                   down this mothering attitude and talk about her feelings.

In this context, perceiving, interpreting, and evaluating the parents through the psychologistic, professionalistic prism of the bonding and grief paradigms allows nurses and social workers to enhance their expertise, or to distinguish their evaluations from common sense, transforming their role into evaluators and emotion managers while transforming parents into the objects of these evaluations.

The routine psychologizing that takes place in the nursery provides staff with a set of institutional schemata that are called into play in life-and-death decisions when parents express beliefs, values, attitudes, or emotions that are grossly at odds with the professionals' point of view.[21] In accounting for these disjunctures of morality and reality, staff typically reframe the parents' perspective as a defense mechanism or as a phase in the grieving process. Parents who continue to express optimism in the face of a very grim prognosis are seen as "not realistic" or experiencing "denial," as in the case of Diana Jones's mother, who continued to insist that her critically ill baby was "a fighter." In the case of a seventeen-year-old African-American woman whose baby had a serious congenital kidney defect (hydronephrosis), the resident was concerned that "the mother can't hear that the baby is not doing well. The other day, they came in and the father asked, 'What's the good news?' " "Yes," responded the nephrologist, "we're not dealing with a situation where she hears what you say. She hears what she wants to hear."

"Sophisticated" parents who are viewed as asking too many questions, particularly about the medical management of their babies, are likely to have their questioning interpreted as a challenge to the physicians' competency.[22] Like Mr. Lopez, discussed in the previous section, these parents are likely to be labeled "intellectualizers." Similarly, Mrs. Parducci, who enjoyed an otherwise positive relationship with the General Nursery staff, was viewed by the attending as having "an almost pathological need to know" when she asked him to read from her baby's chart during the discharge planning conference. To describe a parent as "intellectualizing" implies that a layperson has trespassed on the professional's exclusive terrain of jurisdiction, which demonstrates how fragile are the boundaries between the professional and lay realms. It is educated parents, whose knowledge may overlap that of professionals, who are most likely to encroach on these boundaries. Such parents can be quite threatening to residents' tenuous sense of professional competency. Alternatively, a parent's questions about the medical management of a case may be reframed as somewhat pathological manifestations of anxiety:

RESIDENT: Maybe we should give the parents Valium.

ATTENDING: Why? I spoke to the father before. I remember when my kids were sick—we were very worried, too. I think they're appropriate.

RESIDENT: They're the kinds of parents who are always here, watching for mistakes.

ATTENDING: Well, if we make mistakes, they should point them out to us.

In this case, the resident *decontextualizes* the parents' behavior by separating the parents' response (concern about mistakes, worrying) from the situation or stimulus that provoked it (having a very sick baby).[23] By placing the parents' behavior back in context, the attending provides instructions for responding to the parents as "appropriate."

Although staff encourage parents to talk about and express their feelings to help them resolve their grief, one emotion badly disrupts the nursery's social life: anger directed toward the staff. Consider the example of a sixteen-year-old African-American mother who became angry at the staff's medical management when her baby developed surgical complications that were, by the staff's own admission, iatrogenic. The baby had been transferred to the Randolph Nursery for heart surgery for a serious heart defect (tricuspid atresia). The wound had not healed well and had burst open (dehisced) after the baby had been sent back to the referring nursery. The baby was again transferred to the Randolph Nursery for wound care. According to the resident, the mother had refused to consent to another surgery, saying, "It didn't work last time, so why is it going to work now?" During social service rounds, a resident reported that the mother "has some anger that the baby was transferred back to Mount Sinai Hospital without her being asked." The nurse then reinterpreted the mother's anger as a defense mechanism, suggesting that "maybe it's reaction formation—she's trying to project her guilt about the wound onto someone else." In this case, the nurse *recontextualizes* the mother's anger, or situates it in another context by reframing the mother's anger toward the staff as "really" a defense against her own unconscious guilt. By reinterpreting the mother's behavior in this way, the nurse has, in a single stroke, deflected the attribution of responsibility for the wound from the staff to the mother. By refusing to take parents' anger seriously and at face value, the staff also protect themselves from examining their own role in producing the mother's anger.[24]

Deeply disconcerting to the staff are those occasions when parents reach life-and-death decisions believed to be contrary to what the staff view as the baby's or the parents' own best interest. While some decisions are acknowledged to be inherently problematic ethical "gray areas," other decisions are viewed as having a right answer—a course of action that any reasonable person would take. In these situations of high moral certitude, some professionals become distressed when parents reach decisions that contradict deeply held, taken-for-granted beliefs and presuppositions of staff. In these instances, a psychological grammar of motives is called into play to account for the parents' decision.

Consider, for example, María Sandoval, the baby with Rubinstein-Taybi syndrome (an abnormality accompanied by physical deformities and moderate to severe mental retardation). María's mother, a sixteen-year-old daughter of migrant farmworkers, decided that María should have routine surgery to correct a minor heart defect—a decision that called into question, among other things, the staff's own emotion rules about the kinds of infants it is possible to love. While some members of the Randolph Nursery staff accepted the mother's decision, others questioned her motivation.[25] In an ethics round in which the case was discussed, some residents noted that staff members who saw the baby were "shocked by her appearance," and these residents invoked psychological explanations for the mother's attachment to María and her decision in favor of surgery. As one resident said:

> The usual justification being given is that the mother wants everything done for the baby, and therefore it's appropriate parental interest. The next question is: why is the mother interested in the baby? And I guess one thought that had been raised is that this baby is being hung over her head in terms of guilt about getting pregnant as a young, single woman. If that's the reason . . . that the mother's interested, then I don't think we're addressing the real problem by taking care of the baby's medical problems. The real problem's mother's peace of mind and what's she feeling. So I don't know, I think if she's . . . purely interested, then examining why mother's interested is probably appropriate.

In this case, the resident recontextualizes the mother's interest in María, reframing it as "guilt about getting pregnant as a young, single woman," shifting the locus of the "real problem" from the baby's medical condition to the "mother's peace of mind," a problem calling for psychological rather than medical intervention. The resident also reveals his own moral judgment that being a single parent is something to feel guilty about. By simultaneously invoking the "guilt" schema and the schema of the "teenage mother," the resident combines the schemata of defense mechanisms with those based on gender, class, and marital status. In so doing, he invalidates the mother's choice while reaffirming his own sense of the right thing to do.

In their encounters with parents in life-and-death decisions, members of the nursery staff may experience challenges to their scientific judgment, professional competency, or fundamental beliefs about the right thing to do. It is in these disjunctures of morality or reality that staff invoke psychological explanations for parents' behavior. Psychologizing allows professionals to *neutralize* dissent—that is, to preserve their own worldviews—while faulting or discounting parental judgments.[26] Psychologizing also protects professionals from undertaking the critical scrutiny or self-examination that would occur were they to take parents' views at face value. By invoking psychological accounts, staff do not prevent dissent, but rather blunt its potentially subversive force. Ironically, however, psychologizing by the staff can actually escalate conflict with the parents, who become angered as they find their perceptions invalidated. This is, in fact, what happened in the case of Matthew Reilly—a case that brings together many of the themes of this chapter. Matthew Reilly's stay in the Randolph Nursery epitomizes the processes and dynamics that are set into motion when the judgments of parents and professionals collide.

Case 5: Matthew Reilly   On the first day of his admission to the Randolph Nursery, Matthew Reilly presented the staff with a serious ethical problem. The history began in mid-April, when Matthew was transported from Marysville, a small community forty miles north of the Randolph Nursery, for evaluation of cyanosis (a blue coloring of the skin, indicating insufficient oxygenation of the blood) from a possible heart defect. While at Marysville, Dr. Mark Victor, the cardiology fellow who headed the transport team, had noticed that Matthew also had abnormal features that suggested trisomy 18. According to Dr. Victor, although he talked to Matthew's mother, an intensive-care nurse, about the need to diagnose Matthew's problems, he did not share his suspicions of trisomy 18.

Trisomy 18, or the presence of an extra eighteenth chromosome, is among the most devastating of congenital abnormalities. Most infants with the syndrome die during the first two years of life from respiratory or heart problems, and those who live are profoundly mentally retarded, unable to walk or talk. So catastrophic is this disorder that it is one of the few areas of high moral certitude. In both nurseries I studied, there was a consensus that a diagnosis of trisomy 18 constitutes sufficient grounds for withholding or withdrawing life-saving treatment. While tragic for the family receiving the news, trisomy 18 usually elicits a relatively straightforward decision from the staff: infants with the condition are not treated actively.

The decision concerning Matthew Reilly, however, was not to be unproblematic. When Dr. Steven Miles, the pediatric dysmorphologist, was consulted, he concluded that Matthew lacked some of the abnormal features to warrant a definite clinical diagnosis of trisomy 18:

DR. MILES: It looks like trisomy 18. Now, I don't believe that there have to be 100 percent of the phenotypical features to make a diagnosis, but here some features are lacking. There's a lack of hypoplastic [underdeveloped] nails and overriding fingers that are needed to diagnose trisomy 18 definitively. They are probably latent. So I can't just say, "Go ahead and pull the tubes out." Well, I feel that this is trisomy 18, but I would feel uncomfortable if I were to stick my neck out. . . . *(He mentions some other possible diagnoses.)* . . . Does he have heart disease?

DR. VICTOR: My guess is [he does].

DR. MILES: This is different from the one we had from Northville, which was a classic and had every feature.

DR. VICTOR: Yes, that one was a textbook trisomy 18.

DR. MILES: This one has more than 50 percent of the features. If you want a number, I'd say I'm 60 percent sure . . . I think he's going to turn out to have trisomy 18. What would you do if it was definitely a trisomy 18?

DR. VICTOR: Send him back to Marysville.

DR. MILES: How long will it take to get the chromosome studies?

DR. VICTOR: Till Monday. . . . The major question is what to do with the heart lesion, what to do about the diagnosis until Monday, whether to do an echo and a cath [diagnostic tests for heart defects]. My feeling is not to run up bills if it's a trisomy 18, since chances are the baby will be dead in six months.

DR. MILES: You can present it to the family that there's a 50 to 60 percent chance that the baby is a trisomy 18. This is a hard thing to thrash out in a parental conference.

The uncertainty surrounding Matthew's diagnosis now raised a difficult ethical dilemma: whether to conduct an extensive cardiac diagnostic evaluation before the results of the chromosome studies needed to make a definite diagnosis would be obtained on Monday. Dr. Victor had "no problem" maintaining Matthew on the respirator or obtaining an echocardiogram, a relatively simple test, to make a preliminary diagnosis. The difficult decision was whether to perform a full cardiac catheterization, a costly and invasive procedure, without knowing whether Matthew had trisomy 18. As Dr. Victor explained, a wrong decision in this case raised the possibility of two worst-case scenarios: "What if he has a heart lesion that needs immediate surgery?" he asked. "If we go ahead and cath the baby and then do the surgery, what if we find out it's a trisomy 18 after all? On the other hand, if we don't do anything and the baby dies, then what if we find out it isn't a trisomy?"

When Dr. Mann, the chief of cardiology, performed an echocardiogram to make a tentative diagnosis of Matthew's heart defect, he offered a way out of the impasse: he asked Dr. Victor to find out how long Mrs. Reilly had been married and whether she could have more children. If Matthew were the product of a "precious pregnancy," then he should be treated aggressively. After Dr. Victor reported that Mrs. Reilly had no trouble getting pregnant and that she had had a previous abortion, he and Dr. Mann decided to continue to support Matthew on the respirator until the results of the chromosome studies came back the following Monday. Until they knew whether or not Matthew had trisomy 18, the staff would not do anything "heroic."

Much to the staff's dismay, the chromosome studies were inconclusive. Meanwhile, the Reillys had arrived at the Randolph Nursery. In my interview with Mr. Reilly, I asked what the doctors had told him. He seemed almost fatalistic, accepting the decision as one made by physicians.

MR. REILLY: Well, the little fellow has a heart defect, but they're waiting for the test results before they decide what to do. They think the baby might have a genetic defect, an extra chromosome. They call it trisomy 18. What that means is that normally babies have forty-six chromosomes, and this one has forty-seven. When it's this particular extra chromosome, it's associated with severe retardation.

INTERVIEWER:	When will they know for sure?
MR. REILLY:	They did a chromosome study on Friday, but it wasn't conclusive. They got a picture of the chromosomes, and they thought they saw forty-seven chromosomes in three cells, but in the fourth one they thought they saw forty-six. So yesterday they repeated the test. Tomorrow, they will get a picture, but they may not know for sure until the end of the week.
INTERVIEWER:	What happens then?
MR. REILLY:	If it's trisomy, they don't do anything. They won't mess around with the heart, and I guess the baby will die, and we'll go back to Marysville.
INTERVIEWER:	Are you in agreement with that?
MR. REILLY:	It's not my decision. They don't do anything in cases like these. If it's a trisomy, it's a trisomy, and that's all there is to it.

Mr. Reilly had begun to become attached to Matthew and had found grounds for optimism: "So thank God we can have more kids. But I'm kind of hoping for this one. He looks so cute. And he seems to be responding pretty well. They got him off the respirator, and he's active. He was active before he was born, too. His mother felt him kicking. That's a hopeful sign."

Although Mr. Reilly seemed pleased with the nursery, he reported a friend's negative experiences with it. Such comments were not unusual. Indeed, several families in both nurseries told me of friends who had warned them of "experimentation" at teaching hospitals. Although the precise incidents varied, this may reflect a mistrust of university-based teaching hospitals in parts of the community.

INTERVIEWER:	Are you satisfied with the care you're getting?
MR. REILLY:	Yes, all the nurses and doctors have been great. Some of the doctors have what the nurses call a "God complex," but Dr. Miles was very down-to-earth. They're all very open. One of my friends had a very bad experience here, and we were a little wary. But we've been satisfied.
INTERVIEWER:	What happened to your friend?
MR. REILLY:	They had a baby here that they were sort of experimenting on.
INTERVIEWER:	Could you say a little more about that?
MR. REILLY:	Well, in some of these places, they like rare diseases. This was a baby who couldn't fight off infection, and they told my friend he wasn't going to make it. Well, now the baby is doing just fine—he's a great baby.

Looking at the interview in retrospect, it is possible to discern signs of impending trouble in Mr. Reilly's optimism about Matthew and his apprehensions about the nursery's proclivity to give ominous diagnoses of rare diseases. At the time, however, there was little reason to suspect that the Reillys would soon embark on a collision course with the Randolph Nursery staff.

On Wednesday, the staff received the preliminary results of the chromosome studies. Still ambiguous, the studies suggested that Matthew had an extra chromosome, although it was unclear whether the diagnosis was trisomy 18, trisomy 18–22 (which carries an equally ominous prognosis), or an extra Y chromosome. One of the residents, Dr. Lee, had been present during a conversation between the Reillys and Dr. Miles, the pediatric dysmorphologist. According to Dr. Lee, Matthew's parents had asked Dr. Miles for his opinion about Matthew's diagnosis and prognosis, and he told them that he suspected Matthew had trisomy 18 on the basis of the preliminary chromosome studies and Matthew's abnormal features. For the first time, the Reillys directly challenged the validity of the diagnosis and the chromosome studies and offered alternative interpretations of the clinical findings. The resident attributed their response to denial.

INTERVIEWER: How did the parents respond?

DR. LEE: Well, there's a lot of denial going on. Mrs. Reilly showed us a picture of the baby and said that some of his features were family features. She raised the question that maybe the chromosome studies were wrong, and said, "It's not that I question you, but I can't help but have some doubts about the diagnosis." . . . This is an interesting case for you. At first, on Monday, the mother was saying, "I don't want anything done for the baby if he's a trisomy," but in the past week she's become attached. She feels the baby looks so well, and he's responding so well to treatment, that she just can't believe he has trisomy 18.

Much to the surprise of many members of the nursery staff, Matthew did *not* have trisomy 18. The final results of the chromosome studies suggested that in fact he had an extra Y chromosome. Because the presence of an extra Y chromosome is not necessarily accompanied by serious mental retardation, Matthew was sent to cardiac catheterization. Matthew was to have surgery to correct his heart problem (a large ventriculo-septal defect) after his heart failure stabilized. When I interviewed Mrs. Reilly, she was indignant. She had known all along that Matthew could not be seriously retarded, but the staff had refused to believe her, insisting that he had trisomy 18. She was frustrated by the high turnover of staff members, each having a different opinion, and she was even angrier that the staff had, in her words, "presumed [Matthew] was guilty until he was innocent" and had "branded [him] as a loser from the very first." Mrs. Reilly believed that she had also been unjustifiably labeled as a "denying parent."

INTERVIEWER: This must have been an ordeal for you.

MRS. REILLY: Yes, it has. Every day we see a new person with a new story. First, they told us he had trisomy 18, but now they say it's XYY. From the first, even in Marysville, they told us Matthew was a trisomy. They presumed he was guilty until he was innocent. Now they're saying it's not a trisomy after all, that it's XYY, and they were wrong all along. I told them that the features, the chin and the cleft palate, were all Reilly family features, and I showed them a picture of John [her husband] when he was a baby. Dr. Miles now agrees with me. I knew all along he wasn't a trisomy. I could feel him kicking in the womb, and I knew a severely retarded baby wouldn't do that. Then every time one of us would come up to the crib, he would move around and look up at us and give us eye contact. A severely retarded baby wouldn't do that, either.

INTERVIEWER: How did the nurses respond?

MRS. REILLY: Well, at first the nurses were supportive. But once they heard Matthew was a trisomy, they tried to get me to accept that he would be retarded, that he would die. And when I didn't go along with this, they began to treat me like "the denying parent."

INTERVIEWER: So you feel you got labeled?

MRS. REILLY: Yes, and Matthew was, too. He was branded as a loser from the very first. Here they're more interested in the diagnosis, in what the tests can establish, than in the person. But we were afraid this would happen from the first. We had some friends who had a terrible experience here. Their little boy had been diagnosed as having an immune system disorder. They were told he would have to go home in a tent and that he would die. But now he's two years old and doing fine.

INTERVIEWER: So what do you think can be learned from this?

MRS. REILLY: We were talking to Steven Miles about this. He said he had learned a lot. I guess the main thing is: don't presume he's guilty until he's proved innocent. Give him the benefit of the doubt.

Not only did Mrs. Reilly challenge the nursery staff's diagnosis and their decision rules, and not only did she raise questions about the staff's biases against both her and Matthew, but she also raised questions about the medical management of the case, suggesting that the staff's biases against retarded babies may have led them to neglect Matthew's medical care, even to the extent of producing iatrogenic brain damage.

INTERVIEWER: So what do you see as Matthew's future now? What kind of care do you think he'll need?

MRS. REILLY: He'll need to have surgery for the cleft palate. And heart surgery, too. But otherwise I think he'll be normal. There's no relationship between an extra Y chromosome and intellectual function. The only thing I'm really worried about is that he'll be retarded because of some hypoxic [oxygen-deficient] episode that they neglected. One day I walked in and I noticed his blood gases [measures of respiratory function] had slipped, and they hadn't even noticed it or corrected it. They didn't do the cath because they thought he was a loser and would be retarded. As it turned out, it was for the better to wait.

How did the staff respond to the Reillys' concerns? A few members of the nursery staff—two nurses, Dr. Miles, and one of the residents—had become close to the family. They identified with the parents and were sympathetic to their point of view. These staff members had previously been critical of some policies and practices in the nursery, and the Reillys mobilized these professionals' dormant concerns. Dr. Miles, for example, believed that the staff were indeed biased against infants with genetic defects. Dr. Jonathan Wilder, the resident who was sympathetic to the family, believed that the staff had misdiagnosed Matthew's disorder. In a conversation with a nurse, he described Mrs. Reilly's refusal to let the staff withdraw from Matthew:

DR. WILDER: No one saw the baby as a person. But Mrs. Reilly is saying, "This is a person," and she is demanding that we treat Matthew like one. I think a lot of people resent the extra attention she's demanding.

NURSE: Susan [another nurse] knows the parents really well. Mrs. Reilly complained to her one day that a nurse was sitting there, reading a magazine. I don't know if we really neglected him.

DR. WILDER: Everyone in the nursery has to deal with her . . . , and she is one attractive woman. . . . And she is sophisticated, too. . . . I'm telling you, with her attitude, had she not been tall and attractive, had she come in dressed in hippie clothes and talked the way she did about bonding with the baby in utero, we would say she was a flake.

Most members of the nursery staff, like the attending quoted next were not entirely sympathetic to the parents' perspective. The staff became divided between a minority of doctors and nurses who agreed with the parents and the majority who still felt that Matthew had a poor prognosis. This became apparent during an exchange between Dr. Wilder and an attending during rounds:

DR. WILDER: I think this baby is a good social lesson to all of us. We had just about signed him out due to a heart lesion in the face of trisomy. The parents led the way in terms of enthusiasm for the baby, and now things are going well.

ATTENDING: I disagree. I don't think you can be that optimistic, given the multiple malformations and the grossly abnormal neurological exam. The outcome is unknown, but there's a strong likelihood of serious mental malfunction.

Not surprisingly, most members of the nursery staff were deeply discomfited by the Reillys' anger, and the perceptions of medical and social mismanagement of the case evoked powerful responses. Some staff acknowledged that there may have been more than a grain of truth in some of the parents' contentions, some disagreed, and some responded by psychologizing or blaming physicians in other services, as in this discussion of the Reillys in social service rounds:

SOCIAL WORKER: Well, it's uproar time. Yesterday, she was unloading on Maria [another social worker]. Mark Victor was saying that Mama is quite satisfied with the idea of the doctors falling on their faces. Yesterday, she was smiling. Maria said it was quite an angry smile.

NURSE: Well, she's wrong if she thinks she's going to have a normal baby.

SOCIAL WORKER: I talked to Steven Miles this morning, and he's treating it as a group of congenital symptoms with an unknown origin. The mother seems to be convinced that the features are familial.

RESIDENT 1:   Over the baby's bed, she has a picture of the baby's father to let us know they resemble each other. I don't really think they look all that much alike.

RESIDENT 2 (DR. LEE):   No way! We had a long talk last night with Mom— Bob [the fellow] and I. She thinks everything is familial. She also said that someone had told her that the cleft palate could be from the uterine posture. I doubt it.

SOCIAL WORKER: What approach are you taking to these parents?

DR. LEE: Well, Steven [Miles] said, "I can't just shake her and say, 'You're wrong!' "

SOCIAL WORKER: Why is this baby not having a bleak prognosis so disturbing to us?

CHAPLAIN: Yes, what's the difference? You've got parents who are concerned about the baby and are bonding, so what difference does it make how they explain the syndrome?

DR. LEE: Last night, they were upset that no one was in the driver's seat, that there were too many people painting a different picture.

RESIDENT 1: It's important that someone sit down and talk to them, especially since they've postponed the surgery. We should let them know that it's not just because he's funny looking that he's being put on low priority. . . . We should develop a game plan and centralize our information source. . . .

RESIDENT 3 (DR. WILDER): We *did* fall on our face, and it's clear to me that there's something to be learned from this. At first, the staff was impressed that this was a trisomy 18. Then we thought it was a 22, which is almost as bad.

RESIDENT 1: No, from the first, Mark Victor thought it was probably a trisomy, and he told that to the parents on the first day. Part of the blame in this situation rests with the cardiologists. We weren't really in the driver's seat.

DR. WILDER: But I do think that among the housestaff there is an emotional prejudice that we develop whenever we see a child with multiple anomalies, and we may communicate that to other people. At first, we thought this was a defective child that should be let go. Now it's all backward, and we're going all out. I understand why they're mad.

SOCIAL WORKER: So maybe there's some reality to their anger, and we have to separate that from our own reactions to this.

RESIDENT 1: I think maybe they are relieved because with congenital anomalies it's clearly not their fault, whereas with a chromosome disorder they might feel guilty. Maybe that accounts for why the parents are elated.

· · ·

RESIDENT 1: I think it's going to be hard on us and on everyone's feelings. I think we tend to go all out for the good babies, and when we see one that's malformed, we tend to stay away. I noticed those feelings in myself, and I try to avoid them.

RESIDENT 4:   I'm sure he'll grow up to be a neonatologist and prove us all wrong.

RESIDENT 1:   Probably he'll grow up to be a lawyer. *(He laughs.)*

Regardless of their view of Mrs. Reilly or of her son's prognosis, some residents acknowledged that she had correctly identified one critical weakness of nursery professionals: their negative attitude toward babies with multiple abnormalities. Angry parents are viewed as potential litigants, and this was the first time that staff members explicitly acknowledged one source of their anxiety about the parents: the threat of a malpractice suit.

The staff's concern increased over the next few days when, for reasons that were unknown, Matthew's medical condition suddenly began to deteriorate. First, it seemed that his heart failure had worsened and that he would soon need surgery. Then, as his respiratory status deteriorated, he was once again placed on the respirator. Suddenly and inexplicably, Matthew developed what the staff called an "electrolyte crisis" (in this case, a life-threatening imbalance in sodium, potassium, and glucose—chemicals necessary to sustain vital functions), his kidneys failed to function, and he began to have convulsions. The staff responded to this crisis by treating Matthew very aggressively. Dr. Gordon, the attending who had by now assumed responsibility for the case, returned to the nursery at 10 P.M. and remained through much of the night as the staff made desperate attempts to correct the electrolyte imbalance. Dr. Gordon contemplated dialysis for Matthew's kidney failure—a highly aggressive intervention when attempted on a newborn infant. Summoned from her home in the middle of the night, a nurse donated her own blood for a transfusion—also considered a highly aggressive maneuver.

The Reillys' persistent anger at the staff and their intimations of medical mismanagement, now exacerbated by Matthew's sudden, unexplained deterioration, contributed to the perceptible tension in the nursery. Dr. Miles, the pediatric dysmorphologist, speculated that the residents felt guilty about the case. The staff's tension heightened when the Reillys mobilized doctors in the community, who visited the nursery and made inquiries about Matthew's case. Two physicians from Marysville visited the Randolph Nursery over the weekend. The head nurse, the chaplain, and a resident held a conference with the parents to discuss communication problems and designated three physicians to communicate with the parents. The following Thursday a pediatrician from Marysville conferred with Dr. Gordon about Matthew and participated in afternoon rounds when Matthew's case was discussed. A fourth doctor conferred with Dr. Miles about Matthew at the request of friends of the Reillys. The presence of outside physicians raising questions about the medical management of the case and the potential of deteriorating relations with physicians from Marysville, a major source of referrals, undoubtedly further increased the tensions in the nursery.

The threat of a malpractice suit cast a shadow over the Randolph Nursery. I separately asked a resident and a nurse whether Matthew was indeed being treated aggressively, as I had surmised. Both told me that were it not for the parents' attitude, Matthew would not be treated so aggressively; and when I asked about concern over potential litigation, both said, in identical words, "I think that's in the back of everyone's mind." On rounds, Dr. Gordon, the neonatologist, pointed to a picture of Mrs. Reilly holding Matthew that she had placed over the crib and said, "She used this picture yesterday to show that this was a normal baby that made eye contact. We're going to see this picture in court."

Matthew's seizures continued for three days, unresponsive to anti-convulsant drugs. Persistent seizures (status epilepticus) can be a sign of serious brain damage; and on afternoon rounds, Dr. Gordon began to consider discontinuing treatment:

DR. GORDON: I think we have a decision to make tomorrow. If he continues to seize, I think we should seriously consider whether we're doing the right thing. . . . I talked to Frank Maguire [a pediatric neurologist], and his feeling was that we shouldn't continue. I need to continue until all the problems are stabilized (and we have more information).

RESIDENT: Especially since we're dealing with a metabolic problem, because metabolic problems can resolve.

DR. GORDON: But usually when they resolve, the seizures don't continue.

RESIDENT: How about the possibility of cerebral edema from the multiple insults? How long does it take before that resolves?

DR. GORDON: That's the only thing that makes me want to continue. It takes about two days before you can tell if that will go away.

Undoubtedly anticipating parental resistance to the decision, Dr. Gordon began an attempt to diffuse dissent. At rounds, he told the residents that he had already "tried to prepare the parents" for the worst, a practice that staff called "staging information."

DR. GORDON: I've spent a lot of time talking to them yesterday and today. They understand that the child is very sick. They understand quite a bit—the mother is an [intensive-care] nurse. They understand that the longer the seizures and the more metabolic problems, the more the likelihood of neurological damage. Where we left it is that the child will be supported, and we'll see what happens. Meanwhile, we're treating him with phenobarb and dilantin [anticonvulsant drugs] to see if we can stop the seizures. The parents know there's no way to know yet if the child is neurologically damaged. I think they're more realistic today.

For the first time, the staff described the parents as "realistic," since they now appeared to agree that Matthew had a poor prognosis. According to a nurse, "The parents understand that he may not make it. The father broke down and started to cry. He really was quite appropriate." Not only did the parents appear to "accept" the possibility of Matthew's death, but they now also conformed to the staff's normative notions about "appropriate" emotional display. As one of the residents told me, "The parents were here last night and were crying and expressing a lot of grief. They seem to be at a place now where they're accepting the possibility that he may die. I think it's real important that the parents deal with their grief, or it will affect them for a long time to come."

Matthew's condition failed to improve, and Dr. Gordon decided on the following day to discontinue life support. The neurologist was called to the nursery to examine Matthew and to put a note in the chart to document Matthew's grave neurological status. When I saw Mrs. Reilly, she appeared to question the decision.

MRS. REILLY: Talking about decision making, they're talking about making one right now.

INTERVIEWER: About withdrawing support? How do you feel about that?

MRS. REILLY: Well, I've seen them be wrong so many times before. Matthew has always made all the decisions, and I feel he'll let us know this time.

As Dr. Gordon conferred with the parents, I saw him take out the electroencephalogram (EEG) and explain it to Mrs. Reilly, thereby employing a persuasive strategy discussed earlier in the chapter— appealing to the authority of technology. According to the resident who was present at the conference, Dr. Gordon explained that the situation looked very bad. The fact that Matthew's seizures had not resolved meant that he would probably have severe brain damage.

Mrs. Reilly then confronted the doctor, asking whether he was 100 percent certain. Dr. Gordon's response bore an uncanny resemblance to the words of the attending in the case of Silvia Lopez. He told the parents that one could never be 100 percent sure—that over the years he had seen a few cases in which things had resolved—but more often than not, babies who have persistent seizures are very damaged. Using a dramatic analogy, Dr. Gordon told the parents that he feared Matthew would be like Karen Ann Quinlan: he could be weaned from the respirator but would be a "vegetable." He then told the parents that everyone knew that he hated to turn off respirators, that he was hell to be around at such times, and that he sits with babies while they die. The parents reluctantly agreed to the decision to withdraw life support, and Matthew died that afternoon.

In the midst of the emotional devastation that followed Matthew Reilly's death, members of the nursery staff struggled to make sense of their complicated and conflictual relationship with the Reillys. Two weeks after Matthew's death, the chaplain and a nurse continued to elaborate psychological explanations for the parents' attitudes:

CHAPLAIN:	The baby died, and the parents hugged everyone. Then they didn't tell anyone about the funeral.
INTERVIEWER:	Really?
CHAPLAIN:	That's not surprising at all, in view of their attitude toward the staff. They're setting themselves up for a lot of grief that may not resolve itself until they have another baby—if at all.
NURSE:	I would have liked to observe the dynamics between the parents. He was such a good-looking guy, and she was tall and attractive. I wonder how their attitude was conditioned by their own feelings about having a baby with anomalies.
INTERVIEWER:	You mean that their own feelings of stigma led them to think the staff was neglecting Matthew?
CHAPLAIN:	It's called projection.
NURSE:	I think they should spend more time around the nursery and see how we take care of babies that are ugly—like Marcy Smith.

Matthew Reilly's case is as intriguing and complex for the questions it raises as it is for the questions it answers. Was the parents' anger at the staff "really" part of an elaborate web of denial of a prognosis of mental retardation, as some staff members argued? Or, alternatively, did the staff "really" neglect an infant with a prognosis of normal intelligence because they presumed him "guilty" before proving him "innocent," as the parents contended? Profound reality disjunctures such as these leave the researcher torn between conflicting interpretations.[27] Yet even if all the medical facts of the case were before us, the dispute between the Reillys and the nursery staff probably could not be resolved on empirical grounds, and the "truth" would most likely continue to elude us.

While the case of Matthew Reilly contains idiosyncratic features, such as the failure of the chromosome studies to yield a definitive diagnosis, it illustrates the major patterns and processes discussed in this chapter: the efforts of professionals to diffuse dissent. Having reached a decision to discontinue life support and anticipating parental resistance, the staff attempted to preempt dissent and to persuade the parents to adopt their point of view. These strategies got the parents to agree to the decision. However, staff members could not contain more fundamental conflicts with the family over management of the case, conflicts that evoked powerful emotions in all disputants.

The psychological literature on newborn intensive care is replete with examples of parents' emotional responses to the nursery and to the birth of a disabled infant. Yet the same literature has less to say about the emotional responses of staff to angry parents who fail to validate their professional self-conceptions. This body of theory and research has much to say about the defense mechanisms of parents, but little to say about the defenses of staff.

During Matthew's three-week stay in the Randolph Nursery, the Reillys challenged the staff on a number of levels. They challenged the professionals' diagnostic abilities, their competency, their judgments about "appropriate" emotional attachments to infants, and their commitment to the norm of universalism, or doing one's best for all patients—a fundamental precept of professionalism.[28] While some of the professionals agreed with the parents, most of the others invoked psychological explanations that faulted and discounted the parents' perspective. In their efforts to neutralize dissent, staff members only further angered the parents, who turned outside the nursery for support of views they felt were invalidated within it. This cycle of escalating conflict and mutual invalidation reached the predicted conclusion when the Reillys sued the Randolph Nursery for malpractice.

DISCUSSION: DIFFUSING DISSENT AND MAINTAINING BOUNDARIES

In Chapter 4, I discussed professional strategies for producing assent to professional decisions. When these strategies fail to prevent dissent, a number of processes are set into motion. I have described them in this chapter: staff anticipate, deflect, and preempt dissent; they attempt to persuade parents to accept their point of view; and, when that fails, they neutralize dissent by psychologizing. These practices have sociological implications. By producing assent and diffusing dissent, professionals struggle to maintain invisible boundaries in two senses of the word: first, they attempt to maintain boundaries between professional and lay authority; second, they attempt to maintain boundaries between the nursery and the outside world.

Andrew Abbott's recent work in the sociology of professions examines how professions vie for jurisdiction or ownership of problems.[29] Because professions constitute a system, changes in the jurisdiction of one profession usually affect the jurisdiction of other professions. Professionals compete for a clientele, just as they do for cognitive jurisdiction over other problem areas. Clients, then, figure into this model as part of the spoils rather than as active contestants in battles for jurisdiction. They are affected by the system of professions but are not part of it.

The systems model, then, takes the boundaries between professional and lay jurisdiction for granted. I suggest, however, that professionals and clients can also compete for jurisdiction, and for this reason clients can affect the system of professions as well as being affected by it. In fact, as increasingly restive and educated consumers challenge professional authority, professions have lost legitimacy, and the boundary between professional and lay authority has become contested terrain.[30]

Nowhere is the boundary between professional and lay authority more disputed than in life-and-death decisions, for experts are themselves divided on the question of whether the authority for decision making lies in the professional or public domain. In life-and-death decisions, the boundary between professional and lay jurisdiction may be called into question. Embedded in a life-and-death decision are at least two decisions: an explicit substantive decision about what should be done and an implicit procedural decision about who should make the decision. Parents, then, can challenge professional authority on a number of levels: they can challenge the substance of a decision; they can challenge the social structure of doctor-patient interaction; and they can challenge professional prerogatives to dominate the decision-making process. A parent can also make deep incursions into professionals' self-images, their sense of competency, their sense of ethicality, and their emotional rules about the kinds of babies who can be loved.[31] It is not surprising that these challenges are apt to come from "medically sophisticated" parents, often themselves health professionals, whose knowledge is most likely to overlap that of the professionals. In these circumstances, the metaphorical line of demarcation between professional and lay jurisdiction becomes fluid, fragile, and open to dispute.

Members of the nursery staff respond to these micropolitical challenges to professional dominance by neutralizing dissent: they invoke psychological explanations of parents' behavior that discount parental perspectives while defending professionals' worldviews. When they succeed, staff are able to defend their jurisdictional boundaries against parental encroachment. When they fail, as in the case of Matthew Reilly, conflict escalates as parents feel invalidated, ultimately turning to the courts for affirmation of their views.

Through the practices described in this chapter, professionals attempt to maintain another boundary: the boundary between the nursery and the outside world. By preempting, persuading, and psychologizing, members of the nursery staff try to contain dissent, to keep it within the confines of the nursery, thereby avoiding confrontations with the legal system and challenges from political groups. Throughout most of the 1970s, life-and-death decisions remained private matters decided within the nursery in a process dominated by professionals, rather than issues debated in the public arena. Ultimately, however, the outside world could no longer be kept at bay. Unable to resist the incursions of the wider society into the nursery, professionals were forced into confrontations with the legal system, political groups, and legislators. In the wake of the case of Infant John Doe, the nursery became less a walled fortress than an open city under siege, and professional prerogatives to make life-and-death decisions were challenged by the state—an issue I take up in the conclusion to this book.

CHAPTER 6

Beyond the Nursery

Life-and-Death Decisions
and Paradoxes in Public Policy

> We often move in what appear to be erratic jumps, valuing
> life at a rather low level in some circumstances . . . and at a
> high level in other situations. . . . Of course, this does not
> fully explain the value we place on life in different situations;
> why, for instance, the United States will spend a million
> dollars to rescue a single, downed balloonist but will not
> provide a similar sum to provide shore patrols.
>
> —Guido Calabresi and Philip Bobbitt,
> *Tragic Choices*

Is it possible to make just decisions in an unjust society? This question
is more than rhetorical, and the answer is far from trivial.[1] In this
chapter, I would like to answer this question, if circuitously, by presenting some concluding arguments about life-and-death decisions in
neonatal intensive care.

The perspective of this study arose in part out of a critical dialogue
with bioethical analysis, which has come to dominate much of the
professional and public discourse on decision making. Increasingly,
bioethicists are pursuing a more applied project as they are being
requested to serve as consultants to intensive-care nurseries, to publish guidelines for decision making in medical and scientific journals,
and to serve on policy-making commissions. In fact, following the
recommendations of the President's Commission and the American
Academy of Pediatrics, recent "Doe directives" have recommended
that hospitals appoint ethics committees (infant care review committees), thereby giving quasi-legal recognition to bioethicists who serve
on them.[2]

The ventures of bioethicists into the applied realm have been met
with a mixed reception by medical practitioners. Some clinicians have
welcomed the bioethicist's presence; others have viewed the bioethicist as lending legitimacy to decisions they would make in any case;

164

and still others have been more resistant, criticizing bioethics for its lack of relevance to clinical practice. Despite this mixed reception, ethicists have become increasingly important actors in life-and-death decisions and public debates—a tendency that will only increase with time. One recent study asserted that virtually every large hospital in the country now has a bioethicist on its staff.[3]

By facilitating open discussion and examination of the ethical premises underlying life-and-death decisions, bioethics has expanded medicine's reflective horizons. In fact, encouraging health practitioners to become self-reflective is the major contribution of bioethics to American health care. However, as I began to study life-and-death decisions, it became apparent to me that the analyses ethicists provided were insufficient for studying life-and-death decisions. Whether deontological, utilitarian, or contractarian, bioethics assumes that actors reach decisions alone, apart from institutional constraints. In short, bioethics individualizes the decision-making process. This tendency to individualize, personalize, and privatize decisions is a quintessentially Western phenomenon. As Renée Fox and Judith Swazey have noted in their discussion of Chinese medical morality, other, more communitarian ethical approaches, which avoid the individualistic language of rights and contracts, are possible in different social contexts.[4] As I have argued in earlier chapters, life-and-death decisions are not private matters, but rather take place in the context of organizations, institutions, and power relationships.

RECAPITULATION: DECISIONS AND TECHNOLOGY-INTENSIVE MEDICAL SETTINGS

As this project progressed, I began to develop another, more sociologically informed approach that relates life-and-death decisions to the social context in which they take place. I approached these decisions, then, from the standpoint of the sociology of knowledge, and most of this book examines how the organization of the neonatal intensive-care unit as a work environment structures the decisions of those who work within it. To recapitulate briefly: I showed how the decisions of professionals are shaped by the circumstances of their work. Members of the nursery staff, because of their differing daily experiences, come to develop different views of the facts, data, and evidence to be used in reaching life-and-death decisions as well as different views of the right thing to do.

Next I showed how the organization as an ecology of knowledge allocates different sources of information to participants in life-and-death decisions. Physicians, whose contact with patients is limited and technically focused, assess prognosis largely on the basis of sophisticated diagnostic technology. Nurses, who sustain close, continuous contact with patients, have unique access to information gleaned from interactions with infants. These contrasting prognostic assessments lead to conflicts in life-and-death decisions.

Having discussed the decisions of health professionals, I then considered the role of the parents in life-and-death decisions. Members of the nursery staff do not usually follow a policy of informed consent, but rather employ a set of practices to elicit parents' assent to decisions that have already been made. The technology-intensive nature of the nursery, the "steep slope" of its organization (in which those with the least authority have the most patient contact), its dependency on colleagues as a source of referrals, and the geographic separation of parents from their babies often conspire to place parents on the periphery of the life-and-death decision. To the extent that professionals are successful in producing assent, they are able to avoid conflicts with parents. However, when these conflicts cannot be avoided, staff attempt to diffuse dissent in order to maintain boundaries between professional and parental jurisdiction and in order to maintain boundaries between the nursery and the outside world.

In many ways, neonatal intensive care epitomizes the kinds of dilemmas that arise in the high-technology medical settings that have come to proliferate in our times. A culture that rewards science, technology, teaching, and learning, and that devalues interaction with patients, is coupled with a social structure that places barriers between physicians, patients, and parents. While some decisions are relatively unproblematic, all too often outcomes ensue that adversely affect the lives of all concerned.

This study of life-and-death decisions has also been a study in the sociology of organizations, since it relates these decisions to the social context of the intensive-care nursery as a work environment. In suggesting that the decisions of professionals are shaped by the experiences and realities of their work, I have also ventured into the sociology of occupations. I have examined the structure of work in two senses of the term: as a set of activities and as a set of interpretations and practices that make those activities possible.

In this chapter, I move beyond the organization and discuss how decisions in the nursery are shaped by public policy decisions that affect resource allocation outside the nursery. First, I consider some apparent paradoxes in public policy. Next, I discuss how these paradoxes in public policy create dilemmas for those who make life-and-death decisions. In so doing, I address the relationship of a microsocial phenomenon—decision making—to its macrosocial or institutional context. Finally, I suggest some conclusions for those who study life-and-death decisions and those who make them.

PARADOXES IN PUBLIC POLICY

Paradox 1: Investment in Technology Rather Than in Prevention

A first issue is our society's apparently paradoxical decision to lower infant mortality rates by investing its resources in the highly technological interventions of neonatal intensive care rather than in preventive strategies, such as improved access to prenatal care and improved nutrition. These latter changes would in all likelihood prove more cost-effective.

In 1985, the Institute of Medicine's Committee to Study the Prevention of Low Birthweight compared the costs of (1) providing adequate prenatal care in 1980 to the three million women of childbearing age who were receiving public assistance and who had less than a high school education with (2) the savings that could be expected through decreasing the incidence of low birthweight. Providing adequate prenatal care could lower the incidence of low birthweight from 11.5 to 9 percent and could save $3.38 for each additional dollar spent on prenatal care. The costs of a single year of medical care for the infants born to these women were estimated to be more than $188 million ($222 million in 1990 dollars). Adequate prenatal care would reduce these expenditures to about $147 million ($181 million in 1990 dollars), thereby saving more than $40 million in a single year. The committee estimated that the *total* cost of providing prenatal care to one woman would be less than half of the *daily* cost of neonatal intensive care.[5]

The committee's study is highly significant because it corrects what has been identified as a limitation in the literature concerning the effectiveness of neonatal care: the study compares the cost-effectiveness of neonatal intensive care with an alternative—preventive strategies.[6] Yet despite the committee's finding that neonatal intensive care is less cost-effective than prevention, our society continues to invest in technological intervention.

Guido Calabresi and Philip Bobbitt describe this dilemma metaphorically when they ask why we spend $200,000 to rescue a miner from a decaying mine shaft rather than spending $100,000 to prevent the disaster from occurring in the first place by repairing the mine. Their answer is that the more costly route symbolizes the value of saving lives, or, in James Childress's words, the "compassion of the rescuer and the value of the rescued."[7]

When one considers neonatal intensive care, however, it is apparent that interests as well as values are at stake in our decision to invest in technological rather than public health solutions. Impelled by a desire to lower our embarrassingly high infant mortality rate, the federal government made research funds available to hospitals during the 1960s to develop neonatal intensive-care units. Over the years, neonatal intensive-care units have become increasingly profitable—not only to the equipment companies that manufacture sophisticated technologies but to individual hospitals that encourage the use of revenues from neonatal intensive care to subsidize other units.[8] Thus, in an era of shrinking financial resources and public policy pressures toward cost containment, neonatal intensive care has flourished.

In its 1985 report, the Committee to Study the Prevention of Low Birthweight recommended: (1) expanding prenatal services; (2) improving access to prenatal care; (3) providing health education about risk reduction, health behavior modification, family planning, and birth control; and (4) identifying women at high risk.[9] Other commentators on newborn intensive care have also supported this recommendation for developing a policy of prenatal planning.[10]

It is entirely possible, however, that public health alternatives, such as those I have mentioned, might entail other, more fundamental changes. The Committee to Study the Prevention of Low Birthweight alludes to this issue when it acknowledges a number of structural barriers to utilizing prenatal care: highly restrictive Medicaid eligibility regulations; lack of prenatal care providers willing to care for high-risk mothers receiving Medicaid; insufficient preventive programs in settings used by high-risk populations; an atmosphere of service delivery that is inhospitable to the poor; and inadequate transportation and child care.[11] Yet the committee stops short of the conclusion that prematurity is largely an affliction of poverty and that eradicating prematurity may well require nothing less than eliminating poverty. Like other commentators on neonatal intensive care, the committee remains mired in a *proximal* notion of prevention, which is directed largely toward modifying health behaviors, rather than a *distal* notion of prevention, which strikes directly at the roots of prematurity.[12] A broader, distal conception of prevention might include such changes as income redistribution to ensure access to adequate nutrition; increased regulation of occupational safety and industrial pollution to lower the incidence of congenital anomalies; and major changes in the distribution of health care—changes that are hardly likely to take place in the contemporary political climate.

Suffice it to say that the technological solution is the one that has been chosen, and it has been an expensive one. Neonatal intensive care ranks among the most costly of therapeutic modalities. Expensive equipment, high nurse-patient ratios, and third-party reimbursement practices that encourage cross-subsidization all conspire to create costs that strain the imagination. A leading study published in 1980 by Peter Budetti and his colleagues estimated that the national annual expenditures on newborn intensive care were about $1.6 billion, or an average of $8000 per patient—that is, $2.7 billion, or $13,360 per patient, in 1990 dollars. Another group of researchers, comparing expenditures among patients with high-cost hospitalization, found newborn cases to be among the most expensive, averaging $20,000 per patient ($36,400 in 1990 dollars), thereby exceeding the costs of two of the most expensive adult services—for neoplastic disease and circulatory disease. Estimates of the average cost per patient vary widely among studies, but one pattern is clear: the smaller the infant, the higher the cost of care.[13]

Neonatal intensive care has been credited with playing some role in the dramatic reduction in infant mortality that occurred in the 1960s and 1970s.[14] However, other forces may have been at work as well, such as improved perinatal and maternity care, improved maternal health and nutrition, lower fertility rates, legalized abortion, family planning, Medicaid coverage of pregnancy, and federal government involvement in providing greater access to health care among poverty groups and in providing opportunities for oppressed groups and the poor to raise their standard of living.[15]

The effect of neonatal intensive care on morbidity is a highly complex issue that has been given conflicting interpretations. It is not clear whether, as some would argue, mortality is decreasing faster than morbidity, or, alternatively, the proportion of less severely disabled survivors has decreased while that of severely handicapped survivors has remained constant. However, even the most optimistic researchers acknowledge that the *absolute number* of severely disabled survivors is increasing, particularly among the smallest infants.[16]

This suggests that neonatal intensive care may be contributing to the creation of future costs, including those that transcend the economic, to be borne by families, communities, and the disabled themselves. The problem is even more acute when one considers the nature of the patient population served by the intensive-care nursery. The association between poverty and infant mortality has been well documented in the epidemiological literature. U.S. studies have demonstrated that low socioeconomic status is associated with the birth of premature and low-birthweight infants.[17] The greater prevalence of critically ill infants and disabled children among the poor leads to another irony: the future costs of neonatal intensive care will increasingly fall on those least able to bear them.

Paradox 2: Saving Lives While Withdrawing Resources

The problems just described are compounded when one considers yet another paradox in public policy. Even as our society invests its resources in neonatal intensive care, the current fiscal preoccupation with cost containment is also leading to a reduction in social services—services that are necessary to support those disabled children who survive because of neonatology's therapeutic advances.

Nowhere was this paradox more acutely apparent than in the policies of the Reagan administration. For example, in the 1983 Baby John Doe case in Bloomington, Indiana, the parents and physician decided not to treat an infant with Down syndrome and abnormalities of the throat. However, conflicts among the medical staff led to a court case. Although the Indiana courts upheld the parents' decision, the case came to the attention of the Reagan administration. President Reagan had recently seen a documentary film in which a baby with Down syndrome was allowed to die. Outraged by the film and by reports of the Baby Doe case, Reagan instructed the secretary of the Department of Health and Human Services to draft a series of regulations to protect infants in the nursery. Next, Surgeon General C. Everett Koop became a key actor in formulating policy for treating newborn infants. Koop, a pediatric surgeon, was (and still is) an active member of the pro-life movement and has been an outspoken critic of policies, such as those advocated by Duff and Campbell, that withhold treatment from infants on the basis of their anticipated quality of life.[18] Prior to becoming surgeon general, Koop was surgeon-in-chief of Philadelphia Children's Hospital, which was known for its policy of aggressively treating all infants. One of Koop's accomplishments included treating Christopher Wall, a child born with ectopia cordis, a condition in which the heart is outside the chest. After spending 1117 days in the hospital and undergoing fifteen procedures, Christopher was able to go home—the only patient ever to survive with this type of defect—a feat that attests as much to Koop's commitment to the principle of active intervention as it does to his technical prowess.[19]

The Department of Health and Human Services invoked Section 504 of the Rehabilitation Act, which forbids discrimination on the basis of disability. Then the department instituted a number of so-called Doe directives, which required all nurseries to post a federal toll-free hot-line telephone number to encourage the reporting of infant abuse. Hospitals that withheld food or treatment from infants in the nurseries were threatened with a loss of federal funds. Squads of federal officials descended upon nurseries in response to these calls but failed to find actual instances of abuse. Federal regulations have been challenged in the courts by the American Academy of Pediatrics, the American Hospital Association, and the American College of Obstetrics and Gynecology (which viewed the regulations as a threat to professional autonomy) and have been revised several times. In its current regulations, following the 1984 amendments to the Child Abuse Prevention and Treatment Act, the Department of Health and Human Services continues to insist upon aggressive intervention for all infants except those who are already dying, those who are in a coma, and those who are so ill that care would be futile or inhumane. The regulations have been interpreted in different ways by intensive-care nurseries throughout the country. However, their overall effect has been to push physicians toward highly aggressive intervention. (In fact, today's physicians are, if anything, even more aggressive than those described throughout this book.)[20]

Yet while extolling the sanctity of life and deploring discrimination against the disabled *inside* the nursery, the Reagan administration sought to resolve its fiscal crisis by dramatic and unprecedented cut-backs in funding for programs that would support the disabled *out-side* the nursery. Programs to support the education, medical care, and rehabilitation of the disabled in the community were drastically curtailed. To name only a few of the budget cuts in the Reagan years: the federal budget for special education was reduced by 30 percent; eligibility requirements for receiving disability payments were tightened severely; the federal budget for Crippled Children's Services, which treat birth defects and chronic childhood illnesses, was reduced from $496 million to $373 million; the budget for the developmental disabilities program, which funds services for vocational education, employment, and community living for the disabled, was cut by 43 percent; and states like California were forced to freeze their special education funds.[21] Moreover, federal cutbacks in spending on health care for poor populations are believed to be a major factor in the slowing of the decline in infant mortality rates in the 1980s—infant mortality rates that are used to justify the massive infusion of funds into neonatal intensive care.[22]

To be sure, many advocates of a pro-life policy acknowledge that decisions to sustain the lives of all seriously disabled infants entail some social obligation toward the disabled.[23] Koop, for example, notes that:

> It is my hope that in my present and future pursuits I can be instrumental in the creation of a comprehensive service to be made available to concerned physicians and parents to take the sting out of managing a handicapped child. What I envision is a national computer data-bank type service that physicians and parents can tap by telephone to obtain up-to-date diagnostic information . . . , locations of the most competent local diagnostic services, locations of the closest competent therapeutic services, locations of available governmental and private agencies that could be of help to parents and children, and listings of nearby parents who have coped with similar problems in the past. If this service can be made available to parents and physicians alike, I think that the terrible fear that the odds against the handicapped child are too great to make any effort worthwhile can be removed.[24]

Koop is cognizant of the problem, but the hot-line solution he offers, much like the case-management approach to service delivery that flourished during the Reagan years, is one of referral. In urging policies that exploit existing local services rather than creating new ones, the case-management approach assumes that the services already exist. The problem is that services are duplicated and fragmented—a hodgepodge—and clients fall through the bureaucratic cracks. What is needed is more rational and efficient service coordination. Beneath the rhetoric of liberalism, the referral "solution" proposed by pro-life advocates is completely consistent with the contemporary public discourse on cost containment.

Paradox 3: Sanctity of Life, Stigma, and the Political Economy of Disability

Finally, the same social and economic forces that encourage the sanctity of newborn life in the nursery stigmatize the disabled in the society at large. Although the causes for stigma are complex, the stigma we attach to disability arises at least in part from the exclusion of the disabled from the productive economy. The practice of infanticide, while condemned by ecclesiastical authorities, was tacitly condoned and tolerated in Europe from the Middle Ages through the nineteenth century. Historians who have chronicled the practice have noted that it was often motivated by economic factors. Disabled infants were seen as economic liabilities.[25]

In our own society, it has often been noted that the stigma we attach to disability arises at least in part from our obsession with wealth, attractiveness, and productivity—our fetishism of commodities and conformity that, in Paul Hunt's words, puts "attributes and possessions before the person."[26] Stigmatizing the disabled also serves a latent function, allowing them to be exploited in marginal sectors of the economy, such as sheltered workshops, where they are paid less than the minimum wage.

Stigma, then, is a socially created phenomenon. In a society with a different set of values, which integrated the disabled into the economy, the disabled would be viewed as vital members of the community rather than as economic liabilities. Quality of life, too, is a socially (and politically) constructed phenomenon, forged in a crucible of discriminatory beliefs and practices.[27] Norman Fost notes that many of the choices made in the intensive-care nursery would not be necessary in a social context that did not discriminate against the disabled: "If buildings had ramps, if colleges would not exclude them from dormitories on the grounds that they are fire hazards, and if airlines would not require them to be accompanied by adult companions, many such individuals would not see themselves as significantly handicapped."[28]

In short, we create a set of paradoxes. We invest in costly technological interventions that lower mortality but may increase the absolute number of disabled survivors. We mandate saving the lives of disabled newborn infants, but withdraw resources from their care.

FROM DECISIONS TO DILEMMAS: PARADOXES IN PUBLIC POLICY AND LIFE-AND-DEATH DECISIONS

Both the bioethical and the public discourse on neonatal intensive care treat decisions in the nursery as though they are unaffected by social forces outside the nursery.[29] In fact, the political economy and the epidemiology of neonatal intensive care not only raise macrosocial issues of policy but also create a set of social, ethical, and practical dilemmas for those who make life-and-death decisions. When asked about her opinion of modern medicine, one mother I interviewed noted ironically that the very forces that sustain lives in the nursery undermine those lives in the society at large:

MOTHER: I've seen that it is a big business, and many times they try to save people that this kind of society kills.
INTERVIEWER: Can you say a little more about that?
MOTHER: Technology in industrial [society] has destroyed everything natural in this world, and . . . so we pay a big price for technology. And a lot of times, medicine tries to keep alive what the same kind of technology kills. . . . If your baby's sick because the air is dirty, they can do something for making your children better, [but] they cannot give . . . your children clean air. . . . It's a strange situation, because maybe without this kind of technology [my baby] would be dead, and so it's difficult for me to say I don't want the technology. . . . As [a parent], I cannot [say], "Take off the machine." But then you have a baby [who is] no good . . . for this world . . . , and you're alone in this situation, and so it's hard to say. I have not answered a lot of things.

As this mother implies, parents confront life-and-death decisions faced with the prospect of raising disabled children in an era of diminishing social supports. When I asked a father whose baby was hospitalized in the General Nursery what he saw as his baby's future, he answered: "The future? I don't know. He has problems with his liver and paralysis in his hands and body. Who is going to take care of him? We have seven other children at home that need us. We both have to work. How will we give him medical care? Who will take care of him?"

The decreasing number of educational, social, and residential resources to support disabled children also places certain constraints on professional participants in life-and-death decisions, as the following case from my field notes suggests:

> Early in this research, a case took place in one nursery that portended the case of Baby John Doe. An infant was born with Down syndrome and duodenal atresia [an intestinal obstruction]. A very simple surgical procedure was necessary to correct the lesion. The mother of the baby, a teacher, insisted that the surgery not be performed, stating that she could not care for a retarded child who would also have a colostomy. Many members of the nursery staff felt that the surgery should be performed, but were reluctant to seek a court order to perform the surgery. They feared that the mother would abandon the child to a foster home or to an institution, and lamented the fact that the quality of institutional care was far less than optimal.

Those members of the nursery staff who felt that the baby should live confronted the possibility that the mother would then abandon the baby to an institution lacking the resources to provide quality care. A resident who cared for the baby noted:

> The decision was really . . . whether or not the mother was willing to have a Down's baby with a colostomy or let the baby die. Those were . . . the two options . . . , and it presented a lot of interesting questions, because a Down's child with a colostomy is pretty hard to care for. . . . This kid would have had a colostomy and special care, which really limits your options in terms of institutionalized care. You don't really have the option of [adoption], and I'm not really sure about state hospitals.

Given the regulations that followed the Baby Doe controversies, and given the increasing optimism about the prognosis of Down syndrome, it is unlikely that professionals in today's nurseries would even entertain the idea of acceding to the mother's wishes not to treat a baby with Down syndrome and an intestinal obstruction. Moreover, even at the time, the case was highly controversial, and most members of the nursery staff, including the resident I just quoted, viewed the mother's decision as ethically and legally problematic. However, the sociological point of this case is as accurate today as it was then. In this case and others, those who reached life-and-death decisions were brought face-to-face with institutional constraints—constraints that transform decisions into dilemmas. Torn between what they viewed as the child's best interests and pragmatic constraints on institutional care, these decision makers confronted not only a decision but a *dilemma:* a choice between unsatisfactory alternatives.

CONCLUDING REMARKS

In sum, I have suggested how paradoxes in public policy create dilemmas for those who reach life-and-death decisions. This suggests that bioethics should attempt to address the influence of the social context on life-and-death decisions. From a sociological vantage point, the individualistic focus of bioethics lends it a reformist quality, which seeks solutions in disciplined reflection rather than in changes in the social milieu. However, to the extent that the choices of decision makers are constrained by ironies in public policy, changes in the broader context might be necessary for just decisions to ensue. In a society that embraced public health policies to prevent disability and that provided the resources to care for the disabled and to integrate them into the productive economy, it would not be necessary to choose between infants' rights to life and the quality of life of infants and their families.

Given our society's failure to invest in its disabled members, what should be done in the interim? It is my view that decisions should be structured so as to empower parents to be the principal decision makers. We need to direct our attention toward breaking down both the interpersonal and organizational barriers to informed consent. In the long run, however, a truly just solution would require changes in the wider society. If the foregoing analysis is correct, individual decisions cannot easily be extricated from larger questions of distributive justice and public policy questions of resource allocation. In addition to developing a model of the moral agent, then, I would suggest that bioethics begin to nurture a vision of moral organizations, moral institutions, and a moral society.

Field Research and the Sociology of (Sociological) Knowledge

INTRODUCTION:
FIELD RESEARCH AND PRACTICAL DECISIONS

In this appendix, I turn from my discussion of life-and-death decisions to a description and analysis of yet another kind of decision: decisions reached by researchers in field settings. To state that what is conventionally known as "research methods" involves a process of decision making is quite a commonplace observation: one need only look to an introductory methods text for a lengthy exposition of decisions about sampling, testing hypotheses, and evaluating evidence. However, in field research there is another type of decision, far more subtle and perhaps less consciously reached, for which the canons of the "scientific method" provide few guidelines. These concern such matters as what to observe, when to observe, whom to talk to, what to ask (and *not* to ask), how to record information, what information to record, what to believe, what to question, what to delete, and what to present to the reader. These decisions are frequently oriented to the contingencies of the moment and guided not by scientific rules of procedure but by considerations of ethics, etiquette, politics, pragmatism, and "presentation of self." Yet precisely because they are eminently *practical*, the nature of these decisions is sometimes obscure and the criteria on which they are based, elusive. These subtle day-to-day decisions define the contours of the information available to the researcher and, by implication, to the reader—and contribute no less than more "scientific" decisions to what ultimately come to be called "data."

In this appendix I discuss several decisions I made in the course of this research. These include "conventional" methods as well as the more practically based decisions I have just mentioned. I will discuss how the social organization of the intensive-care nurseries I studied and my place in these organizations influenced the practical decisions I made as a participant-observer and shaped the character of the data I collected and the findings I obtained. I am suggesting, then, that research decisions (like the life-and-death decisions that are the subject of this study) may be viewed as a problem in the sociology of knowledge. I focus on the relationship between one type of knowledge (sociological knowledge) and one social context (the social structure of the intensive-care nursery).[1]

My choice to frame both research decisions and life-and-death decisions as problems in the sociology of knowledge assumes that a comparison can be drawn between what are ostensibly two very different sorts of activities. The consequences of each type of decision making are very different, for there is a real and obvious distinction between a decision that culminates in the life or death of another person and one that contributes to the production of a piece of scholarly work. Moreover, the goals of each type of decision making and the auspices under which each is performed are also quite distinct. The researcher's decisions are said to belong to the scientific enterprise (including techniques for data collection and rules of evidence), whereas those discussed in the remainder of this study fall partly within the realm of morality, since they concern the welfare of other people.

As has often been noted, the rules and procedures for solving scientific problems and those involved in resolving ethical dilemmas are very different.[2] Scientific questions, on the one hand, are largely *data-dependent*—that is, a new piece of information can alter a body of existing knowledge—and hence the goal of a research decision is to produce and evaluate such information. Ethical dilemmas, on the other hand, always contain an element that is *data-transcendent*—that is, in any ethical decision, a point is ultimately reached at which the accumulation of additional information will not resolve the dilemma and can provide no assistance in reaching the decision. Even after all the relevant information ("data") has been gathered, the dilemma cannot be resolved without recourse to a set of moral rules or principles.

Nevertheless, despite the significant contrasts between them, there is a sense in which research decisions and life-and-death decisions can indeed be compared. First, most social scientists recognize that many of the decisions reached during the course of their research affect the welfare of their subjects and therefore involve considerations of morality and values. Moreover, these value-based decisions (e.g., decisions about the extent to which subjects should be informed about the purposes of the research) directly affect the nature of the data that are produced. Conversely, a large part of the life-and-death decision— and indeed of any ethical decision reached in a medical context—is devoted to the accumulation of "facts" or information (e.g., information concerning the infant's diagnosis or prognosis). There is therefore a significant ethical dimension in many activities designated as "science" and a significant scientific dimension in many life-and-death decisions. Both decisions are, then, epistemological hybrids, involving questions of fact and value, science and morality.

But there is a second, less obvious sense in which research decisions and life-and-death decisions may not be quite so distinct as might be supposed. Both types of decision making are justified by recourse to a set of principles, procedures, or formalized methods of reasoning. In the case of research decisions, these may be the ideals of the hypothetico-deductive model or analytic induction; and in the case of ethically based decisions, these may be abstract moral or medical principles, such as "Do no harm," or formalized modes of reasoning, such as formalism or consequentialism. Yet in each case, considerations enter into actual decisions that may be quite unrelated to these formal norms and rules of procedure.

Let me give two illustrations. A resident physician feels that a baby who is likely to survive with severe mental and physical handicaps should not receive life-sustaining treatment because caring for this child would pose undue hardships for the family. On the surface, this seems to be a straightforward application of consequentialist ethics (i.e., the decision is based on an assessment of the consequences for the family of a seriously disabled child). But how did the physician infer that the child would bring undue burdens to the family? The physician knows that the parents are poor and have other young children. In addition, the nurses have told the physician that the mother visits the nursery only infrequently and rarely handles the baby when she does visit and that the father has not been seen.

The nurses believe that this is because the parents are so preoccupied with their other children that they cannot allow themselves to become attached to this baby. Thus, the physician has based his or her assessment of the family situation on assumptions about the hardships of "lower-class life" and on assessments by the nurses, which are in turn based on cues gleaned from observations of the parents and assumptions about visiting patterns and behaviors of parents in intensive-care nurseries. It is also an organizational feature of this nursery that physicians frequently rely on secondhand, pre-interpreted information from the nurses. Thus, while the *criteria* on which this decision is based appear to be quite formal, the decision reflects organizational information patterns and *inferences* based on a complex mix of interactional and observational cues and cultural and organizational knowledge.

Consider also the example of a field researcher who is observing a staff conference in which the life or death of a baby is being decided. The researcher has decided to take notes during the conference, since she (or he) believes that attempting to record the participants' actual conversation would provide a more accurate representation of the event than would recording impressions afterward (an empiricist criterion of scientific adequacy). However, during the conference, the participants' attention seems to be riveted on the researcher whenever she writes. The researcher assumes that recording has disrupted the natural flow of the interaction and is concerned that the participants may be inhibited from expressing their opinions spontaneously. The researcher also does not know the participants in the conference very well and is concerned that recording might arouse their suspicions, disrupt future relationships with them, and restrict access to future conferences. So, reluctantly, she puts away the notebook. In the final decision, then, the researcher has made inferences about the participants' behavior and her own future place in the organization and has balanced formalized notions of scientific adequacy against practical political concerns about future research relationships.

Both life-and-death decisions and research decisions, then, are complex, socially organized activities. The actual reasoning in each case reflects not only abstract "scientific" or "ethical" criteria but subtle inferences and practical considerations, which in turn are based on features of the situation, the relationships between the participants, and the setting in which the decision is made. Because both research decisions and life-and-death decisions are *social* actions that take place within a *social* context, both may be approached from the standpoint of the sociology of knowledge.

PRACTICAL DECISIONS AND
METHODOLOGICAL ADEQUACY

For some time, field researchers have been aware that practical considerations enter into decisions about participation, role choice, and recording strategy, and have realized that these decisions affect the nature and quality of the data produced. Thus, by the 1960s, there were already several systematic discussions of problems of role choice, entree into research settings, field relationships, and recording data.[3] Furthermore, sociologists are cognizant of the fact that these practical choices may make the evaluation of evidence problematic. Consequently, attempts have been made to provide guidelines for evaluating evidence by assimilating field research methodology to more established formal scientific models (such as induction or the hypothetico-deductive method).

For example, an early formulation by Becker discusses problems of inference and proof of participant-observation and attempts to assimilate fieldwork to a hypothesis-testing model. The methodologies of analytic induction and grounded theory attempt to generate concepts and theory from data and to verify this emergent theory by means of a search for deviant cases ("theoretical sampling").[4] Yet in these earlier formulations, "methods," "data," and "findings" continued to be treated as separate phenomena. Thus, despite these efforts to refine and formalize field research methodology, and despite the many thoughtful discussions of practical problems in field research, the influence of the practical problems and decisions of the researcher on the findings and conclusions generated in any particular study remained an unanswered question.

Over the past two decades, ethnomethodology has brought an increasing self-consciousness to fieldwork.[5] Ethnomethodologically informed field researchers have contributed to a deepening awareness of the central problem of field research, noted by Cicourel in 1964: that the researcher's practical decisions contribute to what are designated as "data." Decisions about access and entree into field settings, intensity of participation and level of involvement, strategies for establishing rapport, and choice of informants—along with selectivity in perception, observation, memory, recording, and coding—in effect *create* the data by transforming a large (and unknown) potential observational field into a circumscribed and well-defined set of findings and conclusions. Yet because these decisions are not made available to the reader, substantive conclusions may assume less credibility in the eyes of those who read them.[6]

Furthermore, if we accept one definition of science as a set of explicit and publicly articulated procedures that dictate accepting or rejecting propositions from the corpus of knowledge, so too we must conclude that many of the procedures used in field research are neither made explicit nor publicly articulated.[7] To the extent that this is so, the scientific status of any work using field research is compromised. The problem becomes more complex when we realize not only that many researchers fail to follow, record, and present several of the critical decisions they made in the course of their research, but also that we still know very little about the basic cognitive and interactive processes that make these decisions possible. And so it is that the path from a potential observational field to the findings and conclusions that are actually presented soon disappears from sight.

Beginning with the premise that observer and observed are inseparable, researchers working in "reflexive" or "interpretive" ethnographic traditions have proposed a number of strategies to recover some of the steps along this path. These include using: (1) verbatim conversational materials whenever possible, so that readers can follow the researcher's inferences and render alternative interpretations; (2) a combination of research strategies, so that the relative strengths and weaknesses of each are placed in sharp relief; and (3) detailed methodological notes, so that the researcher can follow his or her own activities over time. Thus, the goal of any study should not only be to produce conclusions about the phenomenon under study but to make the method itself, its strengths and its limitations, an explicit object of inquiry.[8]

In keeping with this reflexive project, this research has attempted not only to learn about the life-and-death decisions reached in two intensive-care nurseries but also to learn about the set of decisions reached throughout the course of this study (which are the subject of this appendix). The purpose of this discussion, then, is to make some of the decisions reached in this research available to the reader and, in so doing, to enhance the credibility of the findings presented. I will begin by presenting an "ethnography of the ethnographer," or a narrative account of the decisions made in this research.

FIELD RESEARCH IN TWO INTENSIVE-CARE NURSERIES: AN ANALYTICAL NARRATIVE

There are many ways that field researchers can enter a setting. Some enter with a well-defined theoretical framework and clearly articulated hypotheses. Others, by dint of chance or design, gain access to a setting and enter with only a very general interest in the kind of activities that take place there. Only after spending some time in the field do their interests crystalize. My own experiences fall somewhere between these two extremes—perhaps slightly closer to the first end of the continuum.

Almost two years before undertaking this project, I had developed an interest in the social and ethical issues surrounding new medical technologies. This interest eventually led me to attend a seminar in biomedical ethics at the medical school at the University of California, San Diego. One lecturer in the course discussed the problems of newborn intensive care. After I discussed my interests with the speaker, he directed me to an institution where attempts were being made to discuss ethical issues carefully. Two months later, I met one of the attending neonatologists at "Randolph Hospital" and began my negotiations for undertaking research there the following year.

Although I had a clear research focus (life-and-death decisions), a set of research questions, and a research design, and although I had read the existing literature concerning life-and-death decisions, I had little firsthand exposure to newborn intensive care. I knew little about the daily workings of intensive-care nurseries and even less about the actors and their concerns.

What follows is an account of my sixteen-month odyssey from a nearly complete outsider to a more or less knowledgeable (albeit marginal) member of two intensive-care nurseries. The reader who is conversant with the anthropological and sociological literature on the art and science of field methods may find that much of what I have to say has a familiar ring. Ethnographic accounts of fieldwork follow a canonical script: the researcher begins as something of an "outsider" and ends up assuming some kind of a role within the group under study—that is, she (or he) becomes an "insider." Somewhere along this road, two important things happen. First, the researcher—who has begun as a stranger or even something of an outcast, occasionally mistrusted and rejected—comes to be accepted by and to develop close relationships with members of the group. Second, the researcher acquires considerable cultural knowledge—that is, she comes to be familiar with the inner workings of the social setting, views activities not witnessed before, and acquires some knowledge of how group members view their own lives. No matter how unique my experiences in two intensive-care nurseries may have appeared to me, they followed the general outlines of this scenario.

For several reasons, however, my account (as well as those of other field-workers) is more than a mere "confessional." First, my ever-changing relationships with members of the intensive-care nursery staffs and my ever-shifting stock of knowledge about the nurseries influenced certain crucial decisions I made at various points in the research. Second, a number of factors conspired to make my first months in the Randolph Nursery a particularly trying experience. At least some of my initial difficulties were related to the culture and the social structure of newborn intensive-care units themselves. As I was soon to learn, the intensive-care nursery is a particularly difficult environment for a person without medical training. In certain respects, I began my research in a position not unlike that of a parent who first encounters newborn intensive care, and I ended up as some sort of auxiliary member of the "health care team." My experiences taught me something about these two very different realities.

A Closed Society?

When I arrived at Randolph Hospital, my first act was to call on the director of the nursery and the attending neonatologist, both of whom I had met briefly the year before. Both had already read a version of my research proposal and voiced no objections to what I wanted to do. The director of the nursery introduced me to the head nurse and the social worker. I explained the purposes of my study to them and gave each a copy of my protocol (which the head nurse placed on file in the nursery for interested staff to read). From these initial interviews, I gained a sense of the general staff composition of the nursery and its patient population, a general outline of the decision-making process at the nursery, and an idea of some of the activities that might be important to observe.

During my first month, I began to observe several activities: monthly morbidity and mortality conferences, weekly social service rounds, and monthly ethics rounds. After I had gained clearance from the hospital's Human Subjects Committee, I began to observe daily rounds and to participate more directly in the daily life of the nursery. Before doing this, I introduced myself and explained the purposes of my study to the attending neonatologist for the month, the fellow, the housestaff, and the charge nurse on each shift. Thus, my entree seemed deceptively simple. I had gained access to the setting and had met several of its "gatekeepers." However, as I began to participate regularly in the nursery, I discovered that establishing close working relationships, founded on trust, with the many members of the nursery staff was not so easily accomplished. This fact was dramatically and vividly brought home to me during one of the first decision-making conferences that I observed, one month after beginning my research. Here is how I described the incident in my field notes:

> Bob [the fellow] had told me there would be a decision about whether to "discontinue" [turn off the respirator for] a premature baby who had had an intraventricular hemorrhage. At a first conference, they had decided to call in the neurologist for a "consult" to evaluate the results of a CAT scan [brain scan] that had been done. When the neurologist appeared, the attending proceeded to introduce the various interns and residents to the neurologist. I did not feel it was right to observe without the neurologist being aware of my presence, so when the attending had finished his introductions, I chimed in with "And one sociologist." "Yes," the attending added dryly, "and one sociologist who is doing her Ph.D. thesis on the very difficult life-and-death decisions we have to make in the nursery. So watch out what you say." I tried to make myself inconspicuous, but apparently did not succeed. Much later in the conversation, they were discussing whether the baby had received too much oxygen, which could cause blindness. The attending then turned to me and said, "And for your notes, this is a very difficult ethical problem, the problem of iatrogenesis. I'm not particularly anxious to be called into court, and it is not in my self-interest to have this baby survive." [My interpretation was that the attending was making a didactic point. Because in fact they decided to continue therapy. Later, it turned out that the baby had not in fact received too much oxygen.]

At the same time that he was providing me with helpful information and making an extremely candid revelation about self-interest, this attending was calling attention to my very precarious status as a "guest" in the nursery—and one who might prove harmful. Rarely, however, was my "trustworthiness" called into question. Rather, on a more basic level, it was difficult to establish even rudimentary relationships with members of the intensive-care nursery staff. On more than one occasion, I felt that I had entered a "closed society."

During my first months in the nursery, I devoted much of my time and effort to establishing working relationships with members of the nursery staff, and to this end I frequently engaged them in informal conversations ("impromptu interviews"). The social worker, a resident who had majored in sociology, and several nurses who had had a long-term relationship with the ethicist who had secured my entree into the setting took a special interest in my study. These were my initial informants. They provided medical information and identified cases that might prove relevant to my study. They also provided what I saw as exceptionally candid accounts of the organization, history, and politics of the nursery and their views of the decision-making process. For example, in talking about a baby who had been abandoned by her parents, the nurses felt very strongly that she should not have been kept alive, and they had no hesitation in indicating to me their opposition to aggressive intervention.

For several reasons, of course, my research design required me to go beyond a few informants and to cultivate research relationships with a larger and more diverse group of staff members. First, I needed a representative sense of the various viewpoints that were called into play in a given decision. I also needed a more diverse set of informants to provide information about the organization of the nursery and to provide multiple accounts of decisions I would inevitably miss. Furthermore, I felt that these accounts should come from persons who had been directly involved in the decision making. Since there was no telling in advance who might be the key participants in any decision, this meant I needed to develop relationships with a larger number of potential informants. My research design, then, demanded that my field relationships resemble a "cluster sample" that would be as heterogeneous as possible. But at the same time, this design created a practical dilemma, for it is difficult to develop relationships simultaneously with nurses, interns, residents, fellows, and attendings. The design also carried with it a built-in marginality that was to make me peripheral to each group.

Other barriers also made it difficult to become integrated into the life of the Randolph Nursery—barriers that were intrinsic to the organization of the intensive-care unit. First, the texture and quality of life in a critical-care environment does not invite casual, informal interactions. Especially in the "high-intensive" room, where the most critically ill babies were found, there was a constant flurry of activity. X-ray technicians, lab technicians, respiratory therapists, and other physicians would be filing in and out of the nursery. Nurses would be

making entries on charts, taking vital signs, and administering medications and would be moving quickly when, at frequent intervals, an
alarm sounded on one of the monitors. Housestaff would be coming
in and out to write orders, examine a baby, or perform a procedure.
All this raised the question of exactly how I was to interact and
develop relationships with people who seemed to be almost constantly
engaged in activities on which someone's life depended. Whenever I
entered the "high-intensive" nursery to ask the nurses about a particular baby, I feared our conversation could have potentially disastrous
consequences. More often, I talked to the nurses in the other rooms,
where the babies were less critically ill and the atmosphere less intense. I spent much time in the conference room, talking to nurses and
housestaff as they took their breaks, or joining them at meals. But
during my initial ventures into the nursery, I felt profoundly peripheral and conscious of "getting in the way."

A second feature of life in the intensive-care nursery is its large and
fluctuating cast of characters. As in all teaching hospitals, attendings
and housestaff at Randolph rotated through the nursery in staggered,
one-month intervals. Moreover, the unique and fluctuating exigencies
of staffing critical-care services meant that nursing staff composition
varied from one day to the next, and I encountered new faces in the
nursery every day. On more than one occasion, I introduced myself to
a nurse, and a week later she would ask, "What did you say your
study was about again?" Thus, it took a much longer time to establish
relationships with people who seemed to disappear for days. Even
after I had spent more than three months in the nursery, I had not met
all the nurses.

Third was my transient status in the nursery. Association patterns
in the nursery are organized along a time dimension (as well as along
occupational lines). At one end of this continuum are the attendings
and the nurses, the "permanent inhabitants" of the nursery, who
develop close working relationships with each other based on a lasting
commitment to the nursery and a shared history. Others (e.g., consultants and technicians) work permanently in the hospital but spend
only a fraction of their time in the intensive-care nursery. At the other
end of the continuum are the transients—visitors, researchers, and
housestaff—some of whom return to the nursery and others of whom
vanish, never to be seen again.

In the nursery, then, time is identified with commitment, and this
results in a certain orientation among the more permanent members

of the nursery staff toward the more transient participants in nursery life. On the one hand, the presence of strangers in a teaching hospital is quite routine, and therefore I was never asked why I was there. On the other hand, permanent employees of the nursery are quite naturally disinclined to develop relationships with persons who are soon to leave and whose commitment to the nursery is likely to be less intense than theirs. Since I was myself a transient, my stay in the nursery was apt to be brief and my commitment to the nursery transitory. Indeed, many of the nursery staff seemed to expect that I would depart soon. "Are you finished with your paper?" was a frequently asked question, reflecting not only different research styles but my transient status as well.

In addition to being a transient whose commitment to the nursery was seen as ephemeral, I was a researcher, whose activities were far from essential to the functioning of the nursery. I often suspected that the role of researcher carries with it a certain predatory and exploitative connotation within the grammar of motives in a teaching hospital. I base this inference on two incidents, which I recorded in my field notes as follows:

> Victor, the fellow, had just described a very complex ethical decision he had to make concerning whether to "cath" [perform a cardiac catheterization on] a baby who was suspected to have trisomy 18. . . . I commented, "That's an interesting ethical dilemma," to which he replied, *"Interesting! I* don't find these things interesting—I find them difficult." Victor is right. It is one thing to study life-and-death decisions and quite another thing to make them.

> · · ·

> Today, I was having lunch with Margot [the social worker] and several nurses. Toward the end of the conversation, I casually asked how I was perceived by the staff. Margot said, "You represent the research arm of the university"—a characterization that intimidates even me. She and the nurses seemed genuinely surprised when I said that I hoped that my research would contribute to the life of the nursery and that I intended to present my findings to the nursery staff at the end of the study.

Another organizational feature of the nursery complicated my initial relationships with the housestaff. This concerned the daily life of the house officer and the place of social and ethical issues in the "reward structure" of the nursery. As I was to learn, the mastery of technical knowledge and the ability to perform procedures (e.g., intubating) are rewarded by the attendings and fellows. Consequently, "ethical and social issues" (including my study) come to assume a very low position in the house officer's hierarchy of priorities. Residents and interns could ill afford the luxury—or burden—of talking to me, except in brief moments of respite, at lunch or dinner. I had also begun my research early in the academic year, when, I was later told, most residents are extremely anxious about their performance in the nursery.

Although some of my initial difficulties in establishing research relationships were the result of my research design and the timing of my study, most went to the heart of the nature of the intensive-care nursery as a social environment—an environment that I first perceived as a "closed society."

Cultural Knowledge and the Problem
of "Cognitive Overload"

At our initial meeting, the director of the nursery had suggested to me that important decisions were frequently made in the afternoon, during "sign-off rounds." In these rounds, which were an important part of the social life of the nursery, residents would "sign off" their patients to the house officer on call for the evening, and the group would review babies' progress with the attending and arrive at a treatment plan. As I began to make rounds on a regular basis, I was brought face-to-face with one of the major barriers to cultural understanding: the vast knowledge of medical terminology needed to understand even the simplest interactions in the nursery. I was observing physicians communicating with each other, and much of their talk was presented in numerical data and coded abbreviations that I could hardly expect them to "translate" for my benefit. I often felt like an anthropologist listening to natives speaking in a tongue that shared with English only the rudiments of syntax. Here are two excerpts from my early field notes:

> One patient, according to the resident, is a three-month-old male infant with an omphalocele that was repaired, and he's here "for surgical complications. The problems are (1) wound care and the inability to feed and (2) two bouts of sepsis and intermittent CHF due to fluid overload." Another baby, a twenty-six-week-old preemie who is nine days old, had a pH of 7.41. The $TCPO_2$ electrode showed a PO_2 of ———. The bilirubin was 3.1, and the baby has had spells of apnea and bradycardia.
>
> (Sign-Off Rounds)(Resident)

. . .

This is a case of twins. A is a girl of 1240 g., and B is a boy of 1440 g. B is, according to the resident, "posing big problems medically. We need to see what the CNS status is. The baby has four chest tubes in and had a bilateral collapse—a pneumomediastinum. We did an LP, which suggested a possible bleed. The plan is to do another LP this morning and DC the pavulon."

(Social Service Rounds)

My general strategy was to ask nurses and, more rarely, housestaff to provide medical explanations (especially in the case of babies who, I had been told, might be relevant to my study). But since there were practical limits to the number of questions I felt free to ask, I kept a list of terms and raced to the nearest textbook or medical dictionary at the earliest opportunity. Naturally, there were limits to the degree to which, and on the persons to whom, I was willing to display my ignorance or to admit that I had just spent two hours in their midst having understood little of what had taken place. (Nor did I feel that displays of ignorance would enhance my field relationships.) I frequently turned to several nurses, who patiently drew diagrams and provided simple lessons in pathophysiology (which, incidentally, I knew they were accustomed to doing with parents). Already, then, I had made practical decisions about what seemed "appropriate" to discuss with whom. My dependence on informants for translations introduced new methodological complications. For example, when I questioned an intern about the prognosis for infants with brain hemorrhages, she replied, "They're completely gorked" (medical slang for "vegetables"). I was later to learn that this information was not entirely correct.

Medical knowledge in the nursery is an extremely important form of cultural knowledge, one which affected my ability to process information in profound ways—for it is impossible to understand the basis of a life-and-death decision without at the same time understanding the prognosis of the infant in question. During my first two months in the nursery, "understanding the medicine" involved in decisions seemed an all-consuming effort. In fact, so much of my attention was focused on understanding the *medical* facets of cases that it became difficult to attend to important *social* facets of cases I was observing. In addition, my ability to record field notes accurately was compromised. My initial field experience was one of what I call "cognitive overload," or the inability to attend to and process several channels of information simultaneously, a phenomenon that limited both my ability to observe and my ability to record data.

Note that medical "language" is not merely a vocabulary or a set of terms (so-called "medicalese"), but conveys complex information about diagnosis, prognosis, and treatment. Consider, for example, the information contained in the following excerpt from my field notes:

> There are other clues, besides the resident's statement that Twin B is "posing big problems medically," to indicate that this is a baby that I should watch closely. The use of four chest tubes and the pneumomediastinum [the escape of air into the chest cavity that contains the heart and major blood vessels] are indicative of critical medical status. They have already done a spinal tap [lumbar puncture or LP] that was probably bloody and suggests that the baby may have had a brain hemorrhage, which could indicate mild to severe neurological damage, e.g., spasticity or retardation, at worst. Babies who are on respirators are sometimes given pavulon to paralyze them, which would make it impossible to observe their movements and make a clinical assessment of their CNS [central nervous system] status. So the plan is to do another spinal tap, discontinue [DC] the pavulon, and observe the baby in order to evaluate his neurological status further. The fact that this is a baby who might die or be severely neurologically damaged suggests that a life-and-death decision *might* be made on this baby in the future.

The prognostic and diagnostic medical information conveyed through medical language is necessary not only to understand the basis of life-and-death decisions but to identify the very sick babies who were likely to be the subjects of decisions—and therefore followed closely in rounds. There was another sense, then, in which I inhabited an "overloaded" world: I knew neither which information to listen to closely in rounds nor which babies I should "follow" closely. In other words, I lacked a basis on which to focus my attention.

These early field experiences led me to a profound appreciation of what parents must face in their initial encounters with neonatal intensive care. To be sure, parents and researchers bring very different resources and systems of relevance to the intensive-care nursery. From the outset, I possessed more medical knowledge than did most of the parents. Theirs was a far more intense commitment to the life of a single patient. Understandably, the nurses had a greater commitment to the parents than to me and made serious attempts to provide them with explanations and to integrate them into the life of the nursery. As a researcher, I was expected to fend for myself. But like the parents, I encountered an environment with a constantly shifting set of people, who were seemingly forever preoccupied, spoke a strange language, and used unfamiliar equipment. I felt peripheral, concerned that I might "get in the way," and, like some of the parents, I was often tempted to withdraw from the unit.[9] With parents, then, I shared the experiences of the quintessentially marginal.

The Art of Being in the Right Place
at the Right Time

So far, I have emphasized the experiential side of my social and cultural marginality in the intensive-care nursery and its consequences for my ability to process information. But the marginality I experienced in the early months of my research also affected my ability to collect data concerning life-and-death decisions.

By the end of my first month in the nursery, I had acquired sufficient knowledge of the organization to identify the activities that might prove relevant to my study (e.g., sign-off rounds and ethics rounds). This enabled me to observe those decisions that were reached during the course of the activities I had "sampled" and those that had been scheduled in advance. Nevertheless, I found that I missed several important impromptu conferences in which life-and-death decisions were made. I attribute this problem mainly to the incipient state of my cultural knowledge. As I have noted, I did not know enough about life-and-death decisions to be able to identify those patients who might be the subjects of decision making. Even when I was able to identify babies who were critically ill or likely to be severely disabled, I had not yet acquired a sense of the timing of decisions to be able to predict the days on which decision-making conferences might be held.

I was therefore forced to rely on informants to identify those patients whom I should follow and to inform me of an impending decision. Later, I attempted a new strategy: I placed myself "on call." The secretary put my name and phone number on the front desk and then asked the staff nurses and the housestaff to call me at any time of day or night that a life-and-death decision was going to be made. (Unfortunately, I was usually called *after* a decision had been made.) After a day on which I had not come in, I would inquire about what had taken place in my absence, and I would occasionally be greeted with the proverbial "You should have been here yesterday." When I missed something important, I would attempt to find out who had been most centrally involved in the decision making and would seek out that person to find out what I had missed. Although I always attempted to obtain at least two accounts of the decision making, in these cases the data had been transformed by the memory and perceptions of my informants.

Of course, part of this problem was due to the nature of the phenomenon I had chosen to study. Life-and-death decisions (in contrast, for example, to diagnostic and treatment decisions in a clinic) constitute only a small fraction of the total activities that take place in the setting—a minute segment of its social life. Only rarely are these decisions scheduled in advance, and thus they always contain an unpredictable element. Inevitably, no field researcher who studies a work environment can live in the setting, and certain activities will arise that the researcher will be unable to witness directly. But the fact that many of the decisions I was not able to observe took place at the beginning of my research led me to conclude that much more than "chance" or "bad luck" was involved.

In short, even so deceptively simple an act as "being present" involves a complex form of decision making. Considerable knowledge of the culture and the social structure of the setting is required to decide such matters as what time to come in and which days to stay home. At the outset of my research, I lacked the cultural knowledge necessary to "predict" when decisions would be reached, and consequently I missed some of them. I had not yet acquired the art of being in the right place at the right time.

The Dilemma of Discretion

Access, or official permission to study a field setting, is granted at the point of entree into the setting. However, as I began my research, I found that certain people and activities were less "accessible" to me as a researcher than others. Gaining access to those people and activities required continuous and delicate negotiations with the participants in life-and-death decisions. Among those persons who were less "accessible" were some of the attending physicians. Attendings, who combined their work in the nursery with teaching and research responsibilities, spent relatively little time in the nursery staying for rounds or participating in the care of babies who became critically ill. For this reason, I would approach the attendings in their spare moments and interview them informally about a particular patient or about their general perceptions of life-and-death decisions.

In addition, it was often exceedingly difficult to interview the parents of babies who were likely to be the subjects of life-and-death decisions. Some parents visited the nursery only infrequently. More-over, because the Randolph Nursery functioned as a major referral center, some of the parents lived in outlying areas. On many occa-sions, parents were called to the nursery when their baby became critically ill, a conference was held with them, and they left the nursery in tears after their baby had died. This scenario left little room for me to engage the parents in an hour-long in-depth interview.

Even when there was sufficient time for me to interview the parents, the nature of the consent process posed another formidable barrier. Frequently, I was approaching parents who were unaware that their baby was critically ill or dying or that they would soon be asked to participate in a life-and-death decision (facts that I knew). But the consent form stated explicitly that I was studying decision making. This posed the ethical dilemma of exactly how I was to respond to the question "*What kind* of decision?" and required me to walk a delicate interactional tightrope, attempting not to reveal potentially upsetting information about the medical condition of a child while remaining as candid as possible about the purpose of my research.

As a result of these problems and dilemmas, I interviewed fewer parents than would have been optimal. I approached parents when-ever possible and whenever I deemed it appropriate to do so (I would not approach a parent who was crying or visibly extremely upset). On some occasions, I did not interview parents until after their baby had died or left the nursery. (I also designed two new interview schedules: a shorter form for on-the-spot interviewing and a longer one for retrospective interviews.) These problems of access illustrate how field researchers frequently strike a balance between considerations of "science," on the one hand, and ethical and "human" contingencies, on the other.

I also found my access to two activities in the decision-making process to be particularly problematic. The first of these were resusci-tations at delivery. However, because infants in the Randolph Nur-sery are routinely resuscitated, I actually missed few life-and-death decisions. Much more serious from the standpoint of this research was the fact that I was sometimes denied permission by staff participants to observe decision-making conferences with parents. This created a significant strategic dilemma. On the one hand, because communica-tion between parents and professionals was a major concern of my study, I knew that I would have to observe at least some of these conferences. On the other hand, I did not wish to get too many refusals to observe, which I feared might culminate in my being officially barred from observing conferences with parents.

What ensued was a series of strategic decisions about whether to request permission to observe these conferences, based on my estimate of the likelihood of being granted permission to observe them (this was my implicit decision rule). I requested permission to observe such conferences only if I had met the parents beforehand or if I had a good relationship with at least some of the staff who participated. Thus, my practical decision making about when to request permission to observe these conferences reflected a calculus in which I weighed the need for observational data against assessments of my relationships with the participants and the possible effects of my requests on my ability to observe future conferences.

My access to these persons and activities reflects a common phenomenon in field research: that members of the organization under study may make decisions that limit the researcher's freedom to observe certain activities. But, equally important, my access to these persons and activities also reflected considerable active decision making on my part about when and under what circumstances it was appropriate to venture into areas I perceived as "off-limits."

The problems I have just mentioned reflect what I call the "dilemma of discretion." Researchers frequently make decisions in which they balance the need for data and information against assumptions about field relationships, considerations of etiquette, and, in short, demands for discretion. Nor is this problem confined to field research situations. Georg Simmel, who wrote cogently on the subject, suggests that in contemporary societies, discretion—or the decision "to renounce the knowledge of all that the other does not voluntarily show us"—becomes an abiding preoccupation in daily social interaction.[10] Simmel notes that actors routinely make decisions about comments to avoid, questions to eschew, and subjects not to mention. So formidable is the regard for the privacy and sensibilities of others that a metaphorical "ideal sphere" comes to surround each individual:

> Relationships among men [sic] are thus distinguished according to the question of mutual knowledge of either "what is not concealed may be known" or "what is not revealed must not be known." To act upon the second of these decisions corresponds to the feeling . . . that an ideal sphere lies around every human being. Although differing in size and in various directions according to the person with whom one entertains relations, this sphere cannot be penetrated. . . . Language very poignantly designates an insult to one's honor as

"coming too close": the radius of this sphere marks, as it were, the distance whose trespassing by another person insults one's honor. . . . To penetrate this circle by taking notice constitutes a violation of [the other's] personality.[11]

Like all actors, researchers make decisions dictated by discretion. But discretion poses a particular problem in field research precisely because decisions not to violate subjects' "ideal spheres" may exact a price on the quality of the information obtained. To speak of research subjects as surrounded by "ideal spheres" is to cast the problems of field research in a language that is literary, metaphorical, vague, and imprecise. But that indeed is how I perceived many of my decisions concerning how to observe scenes, record data, and interact with research subjects.

Discretion often guided my choice of methods for recording data. The quality of data is diminished and transformed by memory as one moves from tape-recorded transcriptions of conversations to detailed notes taken in the course of an activity to brief notes jotted down to retrospective recording. At the same time, however, recording data is a social activity that takes place within a social context. Participants deliberating about matters whose legal status is ambiguous may object to having their comments tape-recorded. While I was not required to secure the consent of participants every time I took notes, note taking is far from an unobtrusive activity and can disrupt the spontaneous flow of the interaction being observed. Frequently, I was led to temper my ideals of methodological adequacy in light of these considerations. My choice of recording strategy depended on how sensitive I perceived the occasion to be. I chose to tape-record most of the ethics rounds and formal ethics conferences I attended. Since I knew most of the participants in those conferences, I assumed they were aware of the conferences' importance to my study and therefore would not object to being tape-recorded.

In other situations, I chose to take detailed notes. These were relatively public occasions (e.g., morbidity and mortality conferences) in which many of the participants were not members of the nursery staff and were therefore unaware of my study. I did not consider it appropriate (i.e., discreet) to disrupt such a conference, explain the purpose of my research, and request permission of people I did not know to tape-record the conversation. When decisions were made during rounds, I took detailed notes in shorthand and tried as much as possible to approximate a verbatim recording of the interaction. I did not tape-record impromptu decisions, since this would have disrupted the flow of the interaction and caused me to miss important aspects of the decision. I also routinely took notes during medical and social service rounds, recording topics that I felt might prove important to my research. Taking notes is not a common practice in medical settings, and my note taking did not escape the attention of the participants, but, aside from occasional comments, no one seriously objected.

There was a third set of activities in which my note taking was far less systematic. Staff members allowed me to sit in on conferences with parents with some degree of reluctance, and consequently I rarely took copious notes on these occasions, but instead jotted occasional notes. Although I felt that this decision compromised the quality of data, my access to these conferences was particularly problematic, and I therefore chose to observe them as unobtrusively as possible. In a few instances, I put aside my notebook entirely when topics of a particularly sensitive nature were brought up (e.g., arguments between staff members).

These recording decisions, then, were based on a variety of factors: an assessment of the topics being discussed; the nature of the decisions I was observing; my relationships with the participants in the situation; the possible effects of recording on the interaction; and my access to future activities. The choice of a means of recording reflected a calculus in which I balanced notions of methodological adequacy against considerations of discretion.

Particularly in the early phases of my research, considerations of discretion influenced my decisions about what topics to explore, what questions to ask, and when to probe. There are, of course, no norms or rules that dictate what is appropriate (or inappropriate) to ask whom. Rather, my decisions were based on my perception of the sensitivity of the question and my relationship with the person I was interviewing. On some occasions, I found that in probing what members of the intensive-care nursery staff took for granted, my questioning was interpreted as an assault on their competence. Here is one such instance from my field notes:

Today, Maria [one of the social workers] was describing a family. I asked her what had been her impressions of this family, and she said they were responding "appropriately." For some time, I had been wondering how nurses and social workers decided that parents were responding "appropriately," and I felt I knew Maria well enough to ask, "What do you mean by 'appropriately?' " To which she replied, "Well, you know, they ask appropriate questions." I asked what she meant by "appropriate questions," at which point she said, "Well, questions about how the baby is doing, when he'll be able to go home, how well he can function. I'm not judging them, you know." She seemed quite embarrassed by my attempt to probe and seemed to think that I was questioning the basis of her evaluations—which, in a sense, I was.

The norms of discretion—if they may be said to exist at all—are created only in the breach, so only retrospectively did I learn that I had ventured beyond the pale of discreet interaction. These situations are the avenues by which field researchers learn how to ask "appropriate" questions in a culture and how to identify topics considered sensitive and assumptions taken for granted—while learning about their relationships with particular research subjects. But asking questions is a major tool for gathering ethnographic data and exploring the perceptions of members of the group under study; and avoiding "inappropriate" questions for the sake of maintaining research relationships makes "the goals of the researcher," as Cicourel says, "subservient to the demands of polite discourse."[12]

There is no consensus among sociologists concerning how decisions about observing, recording, and asking questions should be made when relationships with research subjects seem to be at stake. Some field researchers promulgate an etiquette that sharply cautions against the "reactive effects" of recording on the scene.[13] Others (myself among them) take an opposing view. Researchers' answers to these questions—their particular cost-benefit calculi—depend on their notions of methodological adequacy and their assumptions about human relationships. But whether one chooses to err on the side of empiricism or of discretion, choices will inevitably be made in which data that have been directly observed and faithfully recorded are sacrificed in favor of felicitous field relationships.

Acquiring "Cultural Maps"

The problems and dilemmas I have just discussed were most keenly perceptible during, though not entirely confined to, my first months in the Randolph Nursery. Over time, however, as I continued to observe decision-making conferences, to attend social service rounds, and to accompany physicians on their daily rounds, I became familiar with much of the medical terminology employed by members of the nursery staff. This knowledge enabled me to understand the medical basis of most life-and-death decisions and to ask more informed questions.

Once I had observed several life-and-death decisions, I began to acquire a "map," or general outline, of the decision-making process. I could recognize those criteria members of the intensive-care nursery staff accepted as a matter of consensus (e.g., that babies with a prognosis of terminal illness, short life span, or extremely severe mental damage were often not supported) and those that were the subject of some disagreement (e.g., whether to support babies with uncertain prognoses).

I could also recognize many of the conditions associated with these prognoses (e.g., babies with trisomy 18 or severe brain hemorrhages), the diagnostic steps through which the attendings usually proceeded before reaching a decision (e.g., consultations obtaining CAT scans in the case of intraventricular hemorrhages), and some of the problems that occurred with these procedures (e.g., some babies were too critically ill to be transported to CAT scans, and by the time it was possible to transport them, evidence of the extent of the bleed could not be identified). A major test of this emerging cultural knowledge came when I could identify the babies likely to be the subject of life-and-death decisions and knew enough about the timing of these decisions to be able to "predict" with considerable accuracy when a decision was about to be made.

When I had learned to identify the babies whose progress I should follow closely, I became increasingly less reliant on informants to select patients who might be of interest or to inform me when decisions were about to be reached. No longer did I inhabit a "cognitively overloaded world," but rather I had acquired a clear focus for my observations.

There were other areas in which my increasing cultural knowledge provided a focus for my observations and participation. As I acquired a sense of the typical activities and "rhythms" of the social life of the nursery, I learned that there were certain times (e.g., at night) when fellows and housestaff, as well as nurses, were able to talk informally. I used this knowledge as a basis for structuring my participation in the nursery. Typically, I arrived at noon and ate lunch with nurses or housestaff. Then I accompanied physicians on afternoon rounds, and frequently I stayed for dinner and remained in the nursery late at night, when I worked on my field notes and talked to nurses and housestaff in the conference room. There were some occasions, when a very important decision was being reached, when I spent the night in the nursery so as to be present for informal discussions at night and for early morning rounds. My usual schedule enabled me to be present in the nursery during two or three nursing shifts, and thus to have maximal interaction with nurses and housestaff.

These "cultural maps" (especially those of the decision-making process) were not unlike the "scripts" or "schemas" discussed by psychologists who study information processing.[14] These "maps" enabled me to recognize features of a scene as part of a pattern, guided my perceptions, organized my memory of what I had observed, and structured subsequent interpretations.

Evolving Field Relationships

By the end of my third month in the nursery (and increasingly throughout my stay), there were other indications of perceptible changes in my relationships with interns, residents, and some fellows. Without my having to ask, interns or residents would select patients who might be of interest to me, some taking the time to call me when an important decision occurred. Most took great pains to ensure that I was kept abreast of all the developments in life-and-death decisions and that I knew a conference would be held. Some residents invited me to witness procedures to which outside observers were not usually invited (e.g., cardiac catheterizations, cesarean sections, and other deliveries), while others included me in parties and informal gatherings.

My relationship with the nurses followed a somewhat different trajectory. During my fifth month in the nursery, I significantly modified my research design by beginning to conduct in-depth interviews with nurses (and housestaff) and combining this interviewing with my usual activities as a participant-observer. One of the effects of this interviewing was to introduce dramatic transformations into my relationship with the nurses. Eliciting the views of nurses I had not known could not help changing my relationship with them. Those I had previously known only slightly now became informants, selecting patients of potential interest, introducing me to consultants, notifying me of new developments in decision making, and discussing their views of life-and-death decisions in informal conversation. In addition, there were direct statements through which I evaluated my acceptance. For example, one nurse told me, "I think you have been accepted here as much as any nonmedical person is capable of being accepted." Another nurse stated that I was the only sociologist she had known "who was not a complete nerd."

The interviews were only one factor that introduced changes into my field relationships. Simply remaining in the nursery for a long time, allowing physicians and nurses to become accustomed to my presence, was another. I believe no one was prepared for the sheer amount of time I spent in the nursery or for the enthusiasm with which I approached my task: I did not fit the pattern of the usual "transient." This drew the grudging admiration of the stabler members of the nursery staff, including the attendings. The direct statements and changed demeanor just described demonstrated, in word and deed, that I had become accepted by most, if not all, of the intensive-care nursery staff. These changed relationships were to affect decisions I made as a researcher and the nature and quality of data I was to collect.

The Active Participant
and "Hawthorne Effects"

As I became a more established member of the intensive-care nursery, I moved quite naturally toward more active styles of participation. In the face of altered field relationships, considerations of discretion no longer complicated interactions. I did not hesitate to ask to be included in conferences with parents (when I knew the professional participants), and I interviewed considerably more parents than before. As these barriers of discretion disappeared, I came to adopt a more assertive set of questioning strategies. My newly found knowledge of medical culture enabled me to devise questions to elicit information. For example, when housestaff or fellows seemed to disagree with a decision that had been made, I would ask, "What would you do if this were your private patient?" Once I had come to know staff members, there were few topics I hesitated to bring up or questions I refrained from asking. At the end of my stay in the nursery, I broached even the most sensitive of topics, as can be seen in this excerpt from my field notes:

(When Dr. Stuart, one of the neurology fellows, came into the conference room, I asked him why two babies that I saw as having similar diagnoses were receiving different treatment.)

INTERVIEWER: What puzzles me is that [the two babies] seem to have similar cardiac conditions with a relatively poor prognosis, and, according to you, both have sustained neurologic damage, yet the decision making on the babies has been very different. Is there

some kind of investment in [the baby who has continued
to be supported]?

NEUROLOGY FELLOW: Do you mean, is he an experimental guinea pig?

This incident also illustrates another change in my increasingly
assertive questioning strategies: I occasionally shared my observations
and interpretations with those I knew fairly well and solicited their
opinions. I consciously reached this decision to adopt a more assertive
posture on the basis of both methodological considerations and assumptions about field relationships. Using research subjects to comment on the researcher's interpretations can yield valuable information obtainable through no other means. Direct questions enable the
researcher to explore subjects' perceptions and to clarify points that
remain ambiguous. These questions also serve as a validity check to
determine whether professionals' accounts of their motivations, criteria, and actions are consistent with the researcher's observations and
interpretations. They provide a test of what Schutz called "subjective
adequacy," which may lead the researcher to revise inferences and
interpretations in the light of what has been learned.[15] My interpretations rarely met with any hostility, although staff members sometimes
disagreed with them. Direct questions, however, carry an apparent
danger; and on one occasion, I was startled to learn that one of my
interpretations had evidently made its way through the subterranean
culture of the nursery.

In addition to this conscious decision to assume a more active style
of participation, I also found that my closer involvement with members of the nursery staff drew me into other, more active roles and
modes of participation. Some of these I adopted voluntarily; others I
assumed through no choice of my own; still others I actively resisted.

First, on some days when the nursery was particularly busy and
understaffed, I offered to help out in minor ways, such as answering
the phone and relaying messages. Second, I often served as a con-
fidante and source of support for nurses, housestaff, and parents. I
frequently listened as nurses or residents related the many frustrating
aspects of their work in the nursery and their difficulties in dealing
with other staff members. At the end of my study, I learned that this
role was more than an "observer's category" when the chief resident
told me that "many of the residents really appreciated having you
around to support them through very difficult times." Third, I sometimes provided a convenient "sounding board" (a resident's term) for

housestaff and fellows in the throes of a particularly difficult decision.[16] As they explored their own beliefs and attempted to resolve
dilemmas they confronted, I listened attentively.

Fourth, there were several occasions when social workers, nurses,
house officers, or attendings, knowing that I had access to information
concerning life-and-death decisions, asked me what had taken place
during, for example, a conference they had not been able to attend. I
rarely hesitated to share information that was public, which, I rea-
soned, could easily be obtained from someone else. The fact that I
shared information did not escape the attention of one of the social
workers, who introduced me as "an auxiliary member of the staff who
facilitates communication."

Finally, there were times when I functioned in a capacity not dissimilar to that of a "consultant" in a teaching hospital. Nurses who
were designing their own research protocols asked me for suggestions about topics or research design. As commonly happens to field
researchers, there were times when an attending in the midst of a
very difficult decision asked for my advice. (I attribute this partly to
my professional association with the ethicist who had arranged my
entree into the setting.) I vigorously attempted to avoid giving advice concerning how a life-and-death decision should be made,
pointing out that, as a sociologist, I had no special expertise in resolving ethical dilemmas. This strategy usually proved successful.
However, there was one incident when, as physicians were agoniz-
ing over a decision in rounds, it seemed awkward to the point of
callousness to resist assuming the consultant's role. The incident
also illustrates the authority that researchers' words can assume
when they do give advice.

ATTENDING: If the parents say to us that they don't want us to do anything
extraordinary, that's one thing. But [the cardiology fellow]
talked with the mother last night about catheterization, and she
said, "Do everything possible, whatever you think is necessary." This is a very difficult problem. *(He turns to me.)* Well,
what should we do?

INTERVIEWER: I really don't know. I'm really not an ethicist; I'm just a sociologist.

FELLOW: Well, you've been working with [the ethicist], and that's just as
good.

RESIDENT: I heard that the mother really didn't want us to do anything
aggressive, and that she didn't want a baby that would be
damaged.

(The discussion continued as one of the residents asked the attending whether he would make a series of decisions, such as dialyzing the baby, doing an exchange transfusion, or resuscitating the baby in case of cardiac arrest.)

ATTENDING: I'm trying to distinguish between the things which are simpler and the things which mean the condition is worsening. I certainly wouldn't do anything more with drugs. I just don't have any more drugs to give.

RESIDENT: If the UA [umbilical artery] catheter is in trouble, would you fix it?

ATTENDING: We can't maintain him without it—that's standard care. Now, if he deteriorates on the ventilator and we can't bring him around, then we can quit, but that hasn't happened until now. There's also some question if the renal failure is due to acidosis at birth. . . . *(He pauses for a long time and then turns to me.)* Well, what do you think we should do?

INTERVIEWER: What additional information would you need in order to make a decision? It seems there's some confusion about what the parents think.

ATTENDING: Well, I'll go and talk to the mother on the way home.

The incident points to the problems that may occur when researchers, by dint of conscious decision or subtle persuasion, are impelled to adopt more active roles in the group being studied. The consequences of the researcher's participation have been known to sociologists for several decades, since the early Hawthorne (or Western Electric) studies were conducted: namely, that the researcher, in interacting with members of the group under study, may alter the course of events and produce the very phenomena that he or she purports to describe. When deciding how actively I was to participate in the Randolph Nursery, I weighed the possibly improved field research relationships or additional information that might result from more active participation against the possible "Hawthorne effects" that might ensue. It should be apparent, then, that I would resist giving advice, since my words could (and, in one instance, actually did) intervene in the course of a life-and-death decision.

There are other forms of active participation, however, in which the effects of the researcher's actions on the setting are less discernible and can only be inferred. I assume that many of my actions as a participant-observer had little effect on the actions of staff members. Nevertheless, by "facilitating communication," I was aware that I may have provided participants with information they might not otherwise have acquired (even though the information I actually shared was public and readily available). By adopting more aggressive questioning strategies and sharing information, I knew I risked altering the perceptions of members of the nursery staff. Even my presence in the nursery probably stimulated more discussion of life-and-death decisions, may have caused these decisions to assume more importance in the eyes of those who made them, and may have raised the "ethics consciousness" of staff members. Of course, I cannot substantiate or evaluate the actual consequences of my presence on the nature of the decisions reached in the intensive-care nursery.

"Hawthorne effects" notwithstanding, active participation can yield valuable information that can be secured through no other means. Not only is the researcher exposed to activities and able to explore areas that were heretofore inaccessible, but there is also a more experiential dimension in active participation, for it is a commonplace observation among social psychologists that continuous and close interaction fashions bonds of emotional attachment and commonalities in perspective. I became aware, if only for brief moments, that I shared a common facet of experience with each group of participants in life-and-death decisions with whom I could identify.

Sociologists take great pains to warn field researchers about the ostensible perils of "going native" and to caution them against identifying too closely with research subjects. It is frequently noted that through this identification the researcher may become "co-opted" and be led to abandon a more "objective" and critical perspective.[17] One can, of course, question why a detached stance toward research subjects should necessarily be considered "objective" or free of "bias." But there were a number of factors that I feel prevented this sort of co-option from taking place.

By virtue of my research design, I remained, to the very end, marginal to each group of participants in life-and-death decisions. I was, after all, being exposed to groups of participants who brought very different perceptions, concerns, and systems of relevance to life-and-death decisions. Consequently, my identification with each group varied from moment to moment and situation to situation. While these marginal and situational identifications at times produced profound confusion, they also prevented me from becoming too closely identified with any one group. Moreover, my closer involvement with research subjects was largely confined to the later phases of my stay in the nursery. I was to move on to another setting and to reflect on my research experiences after leaving the field. I was also able to contrast my experiences at various points in the research with my field notes, which served as an indelible record of perceptual shifts. For these reasons, I feel that it is appropriate to regard the closer involvement with research subjects that comes on the wings of active participation not as a source of "bias" to be avoided at all costs but as yet another source of information from which much can be learned.

General Hospital

My four months as a participant-observer in the nursery at General Hospital differed dramatically from my field experiences at Randolph Hospital. I entered the setting having spent a year in another nursery and therefore knowing something about neonatal intensive care. My primary purpose was to undertake a comparative study, and for this reason I knew that my stay would be brief. In addition, I entered the setting through a somewhat different channel. One of the attendings at the Randolph Nursery had suggested that the General Nursery might provide a contrast along the dimensions of size, organizational structure, and patient population. I related this to the ethicist who had arranged my entree into the Randolph Nursery, who in turn contacted the director of the nursery at General Hospital. Shortly thereafter, I had a long phone conversation with the director, who said she was delighted to have someone do the research I had promised.

At the time, the General Nursery was in the process of developing a protocol that outlined a set of procedures for making life-and-death decisions, and the director of the nursery was interested in learning if this protocol was being followed in actual practice, or, in her words, "whether we are actually doing what we think we are doing." The director had outlined a specific task and defined my relationship to the nursery.

From the outset, I entered the setting as an "auxiliary staff member" (a role that I had negotiated at Randolph over a period of months). This role was symbolized by my name tag, which designated me as a "research sociologist." During our initial conversation, the director of the nursery suggested that I attend a faculty meeting at which the official protocol for life-and-death decision making was to be discussed. This meeting gave me the opportunity to meet several members of the attending staff. I then introduced myself to the social worker and the discharge planning nurse, both of whom, I later learned, played key roles in decision making. I also introduced myself at this time to the head nurse, the housestaff, and several other nurses.

My participation at General followed the same outlines as my activities at Randolph, but there were minor differences. I arrived at the nursery in the morning and consulted the social worker or discharge planning nurse to determine whether there were any impending life-and-death decisions. Didactic rounds in the Intensive Care Nursery (in which, I had been told, most life-and-death decisions were discussed) began at 9:30 A.M. and lasted about two hours. After attending rounds, I spent the rest of the day talking informally with residents or nurses, interviewing parents, or observing any decision-making conferences that might take place. In addition, I attended rounds in the other nurseries whenever life-and-death decisions were being discussed.[18] During my third month in the nursery, I began interviewing residents, fellows, and nurses. I also undertook a systematic examination of case records. I did this for two reasons: to examine the notes placed in the charts when decisions were reached and to provide case histories to be used in the interviews.

Almost from the first moment I began my research in the General Nursery, I adopted a more active style of participation, similar to the one I had assumed in the later phases of my stay at Randolph. No sooner had I met the social worker than I asked her to include me in conferences with the parents. I also assumed a more assertive set of questioning strategies, and there were few questions I avoided asking or topics I hesitated to discuss.

My decision to adopt this strategy was guided by three considerations. First, I entered the setting with a larger fund of cultural knowledge, which enabled me to ask more informed questions. Second, knowing that I had less time to spend in this setting, I wished to get maximal information as quickly as possible. A third reason was organizational. The social worker and the discharge planning nurse, who took a special interest in my study and became my informants, occupied pivotal roles in the decision-making process. The discharge planning nurse was aware of all the decisions that were being made and participated in many of them. The social worker was one of the few persons working in the nursery who spoke fluent Spanish (in addition, she was highly respected by the physicians and nurses alike). She knew the families better than either the physicians or the nurses did, and she was included in virtually every conference with the parents, where she functioned in the double capacity of social worker and interpreter for the physician. The conferences, then, had fewer "gatekeepers" than those at Randolph, and once I had come to know the social worker, the conferences were more readily accessible. I also interviewed relatively more of the parents than I did at Randolph (despite the fact that most of the parents were Spanish-speaking and I spoke only broken Spanish). My decision to adopt somewhat different modes of interacting with members of the nursery staff probably contributed to the fact that I seemed to move more quickly into easier field relationships with nurses, residents, and attendings.

Because I had entered the General Nursery through a different path, I was far more knowledgeable about newborn intensive care, I assumed a more active role, and I encountered no resistance from staff members, I was able to collect more data in a much shorter span of time. But any brief stay in a setting has obvious disadvantages. Because the General Nursery was almost three times larger than the nursery at Randolph and because of my limited time in the setting, I decided to concentrate my observations and confine my in-depth interviewing to the newborn intensive-care unit, where most life-and-death decisions were made, although on several occasions I did observe decision-making conferences in the other nurseries. Therefore, I came to know only some of the residents and a few of the nurses who worked in the other nurseries. I rarely observed at night, and hence my interaction was confined to those nurses who worked on the day or afternoon shifts. In general, then, I observed far fewer decisions, developed fewer and less intense field relationships, and relied more on informants than I had at the Randolph Nursery.

Undoubtedly, my knowledge of the organization of the decision-making process remained considerably more superficial than the knowledge I had acquired at Randolph, since it is impossible to compare a four-month field experience with one that spanned a year. Contrasting field research in two settings, then, provides a sort of natural experiment that enables us to identify the actions of the researcher, the features of the organization, and the temporal contingencies that fashion very different field experiences.

The Dialectic of Science and Morality

Before leaving this account of my field research in the General Nursery, I want to return to a set of social decisions to which I have already alluded: those involving ethical considerations. I have already noted that researchers may be drawn *nolens volens* into more active modes of participating in the social life of a group, such as sharing information or giving advice, and that these actions may produce "Hawthorne effects," causing the researcher to intervene in the natural course of activities in the setting. I have also noted that even a mere question or interpretation may have a similar effect, by causing research subjects to attend to what may otherwise have gone unnoticed. At the same time, decisions about participation sometimes pose ethical problems—for by assuming a passive role, evading a question, or withholding information, the researcher may actually harm (or at least fail to help) research subjects, be they parents or professionals, when such assistance is most needed. In these instances, the exigencies of unobtrusive research and the demands of one's own morality are the horns of a difficult dilemma.

How researchers reach uneasy resolutions of these dilemmas depends somewhat on their notions of methodological adequacy, more on their particular research ethics, and most of all on the relative weight they attach to each set of considerations. Whenever I was called on to reach such decisions, I attempted to weigh the possible costs to data that would ensue from active intervention against the possible benefits that active intervention might bring to research subjects—assessments that often proved difficult to make. For example, the social worker in the General Nursery frequently asked me to share information or give my impressions of a family I had interviewed. Answering these questions not only portended possible "Hawthorne effects" but also posed problems of confidentiality, for although several families had released me from a pledge of confidentiality, I had promised it to them nonetheless. I usually resolved this dilemma by answering in very general terms ("They seem to be doing okay" or, occasionally, "Maybe you had better talk to them"), so as to do what I hoped would benefit the families, protect their right to confidentiality, and not dramatically alter the chain of events (since the social worker knew the families well and spoke with them frequently).

There were other types of interactions in which I firmly "drew the line" and which I attempted at almost all costs to avoid, such as giving advice or commenting on the substance of life-and-death decisions. Not only might this directly influence the decision, but I also felt that I would be cast in an expert role for which I possessed no special competence. Moreover, although I felt uneasy about some decisions, I was usually sufficiently ambivalent to at least appreciate both sides of an ethical issue. Shortly after beginning my research, I had devised a rule of thumb: to avoid actions that I thought would intervene in a decision *unless* I felt that my failure to intervene would be very damaging to research subjects or unless I had observed an event that I simply could not countenance. Though somewhat vague, this rule usually served me well. There was, however, one incident (already partly described in Chapter 5) in which I was not able to strike a happy and facile compromise between the canons of unobtrusive research, on the one hand, and my personal beliefs, on the other. Reluctantly and after some deliberation, I tacitly intervened. Here is how I described the incident in my field notes:

> Ramon Martinez, a baby who, according to the consensus of the staff, had made little progress and who who was also grossly malformed, had been in the nursery for over two months. Despite occasional comments about discontinuing therapy, the baby continued to be supported because, although the staff was pessimistic about his prognosis, there was some possibility that he might "have a normal brain." Before I interviewed the parents, the social worker had told me that the father was "repelled" by the baby and visited the nursery rarely, but that the mother seemed concerned about Ramon, attentive, and hopeful about his survival. However, when I interviewed the mother, this did not seem to be the case. During the interview, she expressed concern that the baby might be seriously disabled and severely deformed, frequently asking, "What kind of life will he have?" and seemed anxious about the effect of Ramon's stay in the newborn intensive-care unit upon her six other children. When Mr. Martinez joined us, he expressed the same concern, only with more vehemence and apparent bitterness. At the end of the interview, I was moved to ask them if they objected to my sharing this information with the social worker, and they offered no objections. This posed what I saw as a difficult dilemma for me, for not only was I extremely upset and torn by the family's apparent suffering, but, more important, I was concerned that the social worker had been operating on the basis of misinformation about the mother's feelings. So I said, "Both the parents seemed extremely upset. You might want to talk to them."
>
> The family's situation continued to plague me for several weeks. Both parents stopped visiting the nursery entirely. One day, when I was having lunch with the social worker and the discharge planning nurse, the subject of Ramon Martinez came up. I said, "I'm really worried about the family. You know they haven't been to see Ramon for weeks." The social worker replied, "Well, I think people are taking a much too pessimistic view of the baby." [At that time, several of the nurses had commented that Ramon seemed to be more alert and were a bit more optimistic.]
>
> Two more weeks elapsed, and the discussions in rounds seemed to indicate that Ramon had made little progress. A new group of residents had come to the nursery. One day after rounds, I approached the resident who was taking care of Ramon and said, "I'd like to ask you a question. What is the plan on

the Martinez baby?" At that moment, I knew exactly what I was doing; I was aware that there was no plan and that my question might lead the resident to formulate one. That is exactly what happened; the resident proceeded to say that he and the other residents he knew were appalled that a baby they viewed as having a dismal prognosis had been supported for so long. He resolved to speak with the attending that day.

From that point on, events moved in rapid succession. Conferences were held, specialists were consulted, and, within two weeks, a conference was held with the parents in which it was unanimously decided to discontinue life support on the Martinez baby. The parents, as well as physicians and the nurses, who by that time had viewed the baby quite pessimistically, made the decision with considerable relief. The attending said, "If there has been an error, it was to support this baby too long." The social worker said that the staff of the nursery had "listened to the parent who told us what we wanted to hear." Everyone praised the resident for having made a decision which they viewed as difficult but long overdue. To my knowledge, no one was aware of my part in this decision, and, of course, I cannot *prove* that my words had any influence on the decision making. However, it is my feeling that the decision would have been reached much later had I remained silent.

There is much to be learned sociologically from this incident. These events demonstrate, in a sense, that I had acquired a considerable tacit knowledge of the organization, since I was able to intervene in the chain of events unbeknownst to the participants. The incident also suggests something about the power of the researcher to influence the actions of research subjects and the limitations of that power. My overt attempts to share information with the social worker did little to change her belief or alter her perceptions of the family. But my conversation with the resident was quite another matter, illustrating how great is the power of a "mere" question when it mobilizes a subject's dormant concerns. Few researchers would have acted as I did, for if there is one point of consensus among sociologists concerning field methods, it is this: the sociologist is there to study a social scene and not to change it, so whenever possible, do not interfere. Suffice it to say that there are times when the demands of "science" and those of one's own research morality are at loggerheads.

There are other instances in which researchers are forced into an uneasy synthesis of these conflicting demands. For example, in writing up findings, how much information about the setting should a researcher present when such information threatens to reveal the identity of research subjects? Science, of course, dictates the full disclosure of all sociologically pertinent information, but considerations of confidentiality may dictate a different course. Given the fact that I was

observing decisions whose legal status was ambiguous, I was continually led to balance the importance of an ethnographic detail within my
general argument against the likelihood of violating the confidentiality I had guaranteed. The point is simply that, no matter what the
researcher's decision, the data that are observed and presented to the
reader may be irrevocably transformed by the researcher's actions in
the face of a clash between two different and often conflicting systems
of relevance.

RESEARCH DECISIONS, THE SOCIOLOGY OF KNOWLEDGE, AND THE QUALITY OF DATA

The point of this "ethnography of the ethnographer" has been to
illustrate the central theme of this appendix: that the decisions of the
field researcher may be viewed as a problem in the sociology of
knowledge. I have suggested throughout that the social structure of
the newborn intensive-care unit, and my ever-shifting place in it,
contributed to several significant decisions that I made in the course
of this research, and that these decisions in turn left an indelible
imprint on the data I was to observe, record, and ultimately present
to the reader.

Several consequences of these social and practical decisions on the
nature and quality of the data are apparent. First, I interviewed fewer
parents than would otherwise have been desirable: a total of sixteen,
ten parents in the Randolph Nursery and six in the General Nursery.
Second, the information obtained from informally interviewing the
attendings is not exactly comparable to that acquired through the
more formal interviews with housestaff, nurses, and fellows (although
I believe that through informal interviews and observations over a
long period of time, I was able to obtain a reasonably accurate assessment of the opinions of most attendings). Third, those activities that
were not tape-recorded were subject to unspecified transformation
due to selectivity in perception, memory, and recording. Fourth, those
activities that I did not observe directly were transformed by the
memory and perceptions of my informants. It is, of course, impossible
to delineate precisely the effects of these transformations on the data
I collected.

Another well-known problem in field research concerns the representativeness of the data collected.[19] Because field-workers make
practical decisions concerning what and when to observe that limit

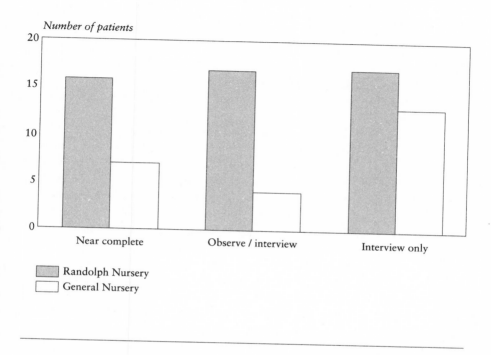

Figure 5. The quality of data collected in Randolph and General nurseries

their ability to investigate certain activities, and because these decisions are based on the contingencies of the moment at hand, they may be guided by ad hoc, rather than representative, sampling. The problem of ad hoc sampling in field research is similar to some of the problems in quota sampling: data may be collected at unrepresentative times and places. Thus, I may have observed only a small and highly unrepresentative fraction of the social life of the nurseries I studied, which may have, in turn, distorted my findings and conclusions. In other words, how representative are my observations of life-and-death decisions in the nurseries I studied?

To obtain an estimate of the quality of the data on which this study is based, I divided the patients in each setting into three groups: (1) those in which I observed all or most of the decision making directly ("near complete"); (2) those in which I collected the data through a combination of direct observation and informant interviews ("observe/interview"); and (3) those in which I studied the decision making only indirectly, through informant interviews ("interview only").[20] The results of this tabulation are presented in Figure 5. Although the quality of data was better in the Randolph Nursery, even in the General Nursery I was able to collect good or reasonable data on a large proportion of patients who were the subjects of life-and-death decisions.

One might ask if there were systematic differences between the "cases" (patients) in which at least some of the data were obtained through direct observation and those cases in which the data were collected through informant interviews. This issue, the question of possible systematic "biases" in sampling, is addressed in the next two figures. Figure 6 asks whether the the kind of decision or the patient's diagnosis affect the quality of data. This graph divides patients in the study population of both nurseries according to the major types of decisions made and examines the quality of data obtained on patients who were the subjects of each kind of decision making. Because my access to the delivery room was limited, I was able to observe relatively fewer resuscitations at birth than other kinds of life-and-death decisions. This limitation notwithstanding, it was possible to study at least one patient who was the subject of each type of decision making through direct observation or through a combination of observation and interviewing.

I also examined the quality of data obtained for patients with several major diagnoses (that is, diagnoses that entered into decision making). As Figure 6 shows, although the quality of data obtained for extremely low-birthweight infants is not as good as those obtained for patients with other diagnoses, it was still possible to obtain good or reasonably accurate data, in which at least some of the decision making was observed directly, for patients in each major diagnostic category. With few exceptions, then, the patients who were followed closely represent a good mix of the major kinds of diagnoses and life-and-death decisions.

There is, however, one significant sampling bias. As Figure 7 suggests, the data concerning the more chronic patients, who were hospitalized for relatively long periods of time, were apt to be complete, whereas the data relating to patients who were hospitalized only briefly were more apt to be collected by means of informant

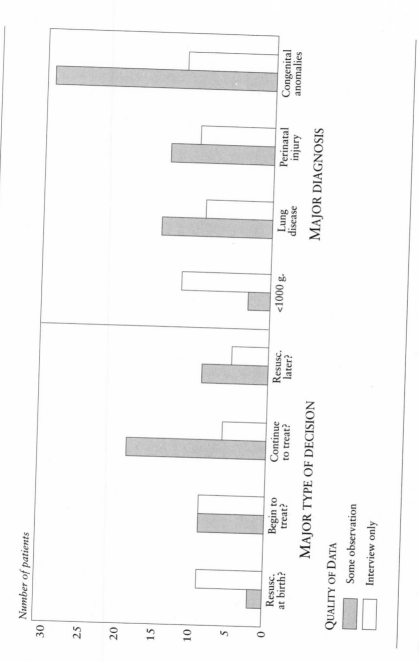

Figure 6. Effect of the decision or diagnosis on the quality of data

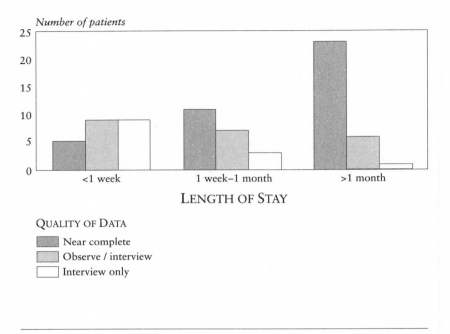

Figure 7. Effect of length of stay on the quality of data

interviews. This is because the shorter the patient's hospitalization, the greater the likelihood that all decision making would take place on a day I was absent from the nursery. Although this pattern may have contributed to a focus on more chronic patients, there are good socio-logical reasons for discussing chronic patients in some detail.

To summarize, largely because of my much longer stay in the Randolph Nursery, the data I collected there were of a substantially higher quality than those I collected at General. Nevertheless, in both settings, there were few "systematic biases" in the data. I was able to collect through direct observation or through observation and inter-viewing data that reflected the major types of decision making, the major diagnostic categories, and the array of decision-making activi-ties in both settings.

Field researchers rarely provide detailed accounts of the many practical decisions reached in the course of their research, and consequently it is often difficult to evaluate the representativeness of the data presented to the reader. This appendix has attempted to speak to this issue. My point is *not* that most field researchers would have reached practical decisions similar to mine. What I *am* suggesting is that all field researchers make decisions guided not only by canons of methodological adequacy but by considerations of politics, pragmatism, ethics, and etiquette. Field research is, then, not only a "scientific" endeavor but a consummately social enterprise. The narrative I have provided is a case study in the sociology of knowledge—only one set of variations on a general theme.

The problems I have addressed stem from the researcher's engagement in the social world. However, practical decisions, ethical dilemmas, and organizational constraints are by no means confined to field research. Rather, they are intrinsic features of any research with human subjects—who, by virtue of their capacity for social interaction, have a way of complicating even the most elegant of research designs. For this reason, methodological adequacy should not be regarded as a goal to be actually attained, but as an elusive vision of a distant desideratum.

Interviewing

During my first few months in the Randolph Nursery, I observed two life-and-death decisions that provoked considerable controversy between the physicians and nurses. After I examined the transcripts of decision-making conferences and informally interviewed physicians and nurses, it appeared that these controversies were not merely idiosyncratic but rather reflected patterned, organizationally rooted differences between the two occupations. In order to go beyond impressions based on observations and informant interviews, I decided to conduct a series of semi-structured, in-depth interviews with fellows, housestaff, and nurses. The goals of the in-depth interviews were (1) to draw more thorough conclusions about the perceptions of staff than could be obtained by observations and informant interviews; (2) to explore in detail the values, beliefs, and modes of prognostic and ethical reasoning participants used in life-and-death decisions; and (3) to pursue theoretical leads and hypotheses that were suggested in the course of observations.

After I conducted pretest interviews, I devised an interview schedule. I conducted interviews with nurses beginning in my sixth month in the nursery and continuing throughout my stay. The following month I began interviewing residents and fellows and continued to interview them throughout my study. Interviewing in the General Nursery followed the same broad outline. I began interviewing nurses and residents in my third month in the nursery, once I had been there

long enough to "collect" cases roughly similar to the ones used in
interviewing the Randolph staff.

I scheduled appointments in advance with respondents. I conducted most interviews with nurses during regular working hours,
although some took place before or after work or occasionally on a
nurse's day off. A nurse who was to be interviewed would usually
request assignment to a patient who was not critically ill (in the
Randolph Nursery). Because I began interviewing residents and fellows after some had already completed their nursery rotations, my
interviews with them followed a somewhat different procedure.
Some interviews took place during house officers' rotations in the
nursery. However, housestaff often preferred to be interviewed during less demanding rotations (e.g., in the clinic). Similarly, I often
interviewed fellows during months when they were away from the
nursery and conducting research, and hence had more flexible
schedules.

Because of the varied and complex exigencies of scheduling, interviews took place in a number of settings: the nursery's conference
room (or any other unoccupied place in the nursery), the head nurse's
office, the examining room of the pediatric clinic, the chief resident's
office, a fellow's office, or, more rarely, the home of a nurse or
resident. The interviews averaged about one hour in length, although
many were considerably longer, and were tape-recorded. Only one
nurse and one fellow refused to have their interviews tape-recorded,
and only two residents declined to answer a question. When promised
confidentiality, nurses, residents, and fellows proved to be exceedingly
enthusiastic, cooperative, and candid respondents.

THE SAMPLE

Table 3 summarizes the design of the samples for nurses, residents,
and fellows in both hospitals. The samples were drawn from a list of
nurses provided by the head nurse in each setting, from a list of
residents provided by the chief resident in Randolph Hospital, and
from a list of residents provided by the director of the General Nursery. There is only one difference in the sampling strategies used in the
two nurseries. I have already mentioned that the General Nursery
is extremely large and is divided administratively into three separate nurseries. Because of my limited time in the General Nursery, I

TABLE 3

SAMPLE DESIGN

Randolph Hospital Nurses

	Total Number	Nonresponse Refusals	Other	Pretest Interviews	Number Interviewed
By Number of Years Worked					
>4	11	0	0	2	6
2–4	11	0	0	2	6
<2	12	0	0	1	6
By Shift					
Day	12	0	0	0	6
P.M.	12	0	0	5	7
Night	10	0	0	0	5
Total	34	0	0	5	18

General Hospital Nurses

	Total Number	Nonresponse Refusals	Other	Pretest Interviews	Number Interviewed
By Number of Years Worked					
>4	8	0	0	0	4
2–4	6	0	0	0	4
<2	3	1	0	0	1
By Shift					
Day	6	0	0	0	4
P.M.	5	0	0	0	2
Night	6	1	0	0	3
Total	17	1	0	0	9
Total, Both Hospitals	51	1	0	5	27

Randolph Hospital Residents and Fellows[a]

Year of Residency	Total Number	Nonresponse Refusals[b]	Others	Total	Pretest	Number Interviewed
Residents						
1	11	1	1	2	0	9
2	5	0	1	1	0	5
3	5	1	0	1	2	4

TABLE 3 *(CONTINUED)*

		Randolph Hospital Residents and Fellows[a]				
Year of Residency	Total Number	Nonresponse Refusals[b]	Others	Total	Pretest	Number Interviewed
Total (Residents)	21	2	2	4	2	17
Fellows[c]	4	0	1	1	0	3
Total (Residents and Fellows)	25	2	3	5	2	20

		General Hospital Residents and Fellows[d]				
Residents						
2[e]	6	0	1	1	0	5
3	4	0	1	1	0	3
Total (Residents)	10	0	2	2	0	8
Fellows[c]	5	0	1	1	0	4
Total (Residents and Fellows)	15	0	3	3	0	12
Total Residents, Both Hospitals	31	2	4	6	2	25
Total Fellows, Both Hospitals	9	0	2	2	0	7
Total Fellows and Residents, Both Hospitals	40	2	6	8	2	32

[a] Attempts were made to interview the total population of residents who rotated through Randolph Hospital during the first six months of the study.

[b] Includes respondents who had left the nursery or were otherwise unavailable while the study was conducted.

[c] Fellows in both hospitals include neonatology fellows who served rotations in the nursery while the study was conducted.

[d] Attempts were made to interview the total population of residents who rotated through the nursery while the study was conducted.

[e] Only second- and third-year residents were interviewed since no first-year residents rotated through the intensive care nursery at General Hospital.

restricted my interviewing to the residents and nurses in the Intensive Care Nursery, where most of the critically ill babies were to be found (and hence most of the life-and-death decisions included in the interview schedule). The nurses in the Intensive Care Nursery, who are registered nurses, are more comparable in terms of background and training to the Randolph nurses than are those in the other General nurseries, many of whom are licensed vocational nurses and nursing assistants. Moreover, the residents in the Intensive Care Nursery also rotated through the other nurseries and were able to provide firsthand accounts of decisions that had occurred outside the Intensive Care Nursery.

In both hospitals, I interviewed a random sample of nurses, stratified by shift and by number of years they had worked in the nursery (Table 3). I adopted this sample design because observations, informal interviews, and pretest interviews in the Randolph Nursery had suggested that nurses' perceptions of patients change over time, and therefore there might be patterned differences in the perceptions of very experienced, relatively experienced, and less experienced nurses, as well as differences by shift. I designed the sample to include half the nurses in each nursery, although the sampling rates within each stratum departed somewhat from this figure. Only one nurse refused to be interviewed, stating that she was "too busy." Altogether, I interviewed a total of twenty-seven, or slightly over half of the fifty-one nurses, in both hospitals.

Table 3 also summarizes the sample design for residents and fellows. I attempted to interview all the residents who rotated through the Randolph Nursery during my first six months there (and all the decisions included in the interview schedule took place during this period). Two residents had left the nursery by the time I conducted the interviews, and two residents refused to be interviewed, one stating that she was "too busy," and the other stating that he "found death and dying very upsetting and prefer[red] not to deal with it." This resulted in an overall response of seventeen out of twenty-one. Similarly, I attempted to interview all the residents who rotated through the Intensive Care Nursery at General Hospital during a three-month period. Because two were unavailable when I conducted the study, I interviewed eight out of ten residents. I interviewed all but two of the nine fellows in both hospitals. I interviewed a total of thirty-two residents and fellows in both hospitals. Thus, I interviewed a total of fifty-eight nurses, residents, and fellows in both nurseries.

INTERVIEW SCHEDULES
AND QUESTIONING STRATEGIES

I developed the interview schedules after pretesting. Although there are slight variations in the design of schedules for nurses, residents, and fellows, the questions followed the same general format: (1) questions designed to elicit respondents' demographic characteristics and professional backgrounds; (2) questions relating to respondents' experiences in the newborn intensive-care unit, including their views of patients, families, and the decision-making process; (3) a series of questions relating to seven patients in each nursery who were the subjects of life-and-death decisions; and (4) a final question in which I asked respondents to provide recommendations for improving the decision-making process.

The interviews consisted of a series of open-ended questions followed by probes. To ensure a certain degree of comparability, I tried to use identical wording when posing the questions and varied the order in which I asked questions only infrequently. I framed the questions so as to encourage respondents to formulate their concerns in their own vocabularies, with a minimum of semantic structuring on my part. By using this semi-structured interview format, I tried to strike a balance between reliability, or providing comparable questions, and validity, or allowing respondents to answer freely, so as to express their actual perceptions.

The most important part of the interview consisted of those questions designed to elicit respondents' views of the decision making concerning seven actual patients in each nursery. I selected these cases according to specific criteria, which are summarized in Tables 4 and 5. I selected the first two cases because staff members in each nursery had perceived them as important, controversial, and highly problematic. I selected the other cases because they corresponded roughly to the prognostic categories used in a survey conducted by Crane.[1] In Crane's study, subjects responded to questions concerning hypothetical cases in four prognostic categories (a salvageable infant with physical damage, a salvageable infant with mental damage, an unsalvageable infant with physical damage, and an unsalvageable infant with mental damage). I found actual patients in each nursery who roughly corresponded to three of Crane's four prognostic categories. There were two reasons for attempting to "replicate" Crane's design as closely as possible. First, the cases she used represent those types of

TABLE 4

DESIGN OF INTERVIEW SCHEDULE, RANDOLPH NURSERY

Case number/Condition	Prognosis		Family			Other issues	Corresponding cases[a]	
	Salvageable?	Intellectual or physical damage	Attitude	Social status	Other		Crane	General
1. Birth defect: chronic lung disease	Uncertain	Uncertain, possible intellectual	Low	—	—	Cost, effect on family	—	—
2. Congenital anomaly: arteriovenous malformation in vein of Galen	Uncertain	Uncertain, possible brain damage indicated by seizure	—	Low	8 other children	Innovative procedure	—	—
3. Congenital anomaly: Down syndrome	Yes	Mental retardation, colostomy after repair of imperforate anus	Low	High	—	—	3A	3
4. Congenital anomaly: Rubinstein-Taybi syndrome	Yes	Mental retardation, corrrectable heart defect	High	Low	Young mother, unmarried	—	3B	4
5. Congenital anomaly: myelomeningocele	Yes	Severe physical damage; brain damage unlikely	Low	—	—	—	2B	5
6. Birth defect: very small premature	Uncertain[b]	Uncertain, possible brain damage	—	—	—	—	—	—
7. Congenital anomaly: trisomy 18	No	Severe mental retardation, short life span	—	—	—	—	1A	7

[a]Parts of this chart have been adapted from Crane (1975: 214–216).
[b]Baby lived but had enlarged ventricle

TABLE 5
DESIGN OF INTERVIEW SCHEDULE, GENERAL NURSERY

Case number/ Condition	Prognosis		Family			Other issues	Corresponding cases	
	Salvageable?	Intellectual or physical damage	Attitude	Social Status	Other		Crane	Randolph
1. Congenital anomaly: central nuclear myopathy (neuromuscular disorder)	No	Severe physical damage, limited lifespan, but normal intellectual function	High	Low	—	Unusual diagnosis	—	—
2. Hydrops fetalis, multiple congenital anomalies	Uncertain	Severe deformities; intellectual function said to be normal until shortly before death	Low	Low	—	Unusual diagnosis	—	—
3. Congenital anomaly: Down syndrome	Yes	Mental retardation and colostomy after repair of imperforate anus	?	Low	39-year-old mother with 14 previous pregnancies	Family situation[a]	3	3
4. Same as table 4, case 4 (hypothetical case taken from Randolph Nursery)								
5. Congenital anomaly: myelomeningocele	Yes	Severe physical damage; brain damage unlikely	Low	—	—	—	2B	5
6. Birth defect: very small premature infant	Uncertain	Uncertain; possible brain damage	—	—	—	—	—	6
7. Congenital anomaly: trisomy 18	No	Severe mental retardation, short life span	—	—	—	—	1A	7[b]

[a] Family situation not comparable to Randolph
[b] More complicated clinical course than case no. 7 at Randolph

patients discussed most frequently in the medical and ethical literature concerning life-and-death decisions in neonatal intensive care. Second, by comparing responses to the hypothetical cases in Crane's study to responses to the actual cases used in this study, we can learn something about decision making in the face of actual or hypothetical dilemmas.

It is, of course, impossible to force the real world to conform to the dictates of an experimental design. Given my very brief stay in the General Nursery, I could not find patients who were identical to those used in the Randolph interviews. The patient with Down syndrome in the General Nursery was hospitalized three months prior to the beginning of my stay in the nursery, and since there are virtually no middle-class families in the General Nursery, the family's social situation differed from that of the patient's family in the Randolph Nursery. The patient at General with trisomy 18 had a slightly more complicated clinical course than did her counterpart in the Randolph Nursery. And despite my repeated requests to physicians and nurses in the General Nursery, they were unable to "produce" a patient even remotely comparable in terms of prognostic and social features to the patient with Rubinstein-Taybi syndrome. Consequently, I used a hypothetical case description with respondents at General. Despite these inevitable compromises with reliability, most cases used in the interview schedules of the two nurseries were roughly comparable, so I could compare responses to similar cases in the two nurseries and approximate the features of a quasi-experimental design.

I began each question concerning the actual cases by reading the patient's name to respondents and then asking them what they knew about the case and how they felt about it. This very open-ended lead question allowed respondents to frame the problems in each case in their own terms and to describe the information base from which they judged the decision making. When respondents were unfamiliar or only vaguely familiar with a particular patient (as was often the case with residents, who served only brief rotations in the nursery), I read a prepared case history that described the patient's clinical course and social situation. These open-ended questions were followed by a series of probes, which were designed (1) to elicit "native categories"; (2) to explore respondents' reasoning processes; and (3) to explore the relative importance attached to certain criteria by posing hypothetical situations.

As I noted in Appendix 1, there were a number of practical problems involved in interviewing the parents, which made it necessary to design three separate schedules. These were (1) a longer interview schedule, to be used when there was sufficient time to interview parents who were in the nursery; (2) a shorter interview schedule, to be used when there was little time to interview parents as a life-and-death decision was being made; and (3) a retrospective interview, to be used when I interviewed parents at home, after their babies had left the nursery or died.

Notes

CHAPTER 1

1. The first estimate appears in Jonsen (1976). The second estimate, given by Budetti et al. (1980), may have varied in subsequent years due to changes in the number of neonatal intensive-care units and fluctuations in the birthrate.

2. Budetti et al. (1980); Budetti and McManus (1982).

3. Jonsen (1976); Jonsen and Lister (1978a).

4. Tooley and Phibbs (1976); Budetti et al. (1980:3).

5. A number of methodological issues suggest the need for caution in interpreting data concerning the effectiveness of neonatal intensive care. Studies of mortality have been criticized on several grounds: Hack et al. (1981) report that 14 percent of the deaths of infants in Cleveland were postponed to the postneonatal period. This suggests that studies of mortality trends that report neonatal deaths in the first twenty-eight days may be biased in an optimistic direction. According to Kitchen and Murton (1985), variations of reporting mortality among infants 501–1000g. may affect the results. Studies vary according to whether they include deaths in the delivery room and neonatal deaths resulting from life-and-death decisions. Together these causes of death account for 29 percent of the deaths in their series, and studies that exclude deaths from these causes will be biased in an optimistic direction. Survival rates differ according to how the weight range is defined: studies that include infants from 501 to 1000g. report higher survival rates than do studies that include infants from 500 to 999g. (Kitchen and Murton, 1985). Researchers have criticized reviews of morbidity based on follow-up studies of individual nurseries, such as Budetti et al. (1980), Stewart, Reynolds, and Lipscomb (1981), and Stewart (1989), on several grounds. Data on the effectiveness of neonatal intensive care have been criticized for the paucity of randomized, controlled clinical trials (Budetti et al., 1980; Sinclair

et al., 1981). Factors affecting the referral of infants to intensive-care nurseries could alter the results (Institute of Medicine, 1985). For example, tertiary-care centers receiving only those infants considered to have a sufficiently favorable prognosis to warrant referral to an intensive-care nursery would be biased in a positive direction (Stewart, 1989). Morbidity (and mortality) data from individual nurseries may vary because units serve populations with differing characteristics (Chalmers and Mutch, 1981; Kiely and Paneth, 1981; Strong, 1983; Kitchen and Murton, 1985). Follow-up studies of the outcome of infants < 1000g. rely upon very small samples (Anspach, 1982; Stewart, 1989). Individual nurseries vary in their policies on the resuscitation of the smallest and most premature infants, and data from those tertiary-care centers that resuscitate the smallest infants may be biased in a negative direction (Stewart, 1989). Follow-up data from different time periods may not be comparable because of changes in technology. By the time follow-up data, particularly concerning the very smallest infants, are published, the infants in those series may have received what are considered outmoded treatments (Anspach, 1982; Strong, 1983; Kitchen and Murton, 1985). Studies vary according to how they operationalize the dependent variable. For example, studies that define "severe impairment" as a developmental quotient (DQ) of less than 80 will have more favorable results than studies that define "severe impairment" as a DQ of less than 70 (Strong, 1983; Stewart, 1989). Finally, studies vary according to the age at which infants are tested, and early testing can miss minor handicaps (Strong, 1983).

6. A variety of evidence supports the contribution of neonatal intensive care to the dramatic reduction in mortality among low-birthweight infants that occurred from 1965 to the early 1980s (Lee et al., 1980; McCormick, 1985). Articles that present and review different types of evidence include Institute of Medicine (1985), McCormick (1985), and Rudolph and Borker (1987). The summary presented here is based on a synthesis of the evidence presented and reviewed in these articles as well as several articles I reviewed independently. Studies employing a variety of research strategies suggest that neonatal intensive care has contributed to a reduction in mortality among premature and low-birthweight infants: (1) Articles based on pooled data from individual nurseries show that mortality has declined dramatically among infants receiving neonatal intensive care from 1965 to 1980 (Budetti et al., 1980; Stewart, Reynolds, and Lipscomb, 1981; Budetti and McManus, 1982; Stewart, 1989). (2) According to birthweight-adjusted mortality analyses, this decline is not due to changes in the birthweight distribution (Budetti and McManus, 1982). Dramatic declines in neonatal mortality occurred while the proportion of low-birthweight infants declined only modestly (Lee et al., 1980; Williams and Chen, 1982). (3) Low-birthweight infants born in hospitals having intensive-care nurseries experience lower mortality and have higher survival rates than infants born in hospitals that do not have neonatal intensive care (Gortmaker et al., 1982; Paneth, Kiely, Wallenstein, et al., 1982; Mayfield et al., 1990; for reviews of this evidence, see Institute of Medicine, 1985; McCormick, 1985; Paneth, 1990). (4) This enhanced survival rate obtains even in comparisons

involving infants transported to regional intensive-care nurseries shortly after birth (Mondanlou, 1980; Paneth, Kiely, Wallenstein, et al., 1982; Ferrara, Schwartz, and Page, 1988). (5) The introduction of NICU's into geographically defined areas has been followed by a decrease in infant mortality for those areas (Usher, 1981; Horwood et al., 1982). (6) Decreases in neonatal mortality in geographically defined regions accompany an increase in the proportion of low-birthweight and very low-birthweight births occurring in nurseries that are tertiary-care centers (McCormick and Shapiro, 1984; McCormick, Shapiro, and Starfield, 1985; Robert Wood Johnson Foundation, 1985). Some qualifications and caveats must be added, however. First, mortality rates for normal-birthweight infants have also been declining (McCormick, 1985). Second, other factors have influenced mortality among premature and low-birthweight infants. Third, since neonatal intensive care seems to offer no advantage for full-term, normal-weight infants, this technology provides only a small marginal benefit to the majority of infants (Paneth et al., 1987; Mayfield et al., 1990; Paneth, 1990).

7. For general discussions of extremely low-birthweight infants—that is, for those < 1000g.—see, for example, Britton, Fitzhardinge, and Ashby (1981); Strong (1983); Stahlman (1984); Walker et al. (1984); Kitchen and Murton (1985); McCormick (1985); Hack and Fanaroff (1986). Infants < 1000g. still have mortality and morbidity rates significantly higher than those of infants of other weight categories (Budetti and McManus, 1982; Paneth et al., 1982; McCormick, 1985; Walker, Vohr, and Oh, 1985). Stewart (1989) reviewed twenty-six outcome studies undertaken in a variety of intensive-care nurseries between 1965 and 1980 for infants < 1000g. She found that during the fifteen-year period, infant mortality fell among the extremely low-birthweight infants. The proportion of able-bodied survivors increased, but the proportion of disabled infants remained constant. Mortality in nurseries for these infants ranged from 33 to 88 percent, with a mean of 64 percent. The proportion of disabled survivors ranged from 2 to 15 percent, with a mean of 7.21 percent. Stewart acknowledged that, since the proportion of disabled survivors remained constant, there was an increase in the absolute number of disabled infants. A close examination of her data concerning infants < 800g. reveals that these infants fared much worse than did the larger extremely low-birthweight infants. In a total of eleven series, the proportion of disabled survivors ranged from 5 to 18 percent, with an average of 7.72 percent of all those born, or 23 percent of all survivors. The relatively high morbidity of infants < 800g. has led many observers to question whether these infants should be treated (e.g., Hack and Fanaroff, 1986).

8. Budetti and McManus (1982); Gustaitis and Young (1986).

9. Klaus and Kennell (1976); Silverman (1979).

10. Wertz and Wertz (1979).

11. Reviewing the outcome of infants < 1000g. admitted to Rhode Island Hospital, Walker et al. (1984) found that the care of those infants was not cost-effective. However, using different economic indicators in a larger community survey, Walker, Vohr, and Oh (1985) found newborn intensive care to

be marginally cost-effective. But care of the very smallest infants was not cost-effective even in this second study.

12. For a discussion of this issue, see Strong (1983). Kirkley (1980) and Schechner (1980) are physicians who have strongly advocated not resuscitating the smallest infants. See a discussion by Singer (1987) of the policies of nurseries in Australia, one of which explicitly does not treat infants < 800g.

13. For accounts of physicians, see, for example, Duff and Campbell (1973); Shaw (1973); for journalists, Lyon (1985); Gustaitis and Young (1986); for ethicists, Weir (1983) (the contributions of ethicists to decision making concerning newborns is discussed in greater detail in Chapter 2); for social scientists, Frohock (1986); Guillemin and Holmstrom (1986) (these studies are *total ethnographies* of neonatal intensive care that treat life-and-death decisions as part of a more general discussion).

14. Calabresi and Bobbitt (1978).

15. Books by legal scholars, journalists, and social scientists include Horan and Delahoyde (1982); Manney and Blattner (1984); Lyon (1985); Frohock (1986); Guillemin and Holmstrom (1986); Gustaitis and Young (1986). Works on the ethics of intensive care include Weir (1983); Shelp (1986). The work of other ethicists is discussed in subsequent chapters. An exhaustive treatment of legal positions is found in Weir (1983).

16. See, for example, Robertson (1975a; 1975b; 1977; 1986); Robertson and Fost (1976); MacMillan (1978).

17. Frader (1985).

18. Examples of surveys conducted during the 1970s include Crane (1975); Shaw, Randolph, and Manard (1977); and Todres, Krane, and Howell (1977). Surveys from the 1980s include Guillemin et al. (1989); Levin (1989).

19. Duff and Campbell (1973); Shaw (1973); Koop reports his policies in Schaeffer and Koop (1979).

20. See, for example, Glantz and Swazey (1979) on the Houle case and Weir (1983) on the Mueller case.

21. Several ethical analyses were written in response to the Baby Doe regulations. Paris and Fletcher (1983) comment critically on the absolute requirement to use nourishment and fluids. Arras (1984) criticizes the ethics of the Infant Doe directives and the President's Commission's "best interests" standard and argues in favor of a standard based on relational potential. Huefner (1986) suggests that the government's response is ethically inadequate and argues in favor of a government policy that uses strengths of Kantian, utilitarian, and Rawlsian ethical systems and reflects the pragmatism of American society. Zaner (1987) outlines the prospects and barriers to ethically relevant research into decisions concerning imperiled infants and embryos. Moreno (1987) provides an excellent ethical and legal analysis of major legal cases concerning newborns, including a discussion of the Baby Doe cases. Churchill and Siman (1986) argue against indiscriminate use of ethical principles in the case of Baby Jane Doe. Cohen (1987) provides an excellent summary of both the ethical and legal arguments concerning the Baby Doe and other legal cases involving disabled infants. Mahowald (1984; 1986) reviews the Baby

Doe developments and argues for an ethic based on the principle of beneficence and the infant's best interest. She suggests that at times it may be in the infant's best interest to die. Wakefield-Fisher (1987) reviews the ethics of the Baby Doe cases. Weir (1983) argues that the Baby Doe regulations present an oversimplified view of decision making. He cautions that physicians may be persuaded to practice defensive medicine in order to save their careers, and he favors a best-interest standard and a decision-making process based on a serial ordering of proxies.

Legal commentaries on the Baby Doe cases and their sequelae include the following. Bopp and Balch (1985) and Bopp (1985), legal activists for the pro-life and disability rights movements, provide comments favorable to government intervention. Haddon (1985) argues in favor of parental authority in life-and-death decisions and against governmental efforts to restrict that authority. Born (1986–87) provides an excellent summary of the background to and the impact of the Child Abuse Amendments. Elkins and Brown (1986) provide an optimistic summary of the clinical and social prospects for infants with Down syndrome and examine the legal issues in the light of the case of Infant John Doe. Rosenblum and Grant (1986) is a summary and discussion of developments after the Baby Doe cases, written from a pro-life standpoint. Shapiro and Barthel (1986) provide an excellent analysis of the Baby Doe regulations and the Child Abuse Amendments, outline potential strengths and weaknesses of infant care review committees, review the experience of a Wisconsin ICRC, and offer what they view as an improved model statue for the Child Abuse Amendments.

22. For a discussion of the role of the state in the Baby Doe controversies, see Reiser (1986).

23. The list of writings concerning the Baby Doe controversies is endless. A number of good accounts of the developments around the Baby Doe cases are Fost (1982); Punch and Simler (1982); Annas (1983a; 1983b; 1984); Wallis (1983); Cimons (1984a; 1984b); Smith (1984); Lyon (1985); Murray (1985a); Rhoden and Arras (1985); Schmeck (1985); Todres (1985); Baker (1986); Bermel (1986); Brahams (1986); Gardell (1986); Holden (1986); Malcolm (1986); Moskop and Saldanha (1986); Stevenson et al. (1986); Taylor (1986a; 1986b); Winslade and Ross (1986); Elias and Annas (1987); Lantos (1987); Moss (1987); York, Gallarno, and York (1990). Discussions of the case of Baby Jane Doe include Gallo (1984) and Levin (1984), as well as Brown (1986), Klaidman and Beauchamp (1986), and Paige and Karnofsky (1986), the last three of which come out of the conference that resulted in the Baby Jane Doe papers. The Baby Doe regulations are to be found in U.S. Department of Health and Human Services (1982; 1983; 1986). The following are some published statements by organizations and persons active in the Baby Doe debates: The Committee on the Legal and Ethical Aspects of Health Care for Children (1983), established early in 1983 by the American Society of Law and Medicine, is highly critical of the proposed "Infant Doe" regulations because they lack concrete clinical guidelines for decision making and have potential negative effects on medical decisions and on the doctor-patient relationship. The com-

mittee endorses the recommendations of the President's Commission (1983). Marcia Angell's (1983) editorial in the *New England Journal of Medicine* typifies the medical profession's highly negative reaction to the proposed regulations. She offers six criticisms: (1) they were issued by an administration that claims to be opposed to government regulation and has shown little regard for the welfare of children in other contexts; (2) they were proposed in the face of considerable expert opposition; (3) they are based on the faulty premise that all life should be supported; (4) they argue that decisions concerning the patient's well-being are outside the authority of the medical profession; (5) they give insufficient attention to parents; and (6) they imply that infants need protection from parents and physicians, when "it is difficult to imagine people who are *less* malicious or indifferent than parents and physicians" (p. 660). Prior to the Supreme Court decisions on the Baby Doe rules, Angell again criticized the regulations for mandating life-sustaining treatment for all newborns irrespective of their quality of life or the views of physicians and parents. She argues, first, that the Baby Doe rules would deny to infants the same rights accorded to incompetent adults—to refuse treatment through surrogates; second, that fear of legal reprisals could inappropriately influence decisions; and third, that decisions should be made by parents and physicians on a case-by-case basis rather than by the government. Three letters to the editor criticize Angell's arguments against the regulations; Angell responds to her critics; and James Strain, chair of the American Academy of Pediatrics, argues that the proposed Child Abuse Amendments, which place authority with the states, are less intrusive (all in Calvert et al., 1986). Carol Berseth (1983), a neonatologist, is highly critical of the Baby Doe ruling because "it inserts an unwelcomed participant into the doctor-patient relationship," undermines "the integrity of the family unit," places ethical decisions "in the hands of one or several minor bureaucrats," and mandates treatments that could cause suffering to parents, staff, and infants (pp. 428–29). She endorses the recommendations of the American Academy of Pediatrics and the President's Commission. William B. Weil (1986), chair of the Bioethics Committee of the American Academy of Pediatrics, discusses the federal Child Abuse and Neglect Amendments of 1984 and raises some critical issues, such as the deleterious effects of fiscal cutbacks on children and whether adult patients also deserve protection.

24. The point about the less-well-publicized dilemmas is made by the President's Commission in its 1983 report. The point about overtreatment is made forcefully by Guillemin and Holmstrom (1986).

25. See, for example, Levin (1985; 1988; 1989); Guillemin and Holmstrom (1986); Rostain (1986).

26. See, for example, Hastings Center (1987) for a discussion of recent nursery policies. I began this fieldwork before the Baby Doe controversies. Throughout the book, I note those decisions that would probably have been made differently following the 1985 federal regulations.

27. See Crane (1975); Shaw, Randolph, and Manard (1977); Todres, Krane, and Howell (1977); Guillemin et al. (1989); Levin (1989).

28. Frankena (1965).

29. Kanter (1977); Freidson (1970).

30. See, for example, McKinlay (1986).

31. Frohock (1986); Guillemin and Holmstrom (1986).

CHAPTER 2

1. Concerning normative ethics, see Frankena (1965). Concerning deontological ethics, see Frankena (1965); Lyon (1985). For definitions of bioethics, see Bok (1977); Jonsen and Hellegers (1977); Ramsey (1977). A good history of bioethics is provided by Jonsen, Jameton, and Lynch (1978).

2. This is meant as a cursory overview of bioethics. Readers wishing more detailed discussions should consult Weir (1984) and Shelp (1986).

3. Jakobovits (1978: 28).

4. Ramsey's only possible exceptions are Lesch Nyhan syndrome, an incurable defect marked by self-mutilation, and very small premature infants, whom he views as receiving experimental treatment (Ramsey, 1978). Arguments about treating and caring for infants are provided in Ramsey (1976; 1978).

5. Koop (1977; 1982: 91).

6. Other advocates of this position include Zachary (1968; 1977); Jakobovits (1978); Kluge (1978; 1980); Sherlock (1979; 1986; 1987); Andrusko (1985); Tiefel (1985). An excellent anthology of pro-life ethical positions is Horan and Delahoyde (1982).

7. Alexander (1949); Schaeffer and Koop (1979).

8. For Singer's ethical writings, see Singer (1975; 1979; 1985); Singer, Kuhse, and Singer (1983); Kuhse and Singer (1985; 1986); and Singer and Kuhse (1988).

9. See Shelp (1986) for an excellent exposition of personhood as a moral concept. Concerning the prerequisites of personhood, see Tooley (1979); Warren (1977); Engelhardt (1973; 1975a; 1975b; 1976; 1986); Singer (1979); Singer and Kuhse (1988).

10. See Shelp (1986) for personhood arguments. Others might disagree. See Warren (1977); Engelhardt (1973).

11. Steinbock (1986) provides an excellent summary and critique of personhood arguments. The quote is from Weir (1984: 181). Steinbock (1986) makes the point about the kidnapper. Concerning the lack of moral equivalence of abortion and infanticide, see John Fletcher (1975). According to Warren (1977), the term *potentiality principle* was first proposed by Michael Tooley. See Kluge (1978; 1980) for statements of this position.

12. Lorber (1975: 300, 52). These criteria include the degree of paralysis, head circumference, curvatures of the spine, serious paralysis, gross congenital anomalies, and a large lesion in the thoracolumbar area (Lorber, 1971, 1975). Lorber (1971; 1972; 1973; 1974; 1978a; 1978b).

13. Zachary (1977); Veatch (1977); Lorber (1975: 52).

14. Campbell and Duff (1979b: 141).

15. Shaw (1977a; 1988).

16. Ramsey (1978: 225). Ramsey does permit quality-of-life judgments by competent patients. Gustafson (1973), for example, disputes the broad definition. On the ambiguity of the arguments, see Smith (1974); Weir (1984).

17. For a statement of this position, see McCormick (1974). McCormick

(1978) also argues that there is no inherent contradiction between the sanctity-of-life and the quality-of-life positions.

18. See Murray (1985b) and Engelhardt (1975a; 1975b) for arguments based on the infant's pain and suffering. Jonsen and Garland (1976a; 1976b) formulated their policy at the Sonoma Conference on the Ethics of Newborn Intensive Care sponsored by the Health Policy Program and the Department of Pediatrics at the University of California, San Francisco. The quote is taken from Jonsen and Garland (1976b: 148). Summaries of the Sonoma conference are found in Culliton (1975). See also Jonsen et al. (1977).

19. Engelhardt (1973), who first used the principle of nonmalificence, allows for nontreatment decisions based on the interests of others, but those who use this principle later exclude the interests of others from consideration. Fost (1983); President's Commission (1983); Weir (1984). For an interdisciplinary endorsement of the best-interest standard, see the Committee on the Legal and Ethical Aspects of Health Care for Children (1983), established early in 1983 by the American Society of Law and Medicine. See also Strain (1983) for an endorsement by the American Academy of Pediatrics.

20. For the criticism concerning its vagueness by Bartholome and a reply by Brody, see Brody and Bartholome (1988). For other criticisms of the best-interest standard, see Arras (1984; 1985). For the position that the interests of society should be considered, see Jones (1984). For the position that the family has legitimate interests and the neonatologist has obligations toward the family, see Strong (1984).

21. Perhaps the most forceful arguments for this position are provided by Fost (1981; 1983). See also Zachary (1977). Strong (1983) summarizes objections to making the parents the principal decision makers.

22. For arguments against medical paternalism, see Shaw (1973; 1977b; 1978; 1988); Duff and Campbell (1976; 1980); Duff (1978a; 1978b; 1979; 1981; 1987); Campbell and Duff (1979a). Shelp (1986) argues that parents should make the decision in a pluralistic society.

23. President's Commission (1983). For an interdisciplinary endorsement of this position, see the Committee on the Legal and Ethical Aspects of Health Care for Children (1983). See also Strain (1983) for an endorsement by the American Academy of Pediatrics. For discussions of ethics committees in practice, see Michaels and Oliver (1986); Fleishman (1987).

24. For discussions of this issue, see Bopp (1985); Bopp and Balch (1985).

25. The debate between ethicists Michael Bayle and Daniel Callahan over the proper role of the state in life-and-death decisions is summarized in Steinfels (1978).

26. Jonsen and Lister (1978b) first raised this issue, but others have raised it subsequently, including Anspach (1982) and Shapiro and Frader (1986).

27. New discussions of the uncertainty problem are in Fischer and Stevenson (1987) and the Hastings Center (1987).

28. On professionals' control of information flow, see West (1983); Mishler (1985); Fisher (1988). Glaser and Strauss (1965) discuss terminally ill patients, Quint (1972), breast cancer patients, Davis (1963; 1972), polio patients, and

Svarstad and Lipton (1976); Lipton and Svarstad (1977), parents of mentally retarded children. For a discussion of the issue of selective information processing and beliefs, see Cicourel (1983).

29. See, for example, Rosenwaike (1971); Budetti and McManus (1982); McCormick (1985).

30. Luker (1984).

31. For a discussion of nursing ethics, see Creighton (1974).

32. Kanter (1977) also argues for this role of organizations.

33. See, for example, Cicourel (1981).

34. See Durkheim's discussion of the collective conscience in Durkheim (1938; 1964).

35. Parsons (1951: 466–77).

36. Scheff (1968; 1972).

37. Fox and Swazey (1974).

38. Fox (1974).

39. Crane (1975).

40. McKilligan's study is described in Hastings Center (1987); other surveys were conducted by Shaw, Randolph, and Manard (1977); Todres, Krane, and Howell (1977).

41. Levin (1989); Guillemin et al. (1989).

42. Kopelman, Irons, and Kopelman (1988).

43. Examples of her research are Levin (1985; 1988; 1989). It could be argued that some of the other studies of decision making, such as Crane (1975), do actually consider how respondents assess both treatments and prognoses, since they ask physicians to choose between levels of treatment.

44. Roth (1963).

45. Glaser and Strauss (1965); Sudnow (1967).

46. Guillemin and Holmstrom (1986).

47. Rostain (1986).

48. For the notion of "thick description," see Geertz (1983).

49. Examples of the sociology of knowledge include Mannheim (1936); Marx and Engels (1947); Schutz (1962; 1967); Berger and Luckmann (1967); Smith (1987; 1990).

50. For a discussion of occupational and organizational treatments of the sociology of knowledge, see Bittner (1967); Freidson (1970); Smith (1987; 1990).

51. Freidson (1970).

52. The term *advisory bureaucracies* is taken from Goss (1961). For a discussion of the autonomy of occupational groups, see Freidson (1970).

53. See Giddens (1984).

CHAPTER 3

1. For discussions of the social and economic effects of long-term cases on parents and professionals, see Anspach (1982: 247–58, 332–88); Guillemin and Holmstrom (1986: 113, 160, 165, 198–225). For discussions of the Karen Ann

Quinlan case, see, for example, Branson and Casebeer (1976); Capron (1976); Levine (1976); Oden (1976); Ramsey (1976).

2. See, for example, Cicourel (1981).

3. For discussions of the issue of prognostic perplexity, see Hemphill and Freeman (1978); Jonsen and Lister (1978b); Anspach (1982: 252–55); Guillemin and Holmstrom (1986: 122–23, 125–30). For discussions of the experimental nature of neonatal intensive care, see Anspach (1982: 252–55); Guillemin and Holmstrom (1986: 97–98, 127, 274).

4. See Chapter 1, notes 6 and 11 for discussions of the morbidity, mortality, and resuscitation of infants < 1000g.

5. For a more detailed discussion of methodological difficulties in the use of follow-up data, see Chapter 1, note 5. For other discussions of difficulties in using follow-up data, see Anspach (1982: 15–17, 253); Guillemin and Holmstrom (1986: 129). Guillemin and Holmstrom (1986: 129) note that nurseries rarely invest heavily in follow-up of their patients and rarely communicate the findings of follow-up studies to staff members. In contrast to these observations, the nurseries I studied, particularly Randolph, placed considerable emphasis on their follow-up studies. Randolph attendings often communicated follow-up findings to residents and nurseries. However, they did so selectively and strategically, usually to support arguments they were making in favor of aggressive intervention.

6. Anspach (1982: 256, 332–87) observes that nurses were often the first to reach pessimistic conclusions about infants' prognoses. Guillemin and Holmstrom (1986: 119–21) corroborate this observation when they note that nurses are usually less committed than physicians to aggressive intervention.

7. Anspach (1982) and Guillemin and Holmstrom (1986) also discuss the work patterns of attendings, residents, and nurses. Anspach (1982: 107, 270–77) and Guillemin and Holmstrom (1986: 29–36, 59, 193–94) discuss residents' limited, short-term, and technically focused contact with patients. Anspach (1982: 278–82, 408–10) and Guillemin and Holmstrom (1986: 46, 55, 56, 59, 173) discuss nurses' continuous contact and social interaction with their patients.

8. For a discussion of typifications, see Schutz (1962). For a discussion of "normal crimes," see Sudnow (1967).

9. Anspach (1982: 266) and Guillemin and Holmstrom (1986: 132, 189–90) discuss the narrow, technical orientation of the nursery staff. I can offer three possible explanations for this difference between the two nurseries observed in this study. First is the very small size of the General sample. Second, the General nurses who were interviewed worked in the intensive portion of the nursery, where the babies are more critically ill, generally more premature, more apt to be given paralyzing drugs, and hence more limited in their capacity to interact. A third reason is organizational. In the General Nursery and in the Randolph "high-intensive" nursery, the very availability of sophisticated monitoring equipment may inhibit the nurses from using other types of information. This interpretation was suggested by one Randolph nurse, who contrasted the types of information she used in the various rooms of the nursery in the following way:

In the intensive room, you're going to see a lot of direct, specific changes. You're going to see the blood pressure dropping down because the kid has a line—an arterial line, usually. They're always on monitors, they're usually intubated [on respirators], so you're drawing blood gases, so you're going to see a lot of specific laboratory data, clinical data that you will know all of a sudden. When you get into [room] 1509, they're all on monitors. But they don't have arterial lines in there, so you have less and less distinct laboratory data to go on, so you go a lot on your observations and what you hear . . . , but you don't have as much information as you do in the other room. And in the other room, 1511, usually they just have peripheral lines for antibiotics, so that you would notice things like feeding. So if a baby starts nippling really poorly and starts looking real pale, and he starts kind of not being real active like he used to, then you kind of think there's some problem there. I think that sometimes you might go a little more on your gut feeling there than you would in the other rooms.

10. For a discussion of the attribution of humanhood to patients, see Anspach (1982: 288–90). Guillemin and Holmstrom (1986: 135–37) also observe that members of the nursery staff frequently "personify" infants.

11. Although numerous studies argue that women are socialized to have an interpersonal orientation, perhaps the best-known argument was made by Carol Gilligan (1982), who suggested that women display a distinct moral reasoning that is oriented to social relationships.

12. For discussions of physicians' tendency to discount the clinical and medical judgments of nurses, see Anspach (1982: 352, 400); Guillemin and Holmstrom (1986: 59, 62, 64).

13. Because some of the interviews concerning Robin Simpson were several pages long, I was obliged to edit some of the responses, including those portions of the interviews that related to Robin's prognosis and the respondents' views of the decisions that were made. When a response has been edited, I have attempted to indicate the gist of the comments I left out. When a portion of a response has been deleted, I have noted this with an ellipsis (. . .). When I was unable to hear a portion of a quotation, I have marked this with a dash (———). These responses to my questions are predictions rendered in retrospect. When confronted with a patient who has already died, it is all too easy to claim one has "known all along" that the patient would never recover. However, memory and retrospective judgment cannot account for the conflicting perspectives on recovery and the different types of knowledge mentioned by the physicians and nurses.

14. Those residents who were critical of or ambivalent toward the decisions that were made (four of the nineteen residents and fellows interviewed) evaluated the decisions in terms of the ethical principles they felt were at issue—for example, the distinction between active and passive euthanasia, or, most commonly, considerations of utility. Their objections were principled rather than prognostic—that is, the salient issue was not Robin's prospects for recovery but the resources expended on her care. Only two residents claimed to have been reasonably certain that Robin's prognosis was poor. By far the largest group of residents and fellows (eleven) said there was insufficient evidence to conclude with reasonable certainty that Robin would not recover. According to most of these physicians (nine), an earlier decision to discontinue treatment would not have been right.

15. The majority of nurses who were interviewed (thirteen) assumed a critical attitude toward some of the decisions that had been made. Some expressed the view that decisions should have been made sooner; others felt that Robin had been treated too aggressively at early points in her clinical course. The nurses' criticisms were based partly on ethical considerations: cost (four), the stress placed on the parents (six), and the parents' lack of involvement in Robin's care (four). However, the most significant issue for these nurses was prognostic. They were considerably more pessimistic than the residents about Robin's neurological status (eight), her psychological integrity (four), and her chances for recovery (nine).

16. For discussions of physicians' disengagement from the consequences of their decisions and their structural disengagement from patients, see Anspach (1982: 409–12); Guillemin and Holmstrom (1986: 190). Anspach (1982: 409–10) observes that nurses are reluctant to care for infants who fail to improve and pose management problems. Guillemin and Holmstrom (1986: 60, 65) make a related point about nurses' problems caring for cases that were difficult and hopeless.

17. See, for example, Reiser (1978).

18. See, for example, President's Commission (1983).

19. This discussion is largely based on Cicourel's (1981) analysis of how larger "macro" conceptions of disease are created by—and also influence—the interaction between patients and physicians in bureaucratic settings. Cicourel notes that the highly schematic information recorded into the physician's progress notes provides the basis for epidemiological findings, which the physician later uses in making a diagnosis and structuring the interaction with the patient. I am proposing a parallel between Cicourel's notion of discourse and interactive cues, which are seldom recorded in patients' charts (which he refers to as "textual summaries"), and hence cannot be validated as prognostic signs (which he calls "larger notions of disease").

20. Hunt (1976).

21. The Apgar score is based on the infant's heart rate, respiratory effort, muscle tone, reflex irritability, and color. Four of the five components of the Apgar score are what I have called "perceptual" (observational) cues.

22. Korones (1976: 55).

23. Foucault (1975).

24. Reiser (1978).

25. Mannheim (1936).

CHAPTER 4

1. Anspach (1982: 412–13) notes that parents are often peripheral to life-and-death decisions. Guillemin and Holmstrom (1986: 169–97) also discuss this issue in detail. See particularly their discussion of how parents are consulted only after the staff has reached a life-and-death decision (Guillemin and Holmstrom, 1986: 192–93), a pattern I also observed in the Randolph and General nurseries. Since, as I discuss in Appendix 1, my access to parents and to conferences between staff and parents was limited, the quality of data presented in Chapters 4 and 5 is not as good as in Chapter 3. However, because

the parents are extremely important actors in life-and-death decisions, I have chosen to discuss them despite limitations in my data. When I was forced to rely upon informants' accounts, I always attempted to obtain at least two, and usually three, accounts.

2. For a summary of arguments about the parents, see Watchko (1983). For a discussion of medical indications policies, see Ramsey (1976; 1978), who originated the concept, and Koop (1977; 1982). For examples of the argument that parents should have the final authority, see Duff and Campbell (1973); Shaw (1973); Shelp (1986).

3. Advocates of limiting parents' roles include Veatch (1977; 1978); President's Commission (1983); Penticuff (1988). Fost (1981) argues that an inherent conflict of interest exists between parents and their baby.

4. For a discussion of bonding, see Klaus and Kennell (1976; 1982).

5. Parsons (1951).

6. For discussion of this issue, see Guillemin and Holmstrom (1986: 134–35).

7. Guillemin and Holmstrom (1986: 187) note that staff paternalistically attempted to protect parents from guilt, and this resulted in two consequences in the nurseries they studied: either presenting the parents with the decision that treatment should be stopped (included in what I call an "assent model") or treating a baby aggressively (a consequence I did not observe in the nurseries I studied).

8. Guillemin and Holmstrom (1986: 66).

9. Rapp (1989: 28–33).

10. Because of the Baby Doe regulations, physicians today may feel obliged to treat this baby.

11. Beeson and Golbus (1979); Beeson (1984); Katz-Rothman (1986). The term *artificial womb* was suggested in an article by Newman (1988).

12. This was the position taken by Beeson (1984); Michaelson (1988).

13. For a discussion of burnout in nursery professionals, see Marshall and Kasman (1982); Marshall, Kasman, and Cape (1982).

14. Hynan (1987: 43).

15. For a discussion of this pattern of "coping through distance," see Newman (1980).

16. Reiser (1978).

17. These transformations are discussed by Reiser (1978); Starr (1982); Freidson (1970).

18. For a discussion of the transiency of the housestaff, see Freidson (1970). Also see Guillemin and Holmstrom (1986: 193–94).

19. Hobbs, Perrin, and Ireys (1985: 86).

20. For a discussion of conflicts between research, teaching, and patient care, see Duff and Hollingshead (1968); Ehrenreich and Ehrenreich (1970); Guillemin and Holmstrom (1986); Guillemin (1988).

21. Wolinsky (1988: 267–69) characterized this pattern as a pyramid. I am grateful to Sydney Halpern for pointing out this parallel.

22. Ehrenreich and English (1979). Abbott (1988: 119).

23. This pattern was also noted by Guillemin and Holmstrom (1986: 55, 56, 173).

24. For a discussion of the issue of second hand information, see Phelby (1982). For a discussion of such forms of collective behavior as rumor generation, see Cicourel (1976).

25. For a discussion of the issue of the barriers between parents and staff created by regionalization, see Guillemin and Holmstrom (1986); Guillemin (1988).

26. For a slightly different discussion of this issue, see Guillemin and Holmstrom (1986: 194), who note that parents of long-term patients were forced to change physicians several times.

27. Guillemin and Holmstrom (1986: 195).

28. For a discussion of hasty judgments made by other staff members, see Bogdan, Brown, and Foster (1982).

29. Benfield, Leib, and Vollman (1978) discuss this absence of psychological harm to parents. Janis and Mann (1977).

30. For a discussion of infant care review committees, see Fleishman (1985; 1987). For criticisms, see Hastings Center (1987).

CHAPTER 5

1. Duff and Hollingshead (1968); Duff and Campbell (1973: 894).

2. For example, see Diamond (1973).

3. Robertson (1975a; 1975b; 1977); Robertson and Fost (1976). For an example of the use of civil statutes, see Shelp (1986). There have been two cases in which criminal prosecution was narrowly averted. One involved an infant with osteogenesis imperfecta (a genetic defect involving multiple bone deformities) who was, according to an account in the popular press, fed intravenous glucose solution rather than infant formula necessary to sustain her life. Nurses reported the case to a New Mexico district attorney, and a criminal investigation ended only when a conflict of interest was perceived in the district attorney's office (Parrish, 1980). Another case, also publicized in the popular press, involved seriously malformed Siamese twins in Danville, Illinois, who could not be separated surgically. The infants were reportedly not resuscitated at birth and were later ordered not to be fed (a practice seen as questionable in some nurseries). Nurses nevertheless gave the twins intravenous glucose solution, and an anonymous report to the legal authorities led to an investigation in which the parents and the obstetrician who had delivered the babies were charged with attempted murder. The charges were dropped for lack of evidence when the nurses refused to link the physicians with the orders not to feed the babies, but civil litigation awarded temporary custody of the boys to the state, and the twins were returned to their parents three months later (Clark, 1981; Weir, 1984); Duff and Campbell (1976; 1980); Shaw (1977b; 1978; 1988); Duff (1978a; 1978b; 1979, 1981; 1987); Campbell and Duff (1979a; 1979b).

4. For a discussion of this issue, see Anspach (1982); Starr (1982).

5. The following are examples of the principal routes by which a decision can enter the legal system: (1) Parents or professionals turn to the courts or the juvenile authorities when they disagree about a life-and-death decision, as in *Maine Medical Center v. Houle* (1974), in which the attending physician and

the pediatric surgeon initiated a neglect case in superior court when the father refused surgery for an infant with multiple physical deformities. (2) Other staff may disagree with the decision and turn to the courts, as when nurses reported a case in which an infant with osteogenesis imperfecta was not given formula to a New Mexico district attorney (Parrish, 1980). (3) Political groups may learn of a case and appeal to authorities. For example, in the Robinson case, in which a baby with spina bifida was not treated, a report by an anonymous nurse to the Family Life League led the Department of Children and Family Services to conduct an investigation (Weir, 1984).

6. For examples of other nurseries, see Guillemin and Holmstrom (1986: 121–22); Rostain (1986).

7. For a discussion of the issue of the undermining of trust, see Millman (1977).

8. For a demonstration of this point, see West (1979).

9. For examples of other nurseries, see Guillemin and Holmstrom (1986).

10. For a discussion of the issue of class, language, and culture conflicts, see Clausen (1985). The phrase "coping through distance" was suggested by Newman (1980). The central contribution of her formulation is to depict withdrawal from the nursery as a coping strategy rather than as a pathological phenomenon, as is suggested by the phrase "disruption of bonding" (Klaus and Kennell, 1976; 1978; 1982).

11. Guillemin and Holmstrom (1986: 177–78) also report that professional parents are likely to come into conflict with members of the nursery staff.

12. The nursery's bias toward aggressive intervention is discussed thoroughly and brilliantly in Guillemin and Holmstrom (1986: 111–42).

13. Stinson and Stinson (1983). Also see Stinson and Stinson (1979).

14. The pattern of the psychologistic framework has been noted by many observers of neonatal units, such as Bogdan, Brown, and Foster (1982); Sosnowitz (1984); Guillemin and Holmstrom (1986); Guillemin (1988). On bonding, see Klaus and Kennell (1976; 1978; 1982); on impairment of bonding, see Giblin, Poland, Waller, and Ager (1988). For a review of the evidence on the effect of bonding on parenting, see McCormick (1985). For examples of criticisms on methodological grounds, see Leventhal (1981); Richards (1989). For an excellent summary of these issues, see McCormick (1985). Concerning liberalized visiting, see Frader (1986).

15. For psychological discussions of parents' reactions to the birth of premature infants, see Solnit and Stark (1961); Drotar et al. (1975); Benfield, Leib, and Reuter (1976); Cramer (1976); Irving, Kennell, and Klaus (1976); Rothstein (1980); Cohen (1982); Richards (1989).

16. Concerning the stage model, see Hobbs, Perrin, and Ireys (1985). For a discussion of guilt, see, for example, Kaplan and Mason (1977).

17. Guillemin and Holmstrom (1986: 175–76, 196–97); Guillemin (1988).

18. Gliedman and Roth (1980: 143–47).

19. For a published statement of this position, see Pemberton (1981).

20. Hochschild (1983).

21. For a discussion of institutional schemata, see Smith (1987). The psychologizing I observed in the Randolph and General nurseries differs somewhat from that observed by Guillemin and Holmstrom (1986: 178), who note:

244 Notes to Pages 145–161

The golden mean of parental behavior is revealed in the typology of difficult parents as articulated by the n.i.c.u. staff during the time of our fieldwork. Parents who broke down emotionally at each visit revealed parental incompetence. Parents who were enthusiastic about their ability to handle a critically ill newborn did not understand the gravity of the situation. Parents, for example, Jehovah's Witnesses, who rejected certain clinical procedures were unreasonable. Parents who demanded more intervention, for example, ligation of patent ductus arteriosus in a baby in total failure, were also unreasonable. Parents who showed no emotion at bedside had psychological problems. Parents who expressed anger or frustration or despair also had psychological problems. Educated parents thought they knew everything; conversely, high-school dropouts were incapable of understanding medical information.

If I interpret this passage correctly, it implies that large numbers of parents whose behavior deviated slightly from an elusive "golden mean" were perceived as deviant and that "appropriate" affect and behavior were beyond the reach of most parents. In the nurseries I studied, many parents were in fact viewed as "appropriate" or "adequate." Parents were encouraged to express virtually all emotions, with the exception of anger, toward the staff. Parents were viewed as "inappropriate" if they failed to "bond" with their babies, if they failed to express sadness when their babies died, or if they challenged staff. In short, not all or even most parents were viewed as having psychological problems, and the interesting question becomes: under what social conditions are negative psychological attributions called into play?

22. See West (1983).

23. For a discussion of what I call "decontextualization," see Smith (1990: 120), who refers to this phenomenon in the context of instructions for perceiving a person as mentally ill.

24. Guillemin and Holmstrom (1986: 196–97) make a parallel point when they note that psychologizing obscures the nursery's own role in producing parents' emotional reactions.

25. Hochschild (1983) first introduced the concept of emotion management, or performing work on one's own emotions. She does make reference to "emotion managers," but she uses the term in the sense of those who manage their own emotions. I am using the term to denote people whose role is to manage the emotions of *others*.

As noted in Chapter 4, the decision to perform the routine surgery may have been made differently today in the wake of the many changes that followed the Baby Doe controversies. Had the decision been made in 1991, it is entirely possible that the staff would not have provided Ms. Sandoval with the option of withholding relatively minor heart surgery from a baby with a prognosis of moderate to severe mental retardation. However, this case dramatically illustrates a social fact that remains true in today's nurseries: staff psychologize when parents reach decisions at odds with those of professionals.

26. For a discussion of morality disjunctures, see Pollner (1987). For a discussion of neutralization, see Sykes and Matza (1957); Millman (1977).

27. For a discussion of reality disjunctures, see Pollner (1987).

28. Universalism, or not giving patients differential treatment because of their status, is one of Parsons's (1951) patterned variables and is, according to Parsons, one of the normative foundations of professional conduct.

29. Abbott (1988).

30. This point is discussed by Haug (1973); Starr (1982). Unlike Haug, who views this loss of legitimacy as a sign of "deprofessionalization," Freidson, in his epilogue to the second edition of *Profession of Medicine* (1970), and Starr (1982) argue that medicine will retain some degree of professional status. However, most observers of contemporary health care agree that the legitimacy of medicine eroded over the past decade.

31. The concept of emotion rules or feeling rules is taken from Hochschild (1983).

CHAPTER 6

1. Calabresi and Bobbitt (1978: 21).

2. President's Commission (1983); Strain (1983); Murray (1985a: 5); Fleishman (1987).

3. For examples of varying receptions, see Lo and Jonsen (1981); Weir (1983); Frader (1985); Gustaitis and Young (1986).

4. For a discussion of this individualization, see Anspach (1989a); Fox and Swazey (1984).

5. Institute of Medicine (1985: 16–17, 213–33).

6. Sinclair et al. (1981).

7. Calabresi and Bobbitt (1978); Childress (1985: 280).

8. Gustaitis and Young (1986: 214).

9. Institute of Medicine (1985: 4–16).

10. Guillemin and Holmstrom (1986); Gustaitis and Young (1986).

11. Institute of Medicine (1985).

12. Other commentators include Guillemin and Holmstrom (1986); Gustaitis and Young (1986).

13. The national estimate is taken from Budetti et al. (1980). Estimates of the cost of neonatal intensive care vary widely. Studies also vary in how they compute the costs of neonatal intensive care. Budetti et al.'s (1980) estimate of the total costs of neonatal intensive care is based largely on data collected earlier by Phibbs, Williams, and Phibbs (1981). According to the Institute of Medicine (1985), Budetti and his colleagues probably underestimated the costs of Level II and Level III nurseries, and for this reason subsequent studies have produced higher estimates.

Schroeder, Showstack, and Roberts (1978) compared expenditures among patients with high-cost hospitalization.

The following is a selective review of the average cost per patient in a number of studies, adjusted to 1990 dollars. This review excludes studies in other countries that did not present exchange rates to U.S. dollars, including: John, Lee, and Li's (1983) Australian study; and Britton, Fitzhardinge, and Ashby's (1981) Canadian study of infants <801g. The Institute of Medicine (1985) notes that adjustments for inflation, such as those presented in the following table, do not reflect changes in medical technology that would raise the cost of some types of medical care. For this reason, these are probably low estimates:

Source	Average Total Cost/Patient for Birthweights (1990 Dollars):			
	All	*<1500g.*	*1000–1499g.*	*<1000g.*
Shroeder, Showstack, and Roberts (1978)	36,400			
Phibbs, Williams, and Phibbs (1981)	14,686 (n=1185) 16,533/ survivor	30,365		36,848 84,339/ survivor
Boyle et al. (1983)[c,d]		22,311 (n=265)	23,287 (n=167) 94,971/ survivor	21,707 (n=98) 163,605/ survivor
Walker, Vohr, and Oh (1985)[a,b]		24,642/ survivor, 1974–75 24,276/ survivor, 1979–80	20,804/ survivor, 1974–75 19,860/ survivor, 1979–80	58,028/ survivor 1974–75 54,474/ survivor, 1979–80
Pomerance et al. (1978)[b,e]				44,874 (n=75) 112,187/ survivor
McCarthy et al. (1979)[a,b,d]				50,328/ survivor
Walker et al. (1984)[a]				112,389/ survivor (n=150)

Explanations of charge computations:
a. Costs = charges
b. Excludes physicians' fees
c. Cost = unit price of service × quantity + physicians' fees + convalescent care
d. Cost includes transport
e. Cost = collected charges @ 94% collection rate

14. Budetti and McManus (1982); Stahlman (1984). But see Chapter 1, note 5, for a discussion of methodological difficulties with data concerning the effectiveness of neonatal intensive care.

15. Budetti and McManus (1982); Levin (1985); Starfield (1985); Rudolph and Borker (1987).

16. A controversial issue is the morbidity-mortality relationship—namely, is the decrease in infant mortality accompanied by an increase in morbidity?

The relationship between neonatal intensive care and morbidity has been given differing interpretations. Two major review articles draw relatively optimistic conclusions from a variety of evidence (Institute of Medicine, 1985; McCormick, 1985). McCormick (1985: 88) summarizes recent trends as follows:

> Recent reviews of outcomes among survivors of neonatal intensive care have documented decreases over time in the proportion of infants with adverse outcomes (Budetti et al., 1980; Stewart, Reynolds, and Lipscomb, 1981). Such reviews must be interpreted cautiously, however, since there is wide variation in the proportion of survivors with adverse outcomes as reported by different studies, and selection factors affecting referral to intensive-care units may affect the results. More recent data based on clinical series (Hack, Fanaroff, and Merkatz, 1979; McCormick, 1981) and population-based morbidity surveys (Shapiro et al., 1983; McCormick, Shapiro, and Starfield, 1985) indicate that the increased survival of low birthweight infants has not been accompanied by an increase in the number with handicaps: the proportion of less severely handicapped survivors has declined, while the proportion of severely handicapped survivors has remained the same. . . . However, concerns remain about the effect of increased survival of the smallest infants (those weighing less than 1000g.) (Phibbs, Williams, and Phibbs, 1981).

Other authors raise qualifications that lend themselves to conflicting interpretations. Some community surveys note an increase in the proportion of affected infants among survivors (Kitchen, Yu, Orgill, et al., 1983), mortality with no change in the proportion of handicap among very-low-birthweight infants (Stanley and Atkinson, 1981; Horwood et al., 1982). Most researchers acknowledge that, particularly among the smallest infants, the absolute number of infants with neurologic handicaps must be rising (Budetti et al., 1980; Chalmers and Mutch, 1981, 1984; Stewart, 1989). This pattern occurs whether, as Budetti et al. (1980) note, mortality is declining faster than morbidity or, as others have reported, morbidity has remained stable (Chalmers and Mutch, 1981, 1984; Stewart, 1989). Although it contradicts their conclusions, this pattern is also consistent with Shapiro et al.'s (1983) finding that the number of infants with severe handicaps has remained the same and that mortality is decreasing faster than morbidity. This pattern has led some to question the claim that investment in neonatal intensive care is cost-effective (Chalmers and Mutch, 1981, 1984). Authors who draw critical conclusions (Chalmers and Mutch, 1981, 1984) cite speculations that this phenomenon may be responsible for the overall increase in cerebral palsy (Paneth et al., 1981) and cite data from Scandinavian countries attributing a rise in cerebral palsy to neonatal intensive care (Hagberg, Hagberg, and Olow, 1984).

17. Rosenwaike (1971); Osofsky and Kendall (1977); Schwartz and Schwartz (1977); McCormick (1985).

18. Duff and Campbell (1973); Koop (1982).

19. Schaeffer and Koop (1979).

20. For a discussion of the Baby Doe case, see, for example, Murray (1985a); Moskop and Saldanha (1986). For a discussion of the impact of the 1984 amendments on contemporary nurseries, see Kolata (1991).

21. Lyon (1985: 258–74).

22. Rudolph and Borker (1987: 7).

23. For example, see Kluge (1978).

24. Koop (1982: 103–4).

25. For discussions of infanticide, see, for example, Langer (1972); Pierzs (1978); Williamson (1978); Darbyshire (1985).

26. Hunt (1966: 159). For a discussion of this issue, see Anspach (1979).

27. For a discussion of this issue, see Gliedman and Roth (1980); Asch (1984); Asch and Fine (1988); Fine and Asch (1988).

28. Fost (1983: 224).

29. Guillemin and Holmstrom (1986).

APPENDIX 1

1. In calling attention to the many practical decisions involved in field research, I by no means intend to suggest that research decisions in survey research are made according to exclusively scientific criteria. Indeed, survey research entails its own set of practical decisions, but a detailed discussion of these is beyond the scope of this appendix. For such a discussion, see Cicourel (1964).

2. For a detailed discussion of these differences, see Frankena (1965).

3. For a discussion of role choice, see Gold (1958). For discussions of entree into research settings, see articles in McCall and Simmons (1969). For a discussion of field relationships, see, for example, Schwartz and Schwartz (1955). Problems of recording data are discussed by McCall (1969).

4. Becker (1958). For discussions of analytic induction, see Manning (1971); Katz (1983). The classic formulation of grounded theory is Glaser and Strauss (1965). Also see, for example, Charmaz (1983). Given the extremely complex interaction between (1) the reading that a researcher has done before undertaking a study and in the course of the research, (2) emerging theoretical concerns, (3) developing cultural knowledge, and (4) the recognition of patterns in observations, it is questionable whether the actual reasoning processes used in any field research study do or even can approximate the ideals of either the hypothetico-deductive model or analytic induction.

5. A fine example of a reflexive approach is provided by Emerson (1983), particularly in his commentary throughout the volume.

6. Cicourel (1964) provides perhaps the earliest and most cogent statement of this issue.

7. This phrase is adapted from a quotation by Kaufmann (1941) as presented in Cicourel (1964).

8. For an example of this approach, see Cicourel (1976).

9. For several reasons, I feel that my initial encounters with the nursery were not unlike those of parents. Those who write about social aspects of neonatal intensive care commonly note that parents sometimes withdraw from the nursery (see Klaus and Kennell, 1976, 1978). Several parents I interviewed expressed their fears of "getting in the way" in the nursery.

Two sociologists who had studied newborn intensive care related similar experiences. One complained that she did not know what to do when she was in the unit. Another, who had studied the same nursery in which I did research, found that she could not get integrated into the unit, and she left after a few months. The experience of profound alienation is by no means unique to sociologists who study newborn intensive care. Bosk (1979: 211), who studied a surgical service, notes, "I know that there were days when I had to force myself to go to the hospital, and other days when I grabbed at any straw as an excuse for a breather."

10. Simmel (1965: 321).

11. Simmel (1965: 320).

12. Cicourel (1964: 100).

13. See McCall (1969: 128–41).

14. For discussions of schemata, see, for example, Rumelhart (1977); Weisberg (1980: 53–59).

15. Schutz (1962; 1967).

16. See Bosk (1979).

17. For example, see Freidson (1970); Millman (1977).

18. The General Nursery was divided administratively into three smaller nurseries: the Intensive Care Nursery, where most of the very critically ill babies were to be found; the Acute Care Nursery; and the Convalescent Care Nursery. The Intensive Care Nursery had a separate attending, residents, and nurses.

19. For a discussion of this issue, see Katz (1983).

20. My unit of analysis is the patient rather than the decision because it is very difficult to define the boundaries of a single decision other than by fiat. If a decision regarding discontinuing treatment was discussed on three occasions, it is impossible to determine whether this is one or three decisions. It was not my intent to collect data concerning every patient in the intensive-care nursery, but rather to study only those patients who were the subjects of life-and-death decisions. I defined a life-and-death situation as one in which the life or death of a patient was verbally discussed and explicitly determined by staff members. This operational definition, like any definition, has its limitations. For example, I did not observe those situations in which the decision making, if it may be characterized as such, was extremely tacit and not verbalized, such as a decision to cease all efforts at resuscitating a baby (one can presumably continue indefinitely) who has not responded and is considered "irreversibly dead." For a discussion of these decisions, see Sudnow (1967).

APPENDIX 2

1. Crane (1975).

Bibliography

Abbott, Andrew.
  1988.   *The system of professions.* Chicago: University of Chicago Press.
Alden, E. R., et al.
  1972.   Morbidity and mortality of infants weighing less than 1000g. in an intensive care nursery. *Pediatrics* 50: 40.
Alexander, Leo.
  1949.   Medical science under dictatorship. *New England Journal of Medicine* 241: 39–47.
Andrusko, Dave.
  1985.   Abortions and infanticide: America's movement away from human rights. *Lincoln Review* 5 (3): 31–39.
Angell, Marcia.
  1983.   Handicapped children: Baby Doe and Uncle Sam. *New England Journal of Medicine* 309 (11): 659–61.
Angell, Marcia.
  1986.   The Baby Doe rules. *New England Journal of Medicine* 10: 642–44.
Annas, George J.
  1983a.   Disconnecting the Baby Doe hotline. *Hastings Center Report* 13 (June): 14–16.
Annas, George J.
  1983b.   Baby Doe redux: Doctors as child abusers. *Hastings Center Report* 13 (October): 26–27.
Annas, George J.
  1984.   The Baby Doe regulations: Governmental intervention in neonatal rescue medicine. *American Journal of Public Health* 74: 618–20.

Annas, George J.
1984–85.   Refusal of lifesaving treatment for minors. *Journal of Family Law* 23: 217–40.

Anspach, Renée R.
1979.   From stigma to identity politics: Political activism among the disabled and former mental patients. *Social Science and Medicine* 13A: 765–73.

Anspach, Renée R.
1982.   Life-and-death decisions in neonatal intensive care: A study in the sociology of knowledge. Ph.D. diss., University of California, San Diego.

Anspach, Renée R.
1987.   Prognostic conflict in life-and-death decisions: The organization as an ecology of knowledge. *Journal of Health and Social Behavior* 28 (3): 215–31.

Anspach, Renée R.
1988.   Notes on the sociology of medical discourse: The language of case presentation. *Journal of Health and Social Behavior* 29 (4): 357–75.

Anspach, Renée R.
1989a.   From principles to practice: Life-and-death decisions in the intensive care nursery. In *New approaches to human reproduction: Social and ethical dimensions,* edited by Linda M. Whiteford and Marilyn L. Poland. Boulder, Colo.: Westview.

Anspach, Renée R.
1989b.   Life-and-death decisions and the sociology of knowledge: The case of neonatal intensive care. In *New approaches to human reproduction: Social and ethical dimensions,* edited by Linda M. Whiteford and Marilyn L. Poland. Boulder, Colo.: Westview.

Areen, Judith.
1987.   Deciding the care of infants with poor prognosis. *Seminars in Perinatology* 1 (3): 254–56.

Arras, John D.
1984.   Toward an ethic of ambiguity. *Hastings Center Report* 14 (April): 25–32.

Arras, John D.
1985.   Ethical principles for the care of imperiled newborns: Toward an ethic of ambiguity. In *Which babies shall live? Humanistic dimensions of the care of imperiled newborns,* edited by Thomas H. Murray and Arthur L. Caplan. Clifton, N.J.: Humana Press.

Asch, Adrienne.
1984.   The experience of disability: Challenge for psychology. *American Psychologist* 39: 529–36.

Asch, Adrienne, and Michelle Fine.
1988.   Shared dreams: A left perspective on disability rights and repro-

ductive rights. In *Women with disabilities: Essays in psychology, culture, and politics,* edited by Michelle Fine and Adrienne Asch. Philadelphia: Temple University Press.

Austin, J. L.
1975.   *How to do things with words.* Cambridge: Harvard University Press.

Australian College of Paediatrics.
1983.   Non-intervention in children with major handicaps: Legal and ethical issues; report of a working party. *Australian Paediatric Journal* 19 (4): 217–22.

Avery, Gordon B.
1987.   Ethical dilemmas in the treatment of the extremely low birth-weight infant. *Clinics in Perinatology* 14 (2): 361–65.

Baker, John G.
1986.   June 19, 1982, letter of Judge John Baker to anonymous person. *Issues in Law and Medicine* 2 (1): 81–83.

Baughman, Lisa Kay.
1987.   Baby Jane Doe's right of privacy from cradle to grave: Infirmities of the 1984 Child Abuse Amendment. *Medicine and Law* 6 (5): 375–84.

Becker, Howard S.
1958.   Problems of inference and proof in participant observation. *American Sociological Review* 23: 652–60.

Beeson, Diane.
1984.   Technological rhythms in pregnancy: The case of prenatal diagnosis by amniocentesis. In *Cultural perspectives on biological knowledge,* edited by Troy Duster and Karen Garrett. Norwood, N.J.: Ablex.

Beeson, Diane, and Mitchell Golbus.
1979.   Anxiety engendered by amniocentesis. In *Birth defects: Original article series 15—Risk, communication, and decision making in genetic counseling,* edited by Charles J. Epstein et al. New York: Alan R. Liss.

Benfield, D. Gary, Susan A. Leib, and Jeanette Reuter.
1976.   Grief response of parents after referral of the critically ill newborn to a regional center. *New England Journal of Medicine* 294: 975–78.

Benfield, D. Gary, Susan A. Leib, and J. H. Vollman.
1978.   Grief response of parents to neonatal death and parental participation. *Pediatrics* 62: 171–77.

Bennett, F. C., N. M. Robinson, and C. J. Sells.
1983.   Growth and development of infants weighing less than 800g. at birth. *Pediatrics* 71: 319–23.

Berger, Peter L., and Thomas Luckmann.
1967.   *The social construction of reality: A treatise in the sociology of knowledge.* Garden City, N.Y.: Doubleday.

Bermel, Joyce.
  1986.   Confusion over the language of the Baby Doe regulations.
                 Hastings Center Report 16 (December): 2.
Berseth, Carol Lynn.
  1983.   A neonatologist looks at the Baby Doe rule: Ethical decisions
                 by edict. *Pediatrics* 72: 428–29.
Berseth, Carol Lynn.
  1987.   Ethical dilemmas in the neonatal intensive care unit. *Mayo
                 Clinic Proceedings* 62 (1): 67–72.
Berseth, Carol Lynn, John D. Kenny, and Roger Durand.
  1986.   Longitudinal development in pediatric residents of attitudes
                 toward neonatal resuscitation. *American Journal of Diseases in
                 Children* 140: 766–69.
Bhat, R., T. K. N. Raju, and D. Vidyaskar.
  1978.   Immediate and long-term outcome of infants less than 1000
                 grams. *Critical Care Medicine* 6: 147–50.
Biklen, Douglas P., and Philip M. Ferguson.
  1984.   In the matter of Baby Jane Doe: Does Reagan really agree with
                 us? *Social Policy* 15: 5–8.
Bittner, Egon.
  1967.   The police on skid row. *American Sociological Review* 32:
                 699–715.
Blalock, Hubert M.
  1960.   *Social statistics.* New York: McGraw-Hill.
Blustein, Jeffrey.
  1988.   Morality and parenting: An ethical framework for decisions
                 about the treatment of imperiled newborns. *Theoretical Medi-
                 cine* 9 (1): 23–32.
Bogdan, Robert, Mary Alice Brown, and Susan Bannerman Foster.
  1982.   Be honest but not cruel: Staff/parent communication on a neo-
                 natal unit. *Human Organization* 64: 10–16.
Bok, Sissela.
  1977.   The tools of bioethics. In *Ethics and medicine: Historical per-
                 spectives and contemporary issues,* edited by Stanley Joel
                 Reiser, Arthur Dyck, and William Curran. Cambridge: M.I.T.
                 Press.
Bopp, James.
  1985.   Protection of disabled newborns: Are there constitutional limi-
                 tations? *Issues in Law and Medicine* 1 (3): 173–200.
Bopp, James, and Thomas J. Balch.
  1985.   The child abuse amendments of 1984 and their implementing
                 regulations: A summary. *Issues in Law and Medicine* 1 (2):
                 91–130.
Born, Mary Ann.
  1986–87.   Baby Doe's new guardians: Federal policy brings nontreatment
                 decisions out of hiding. *Kentucky Law Journal* 75: 659–875.

Bosk, Charles L.
1979.   Forgive and remember: Managing medical failure. Chicago: University of Chicago Press.
Boxall, Jean.
1989.   Preparation for home. In *The baby under 1000g.*, edited by David Harvey, Richard W. I. Cooke, and Gillian A. Levitt. London: Wright.
Boyle, M. H., G. W. Torrance, J. C. Sinclair, and S. P. Horwood.
1983.   Economic evaluation of neonatal intensive care of very-low-birthweight infants. *New England Journal of Medicine* 308: 1330–37.
Bragonier, J. R., I. M. Cushner, and C. J. Hobel.
1984.   Social and personal factors in the etiology of preterm birth. In *Preterm birth: Causes, prevention, and management,* edited by F. Fuchs and P. G. Stubblefield. New York: Macmillan.
Brahams, Diana.
1986.   Severely handicapped newborns and the law. *Lancet* 8487 (April 26): 984–85.
Brahams, Diana.
1988.   No obligation to resuscitate non-viable infant. *Lancet* 8595 (May 21): 1176.
Branson, Roy, and Kenneth Casebeer.
1976.   Obscuring the role of the physician. *Hastings Center Report* 6 (February): 8–11.
Breslau, N., D. Salkever, and K. Smyth-Staruch.
1982.   Women's labor force activity and responsibilities for disabled dependents: A study of families with disabled children. *Journal of Health and Social Behavior* 23: 169–83.
Breslau, N., W. Weitzman, and K. Messenger.
1981.   Psychological functioning of siblings of disabled children. *Pediatrics* 67: 344–53.
Briesemeister, Linda H., and Beth A. Haines.
1988.   The interactions of fathers and newborns. In *Childbirth in America: Anthropological perspectives,* edited by Karen L. Michaelson and contributors. South Hadley, Mass.: Bergin and Garvey.
Britton, S. B., P. M. Fitzhardinge, and S. Ashby.
1981.   Is intensive care justified for infants weighing less than 801 gm. at birth? *Journal of Pediatrics* 99: 937.
Brody, Howard.
1976.   *Ethical decisions in medicine.* Boston: Little, Brown.
Brody, Howard, and William G. Bartholome.
1988.   In the best interests of . . . *Hastings Center Report* 18 (December): 37–40.
Brody, Jane E.
1991.   A quality of life determined by a baby's size. *New York Times,* October 1, 1, 13.

Brown, Lawrence D.
    1986.   Civil rights and regulatory wrongs: The Reagan administration
                 and the medical treatment of handicapped infants. *Journal of
                 Health Politics, Policy, and Law* 11: 231–52.
Buckwald, S., W. A. Zorn, and E. A. Egan.
    1984.   Mortality and follow-up data for neonates weighing 500 to
                 800g. at birth. *American Journal of Diseases of Childhood* 138:
                 779–82.
Budetti, Peter P., and Peggy McManus.
    1982.   Assessing the effectiveness of neonatal intensive care. *Medical
                 Care* 20: 1982.
Budetti, Peter P., Peggy McManus, Nancy Barrano, and Lu Ann Heinen.
    1980.   *The cost-effectiveness of neonatal intensive care.* Washington,
                 D.C.: United States Congress, Office of Technology Assess-
                 ment.
Burt, Robert A.
    1975.   Authorizing death for anomalous newborns. In *Genetics and
                 the law: National symposium on genetics and the law,* edited
                 by Audrey Milunsky and George J. Annas. New York: Plenum.
Butler, J., P. Budetti, P. McManus, S. Stenmark, and P. Newacheck.
    1982.   Health care expenditures for children with chronic disabilities.
                 Paper prepared for Public Policies Affecting Chronically Ill
                 Children and Their Families. Center for the Study of Families
                 and Children, Institute for Public Policy Studies, Vanderbilt
                 University, Nashville, Tenn.
Calabresi, Guido, and Philip Bobbitt.
    1978.   *Tragic choices.* New York: Norton.
Calvert, Richard J., David C. Miller, Ezekiel J. Emanuel, James E. Strain,
    and Marcia Angell.
    1986.   The Baby Doe controversy (letters and response). *New England
                 Journal of Medicine* 315: 707–8.
Campbell, A. G. M., and Raymond S. Duff.
    1979a.   Deciding the care of severely malformed or dying infants. *Jour-
                 nal of Medical Ethics* 5: 65–67.
Campbell, A. G. M., and Raymond S. Duff.
    1979b.   Authors' response to Richard Sherlock's commentary. *Journal
                 of Medical Ethics* 6: 141.
Campbell, A. G. M., and Raymond S. Duff.
    1986.   Treatment decisions for infants and children. *Canadian Medi-
                 cal Association Journal* 135 (5): 447–48.
Caplan, Arthur L.
    1985.   Conclusion. In *Which babies shall live? Humanistic dimensions
                 of the care of imperiled newborns,* edited by Thomas H. Mur-
                 ray and Arthur L. Caplan. Clifton, N.J.: Humana Press.
Caplan, Gerald.
    1960.   Patterns of parental response to the crisis of premature birth.
                 Psychiatry 23: 365–74.

Capron, Alexander Morgan.
  1976.   Shifting the burden of decision making. *Hastings Center Report* 6 (February): 17–19.
Cartwright, Ann.
  1964.   *Human relations and hospital care.* London: Routledge and Kegan Paul.
Chalmers, I., and L. Mutch.
  1981.   Are current trends in perinatal practice associated with an increase or a decrease in handicapping conditions? *Lancet* 8235 (June 27): 1415.
Chalmers, I., and L. Mutch.
  1984.   Investment in neonatal intensive care and the "handicapped survivor" bogey. *Lancet* 8400 (August 25): 469.
Charmaz, Kathy.
  1983.   The grounded theory method: An explication and interpretation. In *Contemporary field research,* edited by Robert M. Emerson. Boston: Little, Brown.
Childress, James F.
  1985.   Protecting handicapped newborns: Who's in charge and who pays? In *Genetics and the law,* vol. 3, edited by Audrey Milunsky and George J. Annas. New York: Plenum.
Churchill, Larry R.
  1985.   Which infants should live? On the usefulness and limitations of Robert Weir's selective nontreatment of handicapped newborns. *Social Science and Medicine* 20 (11): 1097–1102.
Churchill, Larry R., and Jose Jorge Siman.
  1986.   Principles and the search for moral certainty. *Social Science and Medicine* 23 (5): 461–68.
Cicourel, Aaron V.
  1964.   *Method and measurement in sociology.* New York: Free Press.
Cicourel, Aaron V.
  1976.   *The social organization of juvenile justice.* London: Heinemann.
Cicourel, Aaron V.
  1981.   Notes on the integration of micro and macro levels of analysis. In *Advances in social theory and methodology: Toward an integration of micro- and macro-sociologies,* edited by K. Knorr and A. V. Cicourel. London: Routledge and Kegan Paul.
Cicourel, Aaron V.
  1983.   Language and the structure of belief in medical communication. In *The social organization of doctor-patient communication,* edited by Sue Fisher and Alexandra Dundas Todd. Washington, D.C.: Center for Applied Linguistics.
Cimons, Marlene.
  1984a.   "Baby Doe" rule eased, review panels sought. *Los Angeles Times,* January 10, I-8, 9.

Cimons, Marlene.
    1984b.   Medical groups to fight bill on "Baby Doe" cases. *Los Angeles
                 Times,* February 11, I-6.
Clark, Matt.
    1981.   When doctors play God. *Newsweek,* August 31, 48–54.
Clausen, Joy P.
    1985.   A transcultural perspective on the delivery of perinatal health
                 care. In *Bioethical frontiers in perinatal intensive care,* edited
                 by Chandice C. Harris and Fraser Snowden. Natchitoches, La.:
                 Northwestern State University Press.
Clouser, K. Danner.
    1977.   Allowing or causing: Another look. *Annals of Internal Medi-
                 cine* 87: 622–24.
Coburn, Robert C.
    1980.   Morality and the defective newborn. *Journal of Medicine and
                 Philosophy* 5: 340–57.
Cohen, Libby.
    1987.   Euthanasia of handicapped newborns. In *Transitions in mental
                 retardation,* vol. 2, edited by James A. Mulick and Richard F.
                 Antonak. Norwood, N.J.: Ablex.
Cohen, Marcia R.
    1982.   Parents' reactions to neonatal intensive care. In *Coping with
                 caring for sick newborns,* edited by Richard E. Marshall, Chris-
                 tine Kasman, and Linda S. Cape. Philadelphia: W. B. Saunders.
Cohen, Marianna.
    1976.   Ethical issues in neonatal intensive care: Familial concerns. In
                 Ethics of newborn intensive care, edited by Albert R. Jonsen
                 and Michael Garland. Berkeley: Institute of Governmental
                 Studies.
Cohen, R., D. Stevenson, N. Malachowski, R. Arigno, K. Kimble, A.
    Hopper, J. Johnson, K. Uelana, and P. Sunshine.
    1982.   Favorable results of neonatal intensive care for very low birth-
                 weight infants. *Pediatrics* 69: 621–25.
Committee on Fetus and Newborn, Committee of the Section on Perinatal
    Ethics.
    1980.   Estimates of need and recommendations for personnel in neo-
                 natal pediatrics. *Pediatrics* 65: 850–53.
Committee on the Legal and Ethical Aspects of Health Care for Children.
    1983.   Comments and recommendations on the "Infant Doe" pro-
                 posed regulations. *Law, Medicine, and Health Care* 11 (5):
                 203–5.
Cooke, Richard W. I.
    1989.   The cost of intensive care. In *The baby under 1000g.,* edited by
                 David Harvey, Richard W. I. Cooke, and Gillian A. Levitt.
                 London: Wright.
Cooke, Robert E.
    1983.   Ethics on behalf of the mentally retarded. In *Ethical issues in*

the treatment of children and adolescents, edited by Tomas
Silber. Thorofare, N.J.: Slack.

Cramer, B.
1976.   A mother's reactions to the birth of a premature baby. In
             Maternal-infant bonding, edited by Marshall H. Klaus and
             John H. Kennell. St. Louis: C. V. Mosby.

Crane, Diana.
1975.   *The sanctity of social life.* New York: Russell-Sage.

Creighton, Helen.
1974.   Choose life or let die. *Supervising Nurse* 12: 12–13.

Crossley, Mary A.
1987.   Selective nontreatment of handicapped newborns: An analysis.
             Medicine and Law 6: 499–544.

Culliton, Barbara J.
1975.   Intensive care for newborns: Are there times to pull the plug?
             Science 188: 133–34.

Darbyshire, Philip.
1985.   Infanticide: Lambs to the slaughter. *Nursing Times* 81 (33):
             32–35.

Darling, Rosalyn B.
1977.   Parents, physicians, and spina bifida. *Hastings Center Report* 7
             (August): 10–14.

Davis, Allison.
1986.   The view of a disabled woman. *Journal of Medical Ethics* 12:
             75–76.

Davis, Fred.
1963.   *Passage through crisis.* Indianapolis: Bobbs-Merrill.

Davis, Fred.
1972.   *Illness, interaction, and the self.* Belmont, Calif.: Wadsworth.

Dean, John P.
1954.   Participant-observation and interviewing. In *Introduction to
             social research,* edited by John T. Doby. Harrisburg, Pa.:
             Stackpole.

Diamond, Sondra.
1973.   Life-and-death decisions. *Newsweek,* December 3, 12.

Driscoll, J. M., Jr., Y. T. Driscoll, M. E. Steir, et al.
1982.   Mortality and morbidity in infants less than 1000 grams birth-
             weight. *Pediatrics* 69: 21–26.

Drotar, D., A. Baskiewicz, N. Irvin, J. Kennell, and M. Klaus.
1975.   The adaptation of parents to the birth of an infant with a
             congenital malformation: A hypothetical model. *Pediatrics* 56:
             710–17.

Dubler, Nancy N.
1985.   The right to privacy as a protection for the right to refuse care
             for the imperiled newborn. In *Which babies shall live? Human-
             istic dimensions of the care of imperiled newborns,* edited by

Thomas H. Murray and Arthur L. Caplan. Clifton, N.J.: Humana Press.

Duff, Raymond S.
1978a.   A physician's role in the decision-making process: A physician's experience. In *Decision making and the defective newborn,* edited by Chester A. Swinyard. Springfield, Ill.: Charles C. Thomas.

Duff, Raymond S.
1978b.   Deciding the care of defective infants. In *Infanticide and the value of life,* edited by Marvin Kohl. Buffalo, N.Y.: Prometheus.

Duff, Raymond S.
1979.   Guidelines for deciding care of critically ill or dying patients. *Pediatrics* 64: 17–23.

Duff, Raymond S.
1981.   Counseling families and deciding care of severely defective children. *Pediatrics* 67: 315–20.

Duff, Raymond S.
1987.   "Close-up" versus "distant" ethics: Deciding the care of infants with poor prognosis. *Seminars in Perinatology* 11 (3): 96.

Duff, Raymond S., and A. G. M. Campbell.
1973.   Moral and ethical dilemmas in the special care nursery. *New England Journal of Medicine* 289: 890–94.

Duff, Raymond S., and A. G. M. Campbell.
1976.   On deciding the care of severely handicapped or dying persons: With particular reference to infants. *Pediatrics* 57: 487–93.

Duff, Raymond S., and A. G. M. Campbell.
1980.   Moral and ethical dilemmas: Seven years into the debate about human ambiguity. *Annals of the American Academy of Political and Social Science* 447: 19–28.

Duff, Raymond S., and August B. Hollingshead.
1968.   *Sickness and society.* New York: Harper & Row.

Durkheim, Emile.
1938.   *The rules of the sociological method.* New York: Free Press.

Durkheim, Emile.
1964.   *The division of labor in society.* New York: Free Press.

Dyck, Arthur.
1977.   Ethics and medicine. In *Ethics and medicine: Historical perspectives and contemporary concerns,* edited by Stanley Joel Reiser, Arthur Dyck, and William Curran. Cambridge: M.I.T. Press.

Ehrenreich, Barbara, and John Ehrenreich.
1970.   *The American health empire.* New York: Vintage.

Ehrenreich, Barbara, and Deirdre English.
1979.   *For her own good.* Garden City, N.Y.: Doubleday.

Elias, Sherman, and George J. Annas.
1987.   Treatment of handicapped newborns. In *Reproductive genetics*

and the law, by Sherman Elias and George J. Annas. Chicago: Year Book Medical Publishers.

Elkington, J. R.
1970.   Literature of ethical problems in medicine. *Annals of Internal Medicine* 73: 495–98; 662–66; 863–70.

Elkins, Thomas E., and Doug Brown.
1986.   An approach to Down syndrome in light of Infant Doe. *Issues in Law and Medicine* 1 (6): 419–40.

Ellis, T. S., III.
1982.   Letting defective babies die: Who decides? *American Journal of Law and Medicine* 38: 393–423.

Emerson, Joan P.
1970.   Behavior in private places: Sustaining definitions of reality in gynecological examinations. In *Recent sociology,* no. 2, edited by Hans Peter Dreitzel. London: Macmillan.

Emerson, Robert, ed.
1983.   *Contemporary field research.* Boston: Little, Brown.

Engelhardt, H. Tristram.
1973.   Viability, abortion, and the difference between a fetus and an infant. *American Journal of Obstetrics and Gynecology* 116: 429–34.

Engelhardt, H. Tristram.
1975a.   Bioethics and the process of embodiment. *Perspectives in Biology and Medicine* 17: 487–501.

Engelhardt, H. Tristram.
1975b.   Ethical issues in aiding in the death of young children. In *Beneficent euthanasia,* edited by Marvin Kohl. Buffalo, N.Y.: Prometheus.

Engelhardt, H. Tristram.
1976.   *Science, ethics, and medicine.* Hastings-on-Hudson, N.Y.: Institute for Society, Ethics, and Natural Sciences.

Engelhardt, H. Tristram.
1986.   *The foundations of bioethics.* New York: Oxford University Press.

Feldman, Eric, and Thomas Murray.
1984.   State legislation and the handicapped newborn: A moral and political dilemma. *Law, Medicine, and Health Care* 12 (4): 156–63.

Ferrara, Angelo, Melvin Schwartz, and Helen Page.
1988.   Effectiveness of neonatal transport in New York City in neonates less than 2500 grams: A population study. *Journal of Community Health* 13: 3–18.

Fiedler, Leslie A.
1984.   The tyranny of the normal. *Hastings Center Report* 14 (April): 40–42.

Fine, Michelle, and Adrienne Asch, eds.
1988.   *Women with disabilities: Essays in psychology, culture, and politics.* Philadelphia: Temple University Press.

Fischer, Allen F., and David K. Stevenson.
1987.   The consequences of uncertainty: An empirical approach to medical decision making in neonatal intensive care. *Journal of the American Medical Association* 258: 1929–31.
Fisher, Sue.
1988.   *In the patient's best interest.* New Brunswick, N.J.: Rutgers University Press.
Fisher, Sue, and Alexandra Dundas Todd, eds.
1983.   *The social organization of doctor-patient communication.* Washington, D.C.: Center for Applied Linguistics.
Fitzhardinge, P. M., and M. Ramsay.
1973.   The improving outlook for the small prematurely born infant. *Developmental Medicine and Child Neurology* 15: 447–59.
Fleishman, Alan R.
1985.   Caring for babies in danger: The evolution and current state of neonatology. In *Which babies shall live? Humanistic dimensions of the care of imperiled newborns,* edited by Thomas H. Murray and Arthur L. Caplan. Clifton, N.J.: Humana Press.
Fleishman, Alan R.
1987.   Bioethical review committees in perinatology. *Clinics in Perinatology* 14 (2): 379–93.
Fletcher, John C.
1975.   Abortion, euthanasia, and the care of defective newborns. *New England Journal of Medicine* 292: 75–78.
Fletcher, John C.
1978.   Spina bifida with myelomeningocele: A case study in attitudes toward defective newborns. In *Decision making and the defective newborn,* edited by Chester Swinyard. Springfield, Ill.: Charles C. Thomas.
Fletcher, John C.
1982.   Ethics of therapeutic leadership. *Alabama Journal of Medical Sciences* 19 (2): 156–61.
Fletcher, Joseph.
1954.   *Morals and medicine.* Princeton: Princeton University Press.
Fletcher, Joseph.
1972.   Indicators of humanhood: A tentative profile of man. *Hastings Center Report* 2 (November): 1–4.
Fletcher, Joseph.
1974.   Four indicators of humanhood: The enquiry matures. *Hastings Center Report* 4 (December): 6–7.
Fletcher, Joseph.
1978.   Infanticide and the ethics of loving concern. In *Infanticide and the value of life,* edited by Marvin Kohl. Buffalo, N.Y.: Prometheus.
Foot, Philippa.
1977.   Euthanasia. *Philosophy and Public Affairs* 6: 109.

Fost, Norman.
   1981.   Counseling families who have a child with a severe congenital
                anomaly. *Pediatrics* 67: 321.
Fost, Norman.
   1982.   Putting hospitals on notice: Baby Doe and federal funding.
                Hastings Center Report 12 (August): 5–8.
Fost, Norman.
   1983.   Ethical issues in the treatment of critically ill newborns. In
                Ethical issues in the treatment of children and adolescents,
                edited by Tomas Silber. Thorofare, N.J.: Slack.
Foucault, Michel.
   1975.   *The birth of the clinic: An archaeology of medical perception.*
                New York: Vintage.
Fox, Daniel M.
   1986.   Introduction to the Baby Jane Doe papers. *Journal of Health
                Politics, Policy, and Law* 11: 195–97.
Fox, Renée C.
   1974.   Ethical and existential developments in contemporary medi-
                cine. *Milbank Memorial Fund Quarterly* 54: 445–83.
Fox, Renée C.
   1976.   Advanced medical technology: Social and ethical implications.
                Annual Review of Sociology 2: 231–69.
Fox, Renée C., and Judith P. Swazey.
   1974.   *The courage to fail: A social view of organ transplants and
                dialysis.* Chicago: University of Chicago Press.
Fox, Renée C., and Judith P. Swazey.
   1984.   Medical morality is not bioethics: Medical ethics in China and
                the United States. *Perspectives in Biology and Medicine* 27:
                336–60.
Frader, Joel E.
   1979.   Difficulties in providing intensive care. *Pediatrics* 64: 10–15.
Frader, Joel E.
   1985.   Selecting neonatal ethics. *Social Science and Medicine* 20 (11):
                1085–90.
Frader, Joel E.
   1986.   Caring for families. In *Human values in critical care medicine,*
                edited by Stuart J. Youngner. New York: Praeger.
Frankena, William K.
   1965.   *Ethics.* Englewood Cliffs, N.J.: Prentice-Hall.
Freeman, John M.
   1972.   Is there a right to die—quickly? *Journal of Pediatrics* 80: 904–5.
Freeman, John M.
   1973.   To treat or not to treat: Ethical dilemmas of treating an infant
                with a myelomeningocele. *Clinical Neurosurgery* 20: 137.
Freeman, John M.
   1974.   The shortsighted treatment of myelomeningocele: A long-term
                case report. *Pediatrics* 53: 311–13.

Freeman, John M.
 1978.   Ethics and the decision making process for defective children.
                In *Medical wisdom and ethics in the treatment of severely
                defective newborn and young children,* edited by David J. Roy.
                Montreal: Eden Press.
Freeman, John M.
 1986.   Making decisions for the severely handicapped newborn. *Jour-
                nal of Health Politics, Policy, and Law* 11: 285–94.
Freeman, John M., Loretta M. Kopelman, Thomas G. Irons, and Arthur E.
   Kopelman.
 1988.   "Baby Doe" regulations. *New England Journal of Medicine*
                319 (11): 726.
Freeman, John M., Kenneth Shulman, and William Reinke.
 1978.   Decision making and the infant with spina bifida. In *Decision
                making and the defective newborn,* edited by Chester Swin-
                yard. Springfield, Ill.: Charles C. Thomas.
Freidson, Eliot.
 1970.   *Profession of medicine.* 2d. ed. New York: Dodd, Mead.
Freidson, Eliot.
 1972.   *Professional dominance.* Chicago: Aldine.
Frohock, Fred M.
 1986.   *Special care: Medical decisions at the beginning of life.* Chi-
                cago: University of Chicago Press.
Gallo, Anthony.
 1984.   Spina bifida: The state of the art of medical management.
                Hastings Center Report 14 (February): 10–12.
Gamsu, H. R., F. Light, A. Potter, and J. F. Price.
 1979.   Intensive care and the very low birth weight infant. *Lancet* 8145
                (October 6): 736.
Gardell, Mary Ann.
 1986.   June, bioethics, and the Supreme Court. *Journal of Medicine
                and Philosophy* 11 (3): 285–90.
Garland, Michael.
 1976.   Views on the ethics of infant euthanasia. In *Ethics of newborn
                intensive care,* edited by Albert R. Jonsen and Michael Gar-
                land. Berkeley: Institute of Governmental Studies.
Geertz, Clifford.
 1983.   Thick description: Toward an interpretive theory of culture. In
                Field research, edited by Robert M. Emerson. Boston: Little,
                Brown.
Gerber, Paul.
 1982.   Reg. v. Dr. Leonard Arthur: A "post mortem" analysis. *Medi-
                cal Journal of Australia* 1 (7): 285–86.
Gerry, Martin H., and Mary Nimz.
 1987.   The federal role in protecting Babies Doe. *Issues in Law and
                Medicine* 2 (5): 339–77.

Giblin, P. T., M. L. Poland, J. B. Waller, Jr., and J. W. Ager.
1988.   Correlates of parenting on an NICU: Maternal characteristics of family resources. *Journal of Genetic Psychology* 149 (4): 505–14.

Giddens, Anthony.
1984.   *The constitution of society: Outline of the theory of structuration*. Berkeley: University of California Press.

Gilligan, Carol.
1982.   *In a different voice*. Cambridge: Harvard University Press.

Gillon, Raanan.
1986.   Conclusion: The Arthur case revisited. *British Medical Journal* 292 (6519): 543–45.

Glantz, L., and J. Swazey.
1979.   Decisions not to treat: The Saikewiscz case and its aftermath. *Forum in Medicine* 2: 22–32.

Glaser, Barney, and Anselm Strauss.
1965.   *Awareness of dying*. Chicago: Aldine.

Glaser, Barney, and Anselm Strauss.
1967.   *The discovery of grounded theory*. Chicago: Aldine.

Gliedman, John, and William Roth.
1980.   *The unexpected minority: Handicapped children in America*. New York: Harcourt Brace Jovanovich.

Glover, Jonathan.
1977.   *Causing death and saving lives*. New York: Penguin.

Gold, Raymond L.
1958.   Roles in sociological field observations. *Social Forces* 36: 217–23.

Gorski, Sandra L.
1985.   Comment: Premature infants: A legal approach to decision making in neonatal intensive care. *University of San Francisco Law Review* 19: 261–81.

Gortmaker, S., A. Sobol, C. Clark, et al.
1982.   The survival of very low birthweight infants by level of hospital birth: A population study of perinatal systems in four states. *American Journal of Obstetrics and Gynecology* 143: 533–37.

Goss, Mary E. W.
1961.   Influence and authority among physicians in an outpatient clinic. *American Sociological Review* 26: 39–50.

Grassy, R. G., C. Hubbard, S. N. Graven, and R. D. Zachman.
1976.   The growth and development of low birth weight infants born in 1978 receiving intensive neonatal care. *Clinical Pediatrics* 15: 549–53.

Greenstein, Laurie-Jane.
1987.   Withholding life-sustaining treatment from severely defective newborns: Who should decide? *Medicine and Law* 6 (6): 487–97.

Gross, Richard H., et al.
    1983.   Early management and decision making of the treatment of myelomeningocele. *Pediatrics* 72 (4): 450–58.

Grostin, L. A.
    1985.   A moment in human development: Legal protection, ethical standards, and social policy on the selective non-treatment of handicapped neonates. *American Journal of Law and Medicine* 11: 31–78.

Guillemin, Jeanne Harley.
    1988.   The family in newborn intensive care. In *Childbirth in America: Anthropological perspectives,* edited by Karen L. Michaelson and contributors. South Hadley, Mass.: Bergin and Garvey.

Guillemin, Jeanne Harley, and Lynda Lytle Holmstrom.
    1983.   Legal cases, government regulations, and clinical realities in newborn intensive care. *American Journal of Perinatology* 1: 89–97.

Guillemin, Jeanne Harley, and Lynda Lytle Holmstrom.
    1986.   *Mixed blessings: Intensive care for newborns.* New York: Oxford University Press.

Guillemin, Jeanne Harley, I. David Todres, Dick Batten, and Michael A. Grodin.
    1989.   Deciding to treat newborns: Changes in pediatricians' responses to treatment choices. In *New approaches to human reproduction: Social and ethical dimensions,* edited by Linda M. Whiteford and Marilyn L. Poland. Boulder, Colo.: Westview.

Gustafson, James M.
    1973.   Mongolism, parental desires, and the right to life. *Perspectives in Biology and Medicine* 15: 529–51.

Gustaitis, Rasa, and Ernle W. D. Young.
    1986.   *A time to be born, a time to die: Conflicts and ethics in an intensive care nursery.* Menlo Park, Calif.: Addison-Wesley.

Hack, Maureen, Donna DeMontrice, Irwin R. Merkatz, Paul K. Jones, and Avroy A. Fanaroff.
    1981.   Rehospitalization of the very-low-birth-weight infant: A continuum of perinatal and environmental morbidity. *American Journal of Diseases of Childhood* 135: 263–66.

Hack, Maureen, and Avroy A. Fanaroff.
    1986.   Changes in the delivery room care of the extremely small infant (<750g.): Effects on morbidity and outcome. *New England Journal of Medicine* 314: 660–64.

Hack, Maureen, Avroy A. Fanaroff, and Irwin R. Merkatz.
    1979.   The low-birth-weight infant: Evolution of a changing outlook. *New England Journal of Medicine* 301: 1162–65.

Hack, Maureen, Irwin R. Merkatz, Paul K. Jones, and Avroy A. Fanaroff.
    1980.   Changing trends of neonatal and postneonatal deaths in very-

low-birth-weight infants. *American Journal of Obstetrics and Gynecology* 137: 797–800.

Haddon, Phoebe A.
1985.   Baby Doe cases: Compromise and moral dilemma. *Emory Law Journal* 34: 545–615.

Hagberg, B., G. Hagberg, and I. Olow.
1984.   The changing panorama of cerebral palsy in Sweden, 4: Epidemiological trends, 1959–1978. *Acta Pediatrica Scandinavia* 73: 433–40.

Hancock, Emily.
1976.   Crisis intervention in a newborn nursery intensive care unit. *Social Work in Health Care* 1: 421–32.

Hardest choice: Preserving the life of malformed infants.
1974.   *Time,* March 25, 84.

Harvey, David, Richard W. I. Cooke, and Gillian A. Levitt, eds.
1989.   *The baby under 1000g.* London: Wright.

Hastings Center Research Project on the Care of Imperiled Newborns.
1987.   Imperiled newborns: A report. *Hastings Center Report* 17 (December): 5–32.

Haug, Marie R.
1973.   Deprofessionalization: An alternative hypothesis for the future. *Sociological Review Monograph* 20 (December): 195–211.

Hemphill, John Michael, and John R. Freeman.
1978.   Infants: Medical aspects and ethical decisions. In *Encyclopedia of bioethics,* vol. 2, edited by Warren T. Reich. New York: Free Press.

Hentoff, Nat.
1986.   Strange priesthood of bioethics. *Washington Post,* February 20, A19.

Heymann, Philip B., and Sarah Holtz.
1975.   The severely defective newborn: The dilemma and the decision process. *Public Policy* 23: 382–417.

Hirata, T., J. T. Epcar, A. Walsh, et al.
1983.   Survival and outcome of infants 501 to 750 g.: A six-year experience. *Journal of Pediatrics* 99: 937–43.

Hobbs, Nicholas, James M. Perrin, and Henry T. Ireys.
1985.   *Chronically ill children and their families.* San Francisco: Jossey-Bass.

Hochschild, Arlie Russell.
1983.   *The managed heart.* Berkeley: University of California Press.

Holden, Constance.
1986.   High court says no to administration's Baby Doe rules. *Science* 232: 1595–96.

Holder, Angela.
1985.   The child and death. In *Legal issues in pediatrics and adolescent medicine,* 2d ed., by Angela Holder. New Haven: Yale University Press.

Horan, Dennis J.
1977.   Euthanasia as medical management. In *Death, dying, and euthanasia,* edited by Dennis J. Horan and David Mall. Washington, D.C.: University Publications of America.
Horan, Dennis J., and Melinda Delahoyde, eds.
1982.   *Infanticide and the handicapped newborn.* Provo, Utah: Brigham Young University Press.
Horan, Dennis J., and David Mall, eds.
1977.   *Death, dying, and euthanasia.* New York: University Publications of America.
Horan, Dennis J., and Steven R. Valentine.
1982.   The doctor's dilemma: Euthanasia, wrongful life, and the handicapped newborn. In *Infanticide and the handicapped newborn,* edited by Dennis J. Horan and Melinda Delahoyde. Provo, Utah: Brigham Young University Press.
Horwood, S. P., et al.
1982.   Mortality and morbidity of 500-to-1499-gram birthweight infants live-born to residents of a defined geographic region before and after neonatal intensive care. *Pediatrics* 69: 613–20.
Hoskins, E. M., E. Elliot, A. T. Shennan, M. B. Skidmore, and E. Keith.
1983.   Outcome of very low-birth-weight infants born at a perinatal center. *American Journal of Obstetrics and Gynecology* 145: 135–39.
Huefner, Dixie Snow.
1986.   Severely handicapped infants with life-threatening conditions: Federal intrusions into the decision not to treat. *American Journal of Law and Medicine* 12: 171–205.
Hunt, Jane V.
1976.   Mental development of the survivors of neonatal intensive care. In *Ethics of newborn intensive care,* edited by Albert R. Jonsen and Michael Garland. Berkeley: Institute of Governmental Studies.
Hunt, Jane V.
1979.   Longitudinal research: A method for studying the intellectual development of high risk preterm infants. In *Infants born at risk,* edited by T. M. Field, A. M. Sostek, S. Goldberg, and H. H. Shuman. New York: Spectrum Medical and Scientific Books.
Hunt, Paul.
1966.   A critical condition. In *Stigma: The experience of disability,* edited by Paul Hunt. London: G. Chapman.
Hunter, Rosemary S., Nancy Kilstrom, Ernest Kraybill, and Frank Loda.
1978.   Antecedents of child abuse and neglect in premature infants: A prospective study in a newborn intensive care unit. *Pediatrics* 61: 629–35.
Hynan, Michael T.
1987.   *The pain of premature parents.* New York: University Press of America.

In re Quinlan.
1976.   70 N.J. 10, 355 A 2d 647.

Institute of Medicine.
1985.   *Preventing low birthweight.* Washington, D.C.: National Academy Press.

Irving, N., J. Kennell, and M. Klaus.
1976.   Caring for parents of an infant with a congenital malformation. In *Maternal-infant bonding,* edited by Marshall H. Klaus and John H. Kennell. St. Louis: C. V. Mosby.

Jackson, Carol C.
1987.   Severely disabled newborns: To live or let die? *Journal of Legal Medicine* 8: 135–76.

Jakobovits, Immanuel.
1978.   Jewish views on infanticide. In *Infanticide and the value of life,* edited by Marvin Kohl. Buffalo, N.Y.: Prometheus.

Janis, Irving L., and Leon Mann.
1977.   *Decision making.* New York: Free Press.

John, Elizabeth, Kui Lee, and Gloria M. Li.
1983.   Cost of neonatal intensive care. *Australian Paediatric Journal* 19: 152–56.

Johnson, Paul R.
1981.   Selective nontreatment and spina bifida: A case study in ethical theory and application. *Bioethics Quarterly* 3 (21): 91–111.

Jones, Gary E.
1984.   Non-medical burdens of the defective infant. *Philosophy in Context* 14: 29–33.

Jones, Lanie.
1979.   Mimi survives the odds, goes home to mom. *Los Angeles Times,* November 5, I-7.

Jonsen, Albert R.
1976.   Introduction: Ethics and neonatal intensive care. In *Ethics of newborn intensive care,* edited by Albert R. Jonsen and Michael Garland. Berkeley: Institute of Governmental Studies.

Jonsen, Albert R.
1977.   Just what is a newborn baby worth? *Los Angeles Times,* May 26, II-7.

Jonsen, Albert R., and Michael Garland, eds.
1976a.   *Ethics of newborn intensive care.* Berkeley: Institute of Governmental Studies.

Jonsen, Albert R., and Michael Garland.
1976b.   A moral policy for life/death decisions in the intensive care nursery. In *Ethics of newborn intensive care,* edited by Albert R. Jonsen and Michael Garland. Berkeley: Institute of Governmental Studies.

Jonsen, Albert R., and Andre Hellegers.
1977.   Conceptual foundations for an ethics of medical care. In *Ethics and medicine: Historical perspectives and contemporary issues,*

edited by Stanley Joel Reiser, Arthur Dyck, and William Curran. Cambridge: M.I.T. Press.

Jonsen, Albert R., Andrew L. Jameton, and Abyann Lynch.
1978.   History of medical ethics: North America in the 20th century. In *Encyclopedia of bioethics,* vol. 3, edited by Warren T. Reich. New York: Free Press.

Jonsen, Albert R., and George Lister.
1978a.   Life support systems. In *Encyclopedia of bioethics,* vol. 2, edited by Warren T. Reich. New York: Free Press.

Jonsen, Albert R., and George Lister.
1978b.   Newborn intensive care: The ethical problems. *Hastings Center Report* 8 (February): 15–18.

Jonsen, Albert R., R. H. Phibbs, W. H. Tooley, and Michael Garland.
1977.   Critical issues in newborn intensive care. In *Vulnerable infants: A psychosocial dilemma,* edited by Jane Schwartz and Lawrence Schwartz. New York: McGraw-Hill.

Kanter, Rosabeth Moss.
1977.   *Men and women of the corporation.* New York: Basic Books.

Kaplan, David, and Edward A. Mason.
1977.   Maternal reactions to premature birth viewed as an acute emotional disorder. In *Vulnerable infants: A psychosocial dilemma,* edited by Jane Schwartz and Lawrence Schwartz. New York: McGraw-Hill.

Katz, Jack.
1983.   A theory of qualitative methodology: The social system of analytic fieldwork. In *Contemporary field research,* edited by Robert M. Emerson. Boston: Little, Brown.

Katz-Rothman, Barbara.
1986.   *The tentative pregnancy: Prenatal diagnosis and the future of motherhood.* New York: Viking.

Kaufman, S. L., and S. S. Shepard.
1982.   Costs of neonatal intensive care by length of stay. *Inquiry* 19: 167–78.

Kaufmann, Felix.
1941.   *Methodology of the social sciences.* New York: Oxford University Press.

Kessel, S. S., J. Villar, H. W. Berendes, et al.
1984.   The changing pattern of low birthweight in the United States, 1970 to 1980. *Journal of the American Medical Association* 271: 1978–82.

Kett, Joseph F.
1985.   Science and controversy in the history of infancy in America. In *Which babies shall live? Humanistic dimensions of the care of imperiled newborns,* edited by Thomas H. Murray and Arthur L. Caplan. Clifton, N.J.: Humana Press.

Keyserlingk, E. W.
1986. Severely handicapped newborns: Against infanticide. *Law, Medicine, and Health Care* 14 (3–4): 154–57.
Kiely, J. L., and N. Paneth.
1981. Follow-up studies for low-birthweight infants: Suggestions for design, analysis, and reporting. *Developmental Medicine and Child Neurology* 23: 96–99.
Kirkley, William H.
1980. Fetal survival: What price? *American Journal of Obstetrics and Gynecology* 137: 873.
Kitchen, William H., Neil Campbell, John H. Drew, Laurence J. Murton, Robert N. D. Roy, and Victor Y. H. Yu.
1983. Provision of perinatal services and survival of extremely low birthweight infants in Victoria. *Medical Journal of Australia* 2: 314–18.
Kitchen, William H., and Laurence J. Murton.
1985. Survival rates of infants with birth weights between 501 and 1000 g. *American Journal of Diseases of Childhood* 139: 470–72.
Kitchen, William H., Victor Y. H. Yu, Anna A. Orgill, Geoffrey Ford, Ann Rickards, Jill Astbury, Jean V. Lissenden, and Barbara Bajuk.
1983. Collaborative study of very-low-birth-weight infants: Correlation of handicap with risk factors. *American Journal of Diseases of Childhood* 137: 555–59.
Klaidman, Stephen, and Tom L. Beauchamp.
1986. Baby Jane Doe in the media. *Journal of Health Politics, Policy, and Law* 11: 271–84.
Klaus, Marshall H., and Avroy A. Fanaroff.
1973. *Care of the high-risk neonate.* New York: Saunders.
Klaus, Marshall H., and John H. Kennell, eds.
1976. *Maternal-infant bonding.* St. Louis: C. V. Mosby.
Klaus, Marshall H., and John H. Kennell.
1978. Mothers separated from their newborn infants. In *Vulnerable infants: A psychosocial dilemma,* edited by Jane Schwartz and Lawrence Schwartz. New York: McGraw-Hill.
Klaus, Marshall H., and John H. Kennell, eds.
1982. *Parent-infant bonding,* 2d ed. St. Louis: C. V. Mosby.
Klein, M., and L. Stern.
1971. Low birth weight and the battered child syndrome. *American Journal of Diseases of Children* 122: 15–18.
Kluge, Eike-Henner W.
1978. Infanticide as the murder of persons. In *Infanticide and the value of life,* edited by Marvin Kohl. Buffalo, N.Y.: Prometheus.
Kluge, Eike-Henner W.
1980. The euthanasia of radically defective neonates: Some statutory considerations. *Dalhousie Law Journal* 6: 229–57.

Kohl, Marvin, ed.
1978.   *Infanticide and the value of life.* Buffalo, N.Y.: Prometheus.
Kohrman, Arthur F.
1985.   Selective nontreatment of handicapped newborns: A critical
            review essay. *Social Science and Medicine* 20 (11): 1091–95.
Kolata, Gina.
1991.   Parents of tiny infants find care choices are not theirs. *New
            York Times,* September 30, 1, 11.
Koontz, A. M.
1984.   Pregnancy and infant health: Progress toward the 1990 objec-
            tives. *Public Health Reports* 99 (2): 184–92.
Koop, C. Everett.
1977.   The seriously ill or dying child: Supporting the patient and the
            family. In *Death, dying, and euthanasia,* edited by Dennis J.
            Horan and David Mall. New York: University Publications of
            America.
Koop, C. Everett.
1982.   Ethical and surgical considerations in the surgical care of the
            newborn born with congenital anomalies. In *Infanticide and
            the handicapped newborn,* edited by Dennis J. Horan and
            Melinda Delahoyde. Provo, Utah: Brigham Young University
            Press.
Kopelman, Loretta M., Thomas Irons, and Arthur E. Kopelman.
1988.   Neonatologists judge the "Baby Doe" regulations. *New En-
            gland Journal of Medicine* 318: 677–83.
Kopelman, Loretta M., David K. Stevenson, and Allen F. Fischer.
1988.   The second Baby Doe rule. *Journal of the American Medical
            Association* 259: 843–44.
Korones, Sheldon B.
1976.   *High-risk newborn infants,* 2d ed. St. Louis: C. V. Mosby.
Korsch, B. M., E. K. Gozzi, and V. Francis.
1968.   Gaps in doctor-patient communication: Doctor-patient interac-
            tion and patient satisfaction. *Pediatrics* 42: 855–71.
Korsch, B. M., and V. F. Negrette.
1972.   Doctor-patient communication. *Scientific American* 227:
            66–74.
Kraybill, E. N., C. A. Kennedy, S. W. Teplin, and S. K. Campbell.
1984.   Infants with birth weights less than 1000g. *American Journal of
            Diseases in Children* 138: 837–42.
Kuhse, Helga, and Peter Singer.
1985.   *Should the baby live?* Oxford: Oxford University Press.
Kuhse, Helga, and Peter Singer.
1986.   Severely handicapped newborns: For sometimes letting—and
            helping—die. *Law, Medicine, and Health Care* 14 (3–4):
            149–54.

Kumar, Savitri, Endia Anday, Linda Sacks, Rosalind Ting, and Maria
Delivoria-Papadopoulos.
1980.   Follow-up studies of very low birth weight infants (1250 grams
or less) born and treated within a perinatal center. *Pediatrics*
66: 438–44.

Lane v. Candura.
1978.   Massachusetts Appellate Court Adv. Sch. 588.

Langer, William L.
1972.   Checks on population growth: 1750–1850. *Scientific American*
226: 92–99.

Lantos, John D.
1987.   Baby Doe five years later: Implications for child health. *New
England Journal of Medicine* 317: 444–47.

Lantos, John D., Steven H. Miles, Marc D. Silverstein, and Carol B.
Stocking.
1988.   Survival after cardiopulmonary resuscitation in babies of very
low birth weight: Is CPR futile therapy? *New England Journal
of Medicine* 318: 91–95.

Lazarus, Ellen S.
1988.   Poor women, poor outcomes: Social class and reproductive
health. In *Childbirth in America: Anthropological perspectives,*
edited by Karen L. Michaelson and contributors. South Hadley,
Mass.: Bergin and Garvey.

Lee, K. S., N. Paneth, L. Gartner, et al.
1980.   Neonatal mortality: An analysis of the recent improvement in
the United States. *American Journal of Public Health* 80: 15–21.

Lee, Philip R., Albert R. Jonsen, Albert Dooley, and Diane Dooley.
1978.   Social and economic factors affecting public policy and decision
making in the care of the defective newborn. In *Decision making and the defective newborn,* edited by Chester A. Swinyard.
Springfield, Ill.: Charles C. Thomas.

Leventhal, John M.
1981.   Risk factors for child abuse: Methodological standards in case-
control studies. *Pediatrics* 68: 684–90.

Levin, Betty Wolder.
1983.   The cultural context of "Baby Jane Doe" and decision making
for catastrophically ill newborns. Paper presented at the 82d
Annual Meeting of the American Anthropological Association,
Chicago.

Levin, Betty Wolder.
1985.   Consensus and controversy in the treatment of catastrophically
ill newborns. In *Which babies shall live? Humanistic dimensions of the care of imperiled newborns,* edited by Thomas H.
Murray and Arthur L. Caplan. Clifton, N.J.: Humana Press.

Levin, Betty Wolder.
1988.   The cultural context of decision making for catastrophically ill
newborns: The case of Baby Jane Doe. In *Childbirth in Amer-*

ica: *Anthropological perspectives,* edited by Karen L. Michaelson and contributors. South Hadley, Mass.: Bergin and Garvey.

Levin, Betty Wolder.
1989.   Decision making about care of catastrophically ill newborns:
               The use of technological criteria. In *New approaches to human
               reproduction: Social and ethical dimensions,* edited by Linda
               M. Whiteford and Marilyn L. Poland. Boulder, Colo.: West-
               view.

Levin, Betty Wolder.
1990.   International perspectives on treatment choice in neonatal in-
               tensive care units. *Social Science and Medicine* 30 (8): 901–12.

Levin, Betty Wolder, John M. Driscoll, and Alan R. Fleishman.
1990.   Clinicians' attitudes about the aggressiveness of treatment for
               newborns at risk for AIDS: An ethical issue in the NICU. Paper
               presented at the Sixth International Conference on AIDS, San
               Francisco.

Levin, David S.
1984.   John T. Noonan and Baby Jane Doe. *Philosophy in Context* 14:
               35–41.

Levine, Melvin D.
1976.   Disconnection: The clinician's view. *Hastings Center Report* 6
               (February): 11–12.

Lipton, Helene L., and Bonnie Svarstad.
1977.   Sources of variation in clinicians' communication to parents
               about mental retardation. *American Journal of Mental Defi-
               ciency* 82: 155–61.

Lister, David.
1986.   Ethical issues in infanticide of severely defective infants. *Cana-
               dian Medical Association Journal* 135 (12): 1401–4.

Lo, Bernard, and Albert R. Jonsen.
1981.   Bioethics and the lack of clinical relevance. Unpublished manu-
               script.

Lofland, John.
1971.   *Analyzing social settings.* Belmont, Calif.: Wadsworth.

Lorber, John.
1971.   Results of treatment of myelomeningocele. *Developmental
               Medicine and Child Neurology* 13: 179–300.

Lorber, John.
1972.   Spina bifida cystica: Results of treatment of 270 consecutive
               cases with criteria for selection for the future. *Archives of
               Disease in Childhood* 47: 856.

Lorber, John.
1973.   Early results of selective treatment of spina bifida cystica. *Brit-
               ish Medical Journal* 4: 201.

Lorber, John.
1974.   Selective treatment of myelomeningocele: To treat or not to
               treat. *Pediatrics* 53: 307.

Lorber, John.
  1975.   Ethical problems in the management of myelomeningocele and
              hydrocephalus. *Journal of the Royal College of Medicine* 10:
              47–60.
Lorber, John.
  1978a.   The doctor's duty to patients and parents in profoundly hand-
              icapping conditions. In *Medical wisdom and ethics in the treat-
              ment of severely defective newborn and young children,* edited
              by David J. Roy. Montreal: Eden Press.
Lorber, John.
  1978b.   Ethical concepts in the treatment of myelomeningocele. In *De-
              cision making and the defective newborn,* edited by Chester A.
              Swinyard. Springfield, Ill.: Charles C. Thomas.
Luker, Kristin.
  1984.   *Abortion and the politics of motherhood.* Berkeley: University
              of California Press.
Lyon, Jeff.
  1985.   *Playing God in the nursery.* New York: Norton.
Macklin, Ruth.
  1985.   Comment on "The tyranny of the normal." In *Which babies
              shall live? Humanistic dimensions of the care of imperiled new-
              borns,* edited by Thomas H. Murray and Arthur L. Caplan.
              Clifton, N.J.: Humana Press.
MacMillan, Elizabeth S.
  1978.   Birth-defective infants: A standard for nontreatment decisions.
              Stanford Law Review 30: 599–633.
Magnet, Joseph Eliot, and Eike-Henner W. Kluge.
  1985.   *Withholding treatment from defective newborn children.* Co-
              wansville, Quebec: Brown Legal Publications.
Mahowald, Mary B.
  1984.   In the interest of infants. *Philosophy in Context* 14: 9–18.
Mahowald, Mary B.
  1986.   Ethical decisions in neonatal intensive care. In *Human values in
              critical care medicine,* edited by Stuart J. Youngner. New York:
              Praeger.
Maine Medical Center v. Houle.
  1974.   Maine Supreme Court Civil Act. No. 74–145.
Maine. Superior Court, Cumberland.
  1986.   Trial court decision in Houle case. (*Maine Medical Center v.
              Houle.* Docket No. 74–145 1974 Feb 14 [date of decision]).
              Issues in Law and Medicine 2 (3): 237–39.
Malcolm, Andrew H.
  1986.   Ruling on Baby Doe: Impact limited. *New York Times,* June
              11, A16.
Manney, James, and John C. Blattner.
  1984.   *Death in the nursery: The secret crime of infanticide.* Ann
              Arbor: Servant Books.

Mannheim, Karl.
1936.   *Ideology and utopia: An introduction to the sociology of knowledge.* New York: Harcourt Brace Jovanovich.

Manning, Peter K.
1971.   Analytic induction. Paper presented at a seminar session, American Sociological Association, Denver.

Marks, F. Raymond, and Lisa Salkovitz.
1976.   The defective newborn: An analytic framework for a policy dialog. In *Ethics of newborn intensive care,* edited by Albert R. Jonsen and Michael Garland. Berkeley: Institute of Governmental Studies.

Marsh, L. A., T. D. Coleman, and A. L. Jung.
1978.   Financial impact to families of less than 1000g. babies admitted to an NICU. *Pediatric Research* 12: 374–76.

Marshall, Richard E., and Linda S. Cape.
1982.   Coping with neonatal death. In *Coping with caring for sick newborns,* edited by Richard E. Marshall, Christine Kasman, and Linda S. Cape. Philadelphia: W. B. Saunders.

Marshall, Richard E., and Christine Kasman.
1980.   Burnout in the neonatal intensive care unit. *Pediatrics* 65: 1161–65.

Marshall, Richard E., and Christine Kasman.
1982.   Burnout. In *Coping with caring for sick newborns,* edited by Richard E. Marshall, Christine Kasman, and Linda S. Cape. Philadelphia: W. B. Saunders.

Marshall, Richard E., Christine Kasman, and Linda S. Cape, eds.
1982.   *Coping with caring for sick newborns.* Philadelphia: W. B. Saunders.

Marx, Karl, and Friedrich Engels.
1947.   *The German ideology.* New York: International Publishers.

Mason, J. K., and David W. Kaplan.
1986.   Parental choice and selective non-treatment of deformed newborns: A view from mid-Atlantic. *Journal of Medical Ethics* 12: 67–71.

Mather, H. G., D. C. Morgan, and N. G. Pearson.
1976.   Myocardial infarction: A comparison between home and hospital care for patients. *British Medical Journal* 1: 567.

Mather, H. G., N. G. Pearson, and K. L. Q. Read.
1971.   Acute myocardial infarction: House and hospital treatment. *British Medical Journal* 3: 334–38.

Mayfield, J. A., R. A. Rosenblatt, L.-M. Baldwin, et al.
1990.   The relationship of obstetrical volume and nursery level to perinatal mortality. *American Journal of Public Health* 80: 819–23.

McCall, George.
1969.   Data quality control in participant observation. In *Issues in participant observation,* edited by George McCall and J. L. Simmons. Reading, Mass.: Addison-Wesley.

McCall, George, and J. L. Simmons, eds.
1969.   *Issues in participant observation.* Reading, Mass.: Addison-Wesley.
McCarthy, J. T., B. L. Koops, P. R. Honeyfield, and L. J. Butterfield.
1979.   Who pays the bill for neonatal intensive care? *Journal of Pediatrics* 95: 755–61.
McCormick, Marie C.
1985.   The contribution of low birth weight to infant mortality and childhood morbidity. *New England Journal of Medicine* 312: 82–90.
McCormick, Marie C., Sam Shapiro, and Barbara H. Starfield.
1980.   Rehospitalization in the first year of life for high-risk survivors. *Pediatrics* 66: 991–99.
McCormick, Marie C., Sam Shapiro, and Barbara H. Starfield.
1984.   High-risk young mothers: Infant mortality and morbidity in four areas in the United States, 1973–1978. *American Journal of Public Health* 74: 18–23.
McCormick, Marie C., Sam Shapiro, and Barbara H. Starfield.
1985.   The regionalization of perinatal services: Summary of the evaluation of a national demonstration program. *Journal of the American Medical Association* 253: 799–804.
McCormick, Richard A.
1974.   To save or let die. *Journal of the American Medical Association* 229:172–76.
McCormick, Richard A.
1978.   The quality of life, the sanctity of life. *Hastings Center Report* 8 (February): 30–35.
McCormick, Richard A.
1981.   Women, newborns, and the conceived. In *Notes on moral theology,* by Richard A. McCormick, Lanham, Md.: University Press of America.
McKinlay, John.
1986.   A case for refocussing upstream: The political economy of illness. In *The sociology of health and illness,* 2d ed., edited by Peter Conrad and Rochelle Kern. New York: St. Martin's.
McLone, David G.
1986.   The diagnosis, prognosis, and outcome for the handicapped newborn: A neonatal view. *Issues in Law and Medicine* 2 (1): 15–24.
Meier, Paula, and John B. Patton.
1984.   *Clinical decision making in neonatal intensive care.* Orlando, Fla.: Grune and Stratton.
Michaels, Richard H., and Thomas K. Oliver.
1986.   Human rights consultation: A 12-year experience of a pediatric bioethics committee. *Pediatrics* 78 (4): 566–72.
Michaelson, Karen L.
1988.   Childbirth in America: A brief history. In *Childbirth in America: Anthropological perspectives,* edited by Karen L.

Michaelson and contributors. South Hadley, Mass.: Bergin
and Garvey.

Michaelson, Karen L., and contributors, eds.
1988.   *Childbirth in America: Anthropological perspectives*. South
Hadley, Mass.: Bergin and Garvey.

Miller, Arden C.
1985.   Infant mortality in the U.S. *Scientific American* 253 (1): 1–10.

Miller, Herbert C.
1983.   A model for studying the pathogenesis and incidence of low-
birth-weight infants. *American Journal of Diseases of Childhood* 137: 323–27.

Millman, Marcia.
1977.   *The unkindest cut: Life in the backrooms of medicine*. New
York: Morrow.

Milstein, Bonnie.
1985.   The law and bioethics: The applicability of civil rights laws to
health care. In *Bioethical frontiers in perinatal intensive care*,
edited by Chandice C. Harris and Fraser Snowden. Natchitoches, La.: Northwestern State University Press.

Mimz, Mary M.
1988.   *Johnson v. Sullivan* (Note). *Issues in Law and Medicine* 4 (1):
123–25.

Minnesota. County Court, Juvenile Division, County of Redwood.
1986.   Order in the Steinhaus case. (*In re Lance Steinhaus*. No.
J-86-92. 1986 Sep 11 [date of decision]). *Issues in Law and
Medicine* 2 (3): 241–52.

Mishler, Eliot.
1985.   *The discourse of medicine*. New York: Ablex.

Mondanlou, H. D.
1980.   Perinatal transport to a regional perinatal center in a metropoli-
tan area: Maternal vs. neonatal transport. *American Journal of
Obstetrics and Gynecology* 138 (1): 157–63.

Moreno, Jonathan D.
1987.   Ethical and legal issues in the care of the impaired newborn.
Clinics in Perinatology 14 (2): 345–60.

More premature babies survive.
1988.   *The Futurist* 22: 46.

Moseley, Kathryn L.
1986.   The history of infanticide in western society. *Issues in Law and
Medicine* 1 (5): 345–61.

Moskop, John C., and Rita L. Saldanha.
1986.   The Baby Doe rule: Still a threat. *Hastings Center Report* 16
(April): 8–14.

Moss, Kathryn.
1987.   The "Baby Doe" legislation: Its rise and fall. *Policy Studies
Journal* 15: 629–51.

Murray, Thomas H.
    1985a.   The final anticlimactic rule on Baby Doe. *Hastings Center Report* 15 (June): 5–9.
Murray, Thomas H.
    1985b.   Suffer the little children: Suffering and neonatal intensive care. In *Which babies shall live? Humanistic dimensions of the care of imperiled newborns,* edited by Thomas H. Murray and Arthur L. Caplan. Clifton, N.J.: Humana Press.
Murray, Thomas H.
    1985c.   Why solutions continue to elude us. *Social Science and Medicine* 20 (11): 1103–7.
Murray, Thomas H., and Arthur L. Caplan.
    1985a.   Introduction: Beyond Babies Doe. In *Which babies shall live? Humanistic dimensions of the care of imperiled newborns,* edited by Thomas H. Murray and Arthur L. Caplan. Clifton, N.J.: Humana Press.
Murray, Thomas H., and Arthur L. Caplan, eds.
    1985b.   *Which babies shall live? Humanistic dimensions of the care of imperiled newborns.* Clifton, N.J.: Humana Press.
Murton, Laurence J., Lex W. Doyle, and William H. Kitchen.
    1987.   Care of very low birthweight infants with limited neonatal intensive care resources. *Medical Journal of Australia* 146: 78–81.
Nelson, Harry.
    1979.   Pulling the plug on the newborn: An ethical morass. *Los Angeles Times,* April 22, II-1, 4, 5.
Newman, George.
    1986.   Response to Freeman: The Stony Brook perspective. *Journal of Health Politics, Policy, and Law* 11: 295–96.
Newman, Lucile F.
    1980.   Parents' perceptions of their low birth weight infants. *Paediatrician* 9: 182–90.
Newman, Lucile F.
    1988.   The artificial womb: Social and sensory environments of low birthweight infants. In *Childbirth in America: Anthropological perspectives,* edited by Karen L. Michaelson and contributors. South Hadley, Mass.: Bergin and Garvey.
Newman, Neville.
    1983.   The ethical dilemma: Selective non-treatment of newborn infants with major handicaps. *Medical Journal of Australia* 2 (6): 252–53.
Oden, Thomas C.
    1976.   Beyond the ethic of immediate sympathy. *Hastings Center Report* 6 (February) 12–14.
Office of Technology Assessment, U.S. Congress.
    1987.   *Neonatal intensive care for low birth-weight infants: Costs and*

effectiveness. Washington, D.C.: U.S. Government Printing Office.

Orgill, A. A., J. Astbury, B. Bajuk, and V. Y. H. Yu.
1981.   Early neurodevelopmental outcome of very low-birthweight infants. *Australian Paediatric Journal* 15: 193–96.

Orgill, A. A., J. Astbury, B. Bajuk, and V. Y. H. Yu.
1982.   Early development of infants 1000g. or less at birth. *Developmental Medicine and Child Neurology* 57: 823–27.

Osofsky, Howard J., and Norman Kendall.
1977.   Poverty as a criterion of risk. In *Vulnerable infants,* edited by Jane Schwartz and Lawrence Schwartz. New York: McGraw-Hill.

Otten, Alan L.
1983.   Doctors' dilemmas: As medicine advances, Hastings Center tries to solve ethical issues. *Wall Street Journal,* November 23, A1, 18.

Paige, Constance, and Elisa B. Karnofsky.
1986.   The antiabortion movement and Baby Jane Doe. *Journal of Health Politics, Policy, and Law* 11: 255–69.

Paneth, Nigel.
1986.   Recent trends in preterm delivery rates in the United States. In *Prevention of preterm birth,* edited by E. Papiernik, G. Breart, and N. Spira. Paris: Inserm.

Paneth, Nigel.
1990.   Technology at birth (Editorial). *American Journal of Public Health* 80: 791–92.

Paneth, Nigel, J. L. Kiely, Z. Stein, and M. Susser.
1981.   The incidence of cerebral palsy: Which way are we going? *Developmental Medicine and Child Neurology* 23: 111–12.

Paneth, Nigel, J. L. Kiely, S. Wallenstein, et al.
1982.   Newborn intensive care and neonatal mortality in low birth-weight infants: A population study. *New England Journal of Medicine* 307: 149–55.

Paneth, Nigel, J. L. Kiely, S. Wallenstein, et al.
1987.   The choice of place of delivery. *American Journal of Diseases of Childhood* 141: 60–64.

Pape, K. E., R. J. Buncic, S. Ashby, and P. M. Fitzhardinge.
1978.   The status at two years of low-birth-weight infants born in 1978 with birth weights of less than 1000g. *Journal of Pediatrics* 92: 253–60.

Paris, John J.
1985.   Religious traditions in bioethical decision making: Considerations on the sanctity of life. In *Bioethical frontiers in perinatal intensive care,* edited by Chandice C. Harris and Fraser Snowden. Natchitoches, La.: Northwestern State University Press.

Paris, John J., and Anne B. Fletcher.
1983.   Infant Doe regulations and the absolute requirement to use

nourishment and fluids for the dying infant. *Law, Medicine, and Health Care* 11 (5): 210–13.

Paris, John J., and Anne B. Fletcher.
1987.   Withholding of nutrition and fluids in the hopelessly ill patient. *Clinics in Perinatology* 14 (2): 367–77.

Parnel, Wickham, Judy Hanstein, Jack R. Phillips, Ruth F. Henry, Cathy Itri, Werner Rein, Howard Monohan, Wallace Ring, Alfred Harrison, Helen Harrison, James L. Cain, and Frederic Kleinberg.
1979.   Comments on Stinson and Stinson. *Atlantic* 233: 31, 34.

Parrish, Michael.
1980.   The quality of mercy. *New West* 5: 13–22.

Parsons, Talcott.
1951.   *The social system.* New York: Free Press.

Parsons, Talcott.
1964.   Definitions of health and illness in the light of American values and social structure. In *Patients, physicians, and illness,* 2d ed., edited by E. Gartley Jaco. New York: Free Press.

Parsons, Talcott, and Renée Fox.
1952.   Illness, therapy, and the American urban family. *Journal of Social Issues* 13 (4): 31–44.

Paulus, Sharon M.
1985.   In re L. H. R. (Note). *Issues in Law and Medicine* 1 (3): 233–36.

Pemberton, Patrick J.
1981.   Parental attitudes towards the mode of death of their newborn infants. *Australian Paediatric Journal* 17: 281–82.

Penticuff, Joy Hinson.
1988.   Neonatal intensive care: Parental prerogatives. *Journal of Perinatal and Neonatal Nursing* 1: 77–86.

Pharoah, P. O. D., and E. D. Alberman.
1981.   Mortality of low birthweight infants in England and Wales. *Archives of Disease in Childhood* 56: 86–89.

Pharoah, P. O. D., T. Cooke, L. Rosenbloom, and R. W. I. Cooke.
1987.   Effects of birth weight, gestational age, and maternal obstetric history on birth prevalence of cerebral palsy. *Archives of Disease in Childhood* 62: 1035–40.

Phelby, Derek F. H.
1982.   Changing practice on confidentiality: A cause for concern. *Journal of Medical Ethics* 8: 12–24.

Phibbs, Ciaran S., Ronald L. Williams, and Roderick H. Phibbs.
1981.   Newborn risk factors and costs of neonatal intensive care. *Pediatrics* 68: 313–21.

Philips, Joseph B., III, Helen Dickman, Michael Resnick, Robert Nelson, and Donald Eitzman.
1984.   Characteristics, mortality, and outcome of higher-birth weight infants who require intensive care. *American Journal of Obstetrics and Gynecology* 149: 875–79.

Pierzs, M.
1978.   *Infanticide: Past and present.* New York: Morton.

Poland, Ronald L., and Bruce A. Russell.
    1987.   The limits of viability: Ethical considerations. *Seminars in Perinatology* 11 (3): 257–61.
Pollner, Melvin.
    1987.   *Mundane reason: Reality in everyday and sociological discourse.* Cambridge, England: Cambridge University Press.
Pomerance, Jeffrey J., B. S. Schiffrin, and J. L. Meredith.
    1980.   Womb rent. *American Journal of Obstetrics and Gynecology* 137: 486–90.
Pomerance, Jeffrey J., Christinia T. Ukrainski, Tara Ukra, Diane H.
    Henderson, Andrea H. Nash, and Janet L. Meredith.
    1978.   Costs of living for infants weighing 1000 grams or less at birth. *Pediatrics* 61: 908–10.
Post, Stephen G.
    1987.   Family ethics in caring for newborns with impairments. *Health Progress* 68: 57–61.
Post, Stephen G.
    1988.   History, infanticide, and imperiled newborns. *Hastings Center Report* 18 (August/September): 14–33.
Powell, T. G., P. O. D. Pharoah, and R. W. I. Cooke.
    1986.   Survival and morbidity in a geographically defined population of low birthweight infants. *Lancet* 8480 (March 8): 539–43.
President's Commission for the Study of Ethical Problems in Medicine and
    Biomedical and Behavioral Research.
    1983.   *Deciding to forego life-sustaining treatment.* Washington, D.C.: U.S. Government Printing Office.
Pro and con: Should Uncle Sam protect handicapped babies? (Interviews
    with Dr. C. Everett Koop and Dr. Harry Jennison).
    1984.   *U.S. News and World Report,* January 16, 63–64.
Punch, Linda, and Sheila L. Simler.
    1982.   "Baby Doe" thrusts administrators into middle of life-death decision. *Modern Health Care,* July, 72–74.
Qui, Ren Zong.
    1987.   Economics and medical decision making: A Chinese perspective. *Seminars in Perinatology* 11 (3): 262–63.
Quilligan, E. J., and R. H. Paul.
    1975.   Fetal monitoring: Is it worth it? *Obstetrics and Gynecology* 45: 96–100.
Quint, Jeanne C.
    1972.   Institutionalized practices of information control. In *Medical men and their work,* edited by Eliot Freidson and Judith Lorber. Chicago: Aldine.
Rachels, James.
    1979.   Killing and starving to death. *Philosophy* 54: 159–71.
Ragatz, Stephen C., and Patricia H. Ellison.
    1983.   Decisions to withdraw life support in the neonatal intensive care unit. *Clinical Pediatrics* 22 (11): 729–35.

Rajopalan, R., G. Stickle, R. Kairam, and J. Driscoll.
1984.   Some clinical determinants of the cost of neonatal intensive
             care. Unpublished paper.
Ramsey, Paul.
1976.   Prolonging dying: Not medically indicated. *Hastings Center
             Report* 6 (February): 14–17.
Ramsey, Paul.
1977.   The nature of medical ethics. In *Ethics and medicine: Historical
             perspectives and contemporary issues,* edited by Stanley Joel
             Reiser, Arthur Dyck, and William Curran. Cambridge: M.I.T.
             Press.
Ramsey, Paul.
1978.   *Ethics at the edges of life.* New Haven: Yale University Press.
Raphael, D. D.
1988.   Handicapped infants: Medical ethics and the law. *Journal of
             Medical Ethics* 14 (1): 5–10.
Rapp, Rayna.
1988.   The power of "positive" diagnosis: Medical and maternal
             discourses on amniocentesis. In *Childbirth in America: Anthro-
             pological perspectives,* edited by Karen L. Michaelson and con-
             tributors. South Hadley, Mass.: Bergin and Garvey.
Rapp, Rayna.
1989.   Chromosomes and communication: The discourse of genetic
             counseling. In *New approaches to human reproduction: Social
             and ethical dimensions,* edited by Linda M. Whiteford and
             Marilyn L. Poland. Boulder, Colo.: Westview.
Reich, Warren T., and David L. Ost.
1978.   Ethical perspectives on the care of infants. In *Encyclopedia of
             bioethics,* vol. 2, edited by Warren T. Reich. New York: Free
             Press.
Reiser, Stanley Joel.
1978.   *Medicine and the reign of technology.* Cambridge, England:
             Cambridge University Press.
Reiser, Stanley Joel.
1986.   Survival at what cost? Origins and effects of the modern contro-
             versy on treating severely handicapped newborns. *Journal of
             Health Politics, Policy, and Law* 11: 198–213.
Reiser, Stanley Joel, Arthur Dyck, and William Curran, eds.
1977.   *Ethics and medicine: Historical perspectives and contemporary
             issues.* Cambridge: M.I.T. Press.
Rhoden, Nancy K., and John D. Arras.
1985.   Withholding treatment from Baby Doe: From discrimination to
             child abuse. *Milbank Memorial Fund Quarterly/Health and
             Society* 63: 18–51.
Richards, Martin.
1989.   The social and emotional needs of the parents and baby. In *The

baby under 1000g., edited by David Harvey, Richard W. I. Cooke, and Gillian A. Levitt. London: Wright.

Riga, Peter J.
1984.   Death and the care of defective neonates. In *The death decision,* edited by Leonard J. Nelson. Ann Arbor: Servant Books.

Roberton, N. R. C.
1979.   Intensive care and the very-low-birthweight infant. *Lancet* 8138 (August 18): 362.

Roberts, John L.
1982.   Adapting to the NICU: The houseofficer's perspective. In *Coping with caring for sick newborns,* edited by Richard E. Marshall, Christine Kasman, and Linda S. Cape. Philadelphia: W. B. Saunders.

Robertson, John A.
1975a.   Discretionary non-treatment of defective newborns. In *Genetics and the law: National symposium on genetics and the law,* edited by Audrey Milunsky and George J. Annas. New York: Plenum.

Robertson, John A.
1975b.   Involuntary euthanasia of defective newborns: A legal analysis. *Stanford Law Review* 27: 213–69.

Robertson, John A.
1977.   Involuntary euthanasia of defective newborns: A legal analysis. In *Vulnerable infants: A psychosocial dilemma,* edited by Jane Schwartz and Lawrence Schwartz. New York: McGraw-Hill.

Robertson, John A.
1986.   Legal aspects of withholding treatment from handicapped newborns: Substantive issues. *Journal of Health Politics, Policy, and Law* 11: 215–29.

Robertson, John A., and Norman Fost.
1976.   Passive euthanasia of defective newborn infants: Legal considerations. *Journal of Pediatrics* 88: 883–89.

Robert Wood Johnson Foundation.
1985.   *Special report: The perinatal program—What has been learned.* Princeton, N.J.: Robert Wood Johnson Foundation.

Rosenblum, Victor G., and Michael L. Buddle.
1982.   Historical and cultural considerations of infanticide. In *Infanticide and the handicapped newborn,* edited by Dennis J. Horan and Melinda Delahoyde. Provo, Utah: Brigham Young University Press.

Rosenblum, Victor G., and Edward B. Grant.
1986.   The legal response to Babies Doe: An analytical prognosis. *Issues in Law and Medicine* 1 (5): 395–404.

Rosenthal, Elizabeth.
1991.   As more tiny infants live, choices and burdens grow. *New York Times,* September 29, 1, 16.

Rosenwaike, Ira.
1971.   The influence of socioeconomic status on incidence of low birth-weight. *H.S.M.H.A. Report* 86: 642–49.
Ross, Catherine E., and Raymond S. Duff.
1978.   Quality of outpatient pediatric care: The influence of physicians' background, socialization, and work/information environment on performance. *Journal of Health and Social Behavior* 19: 348–60.
Rostain, Anthony.
1986.   Deciding to forgo life-sustaining treatment in the intensive care nursery: A sociologic account. *Perspectives in Biology and Medicine* 30: 117–34.
Roth, Julius.
1963.   *Timetables.* Indianapolis: Bobbs-Merrill.
Rothstein, Peter.
1980.   Psychological stress in families of children in a pediatric intensive care unit. *Pediatric Clinics of North America* 27: 613–20.
Roy, David J., ed.
1978.   *Medical wisdom and ethics in the treatment of severely defective newborn and young children.* Montreal: Eden Press.
Rudolph, Claire S., and Susan R. Borker.
1987.   *Regionalization: Issues in intensive care for high risk newborns and their families.* New York: Praeger.
Rue, Vincent M.
1985.   Death by design of handicapped newborns: The family's role and response. *Issues in Law and Medicine* 1 (3): 201–25.
Rumelhart, David E.
1977.   *Introduction to human information processing.* New York: Wiley.
Saigal, S., P. Rosenbaum, B. Stoskopf, and R. Milner.
1982.   Follow-up of infants 501–1500 grams of a geographically defined region with perinatal intensive care facilities. *Journal of Pediatrics* 100: 606–13.
Salkever, D.
1980.   Children's health problems: Implications for parental labor supply and earnings. In *Economic aspects of health,* edited by Victor Fuchs. Chicago: University of Chicago Press.
Schaeffer, Francis A., and C. Everett Koop.
1979.   *Whatever happened to the human race?* Old Tappan, N.J.: Revell.
Schechner, Sylvia.
1980.   For the 1980's: How small is too small? *Clinics in Perinatology* 7: 142.
Scheff, Thomas.
1968.   *Being mentally ill.* Chicago: Aldine.

Scheff, Thomas.
  1972.   Decision rules, types of error, and their consequences in medi-
              cal diagnosis. In *Medical men and their work,* edited by Eliot
              Freidson and Judith Lorber. Chicago: Aldine.
Schmeck, Harold M.
  1985.   Life, death, and the rights of handicapped babies. *New York
              Times,* June 18, C1, 3.
Schneider, Edward D., ed.
  1985.   *Questions about the beginning of life: Christian appraisals of
              seven bioethical issues.* Minneapolis: Augsburg.
Schroeder, Steven, J. A. Showstack, and H. E. Roberts.
  1978.   *High cost hospitalization: A descriptive study.* HRA Contract
              No. 230-77-0035.
Schutz, Alfred.
  1962.   *The problem of social reality.* Vol. 1 of *Collected papers.* The
              Hague: Martinius-Nijhoff.
Schutz, Alfred.
  1967.   *The phenomenology of the social world.* Evanston: Northwest-
              ern University Press.
Schwartz, Jane, and Lawrence Schwartz, eds.
  1977.   *Vulnerable infants: A psychosocial dilemma.* New York:
              McGraw-Hill.
Schwartz, Morris, and Charlotte Green Schwartz.
  1955.   Problems in participant-observation. *American Journal of Soci-
              ology* 60: 344–50.
Seidler, Eduard.
  1987.   Recent developments in perinatal and neonatal ethics: A Euro-
              pean perspective. *Seminars in Perinatology* 11 (3): 210–15.
Sellers, James.
  1985.   On turning it over to the parents (Editorial). *Christian Century*
              102 (7): 204.
Shall this child die?
  1973.   *Newsweek,* November 12, 70.
Shapiro, Robyn S., and Richard Barthel.
  1986.   Infant care review committees: An effective approach to the
              Baby Doe dilemma? *Hastings Law Journal* 37: 827–62.
Shapiro, Robyn S., and Joel E. Frader.
  1986.   Critically ill infants. In *Medicolegal aspects of critical care,*
              edited by Katherine Benesch et al. Rockville, Md.: Aspen.
Shapiro, Sam, Marie C. McCormick, and R. Nesbitt.
  1968.   *Infant, perinatal, maternal, and childhood mortality in the
              United States.* Cambridge: Harvard University Press.
Shapiro, Sam, Marie C. McCormick, Barbara H. Starfield, and Barbara
      Crawley.
  1983.   Changes in infant morbidity associated with decreases in neo-
              natal mortality. *Pediatrics* 72: 408–15.

Shapiro, Sam, Marie C. McCormick, Barbara H. Starfield, Jeffrey P.
Krisher, and Dean Bross.
1980.   Relevance of correlates of infant deaths for significant morbid-
             ity at 1 year of age. *American Journal of Obstetrics and Gyne-
             cology* 136: 363–71.
Shaw, Anthony.
1973.   Dilemmas of informed consent in children. *New England Jour-
             nal of Medicine* 289: 855–90.
Shaw, Anthony.
1977a.   Conditions in newborns that pose special problems. *Contem-
             porary Surgery* 11: 51.
Shaw, Anthony.
1977b.   Defining the quality of life. *Hastings Center Report* 7 (Octo-
             ber): 11.
Shaw, Anthony.
1978.   Who should die and who should decide? In *Infanticide and the
             value of life,* edited by Marvin Kohl. Buffalo, N.Y.: Prome-
             theus.
Shaw, Anthony.
1988.   QL revisited. *Hastings Center Report* 18 (April/May): 10–12.
Shaw, Anthony, Judson G. Randolph, and Barbara Manard.
1977.   Ethical issues in pediatric surgery: A national survey of pedia-
             tricians and pediatric surgeons. *Pediatrics* 60: 588–99.
Shelp, Earl E.
1986.   *Born to die? Deciding the fate of critically ill infants.* New
             York: Free Press.
Sherlock, Richard.
1979.   Selective nontreatment of newborns. *Journal of Medical Ethics*
             5: 139–42.
Sherlock, Richard.
1986.   Selective nontreatment of newborns. In *Bioethical issues in
             death and dying,* 2d ed., edited by Robert F. Weir. New York:
             Columbia University Press.
Sherlock, Richard.
1987.   *Preserving life: Public policy and the life not worth living.*
             Chicago: Loyola University Press.
Silber, Tomas.
1983.   *Ethical issues in the treatment of children and adolescents.*
             Thorofare, N.J.: Slack.
Silverman, William A.
1979.   Incubator-baby sideshows. *Pediatrics* 64: 127–42.
Silverman, William A.
1981.   Mismatched attitudes about neonatal death. *Hastings Center
             Report* 11 (December): 12–16.
Simmel, Georg.
1950.   *The sociology of Georg Simmel,* edited by Kurt Wolf. Glencoe,
             Ill.: Free Press.

Simmel, Georg.
  1965.   Secrecy and group communication. In *Theories of society:*
               Foundations of modern sociological theory, 2d ed., edited by
               Talcott Parsons, Edward Shils, Kaspar D. Naegele, and Jesse R.
               Pitts. New York: Free Press.
Simms, Madeleine.
  1983.   Severely handicapped infants: A discussion document. *New*
               Humanist 98: 15–22.
Simms, Madeleine.
  1986.   Informed dissent: The views of some mothers of severely men-
               tally handicapped young adults. *Journal of Medical Ethics* 12:
               72–76.
Sinclair, J. C., G. W. Torrance, M. H. Boyle, S. P. Horwood, S. Saigal, and
  D. L. Sackett.
  1981.   Evaluation of neonatal intensive care programs. *New England*
               Journal of Medicine 305: 489.
Singer, Peter.
  1975.   *Animal liberation.* New York: Avon.
Singer, Peter.
  1979.   Unsanctifying human life. In *Ethical issues relating to life and*
               death, edited by John Ladd. New York: Oxford University
               Press.
Singer, Peter.
  1985.   Neonatal intensive care: How much and who decides. *Medical*
               Journal of Australia 142: 335–36.
Singer, Peter.
  1987.   A report from Australia: Which babies are too expensive to
               treat? *Bioethics* 1 (3): 275–83.
Singer, Peter, and Helga Kuhse.
  1988.   Resolving arguments about the sanctity of life: A response to
               Long. *Journal of Medical Ethics* 14 (4): 198–99.
Singer, Peter, Helga Kuhse, and Cora Singer.
  1983.   The treatment of newborn infants with major handicaps: A
               survey of obstetricians and paediatricians in Victoria. *Medical*
               Journal of Australia 2 (6): 274–78.
Smith, David H.
  1974.   On letting some babies die. *Hastings Center Report* 2: 37–46.
Smith, David H.
  1978.   Death, ethics, and social control. In *Medical wisdom and ethics*
               in the treatment of severely defective newborn and young chil-
               dren, edited by David J. Roy. Montreal: Eden Press.
Smith, Dorothy E.
  1987.   *The everyday world as problematic: A feminist sociology.* Bos-
               ton: Northeastern University Press.
Smith, Dorothy E.
  1990.   *The conceptual practices of power: A feminist sociology of*
               knowledge. Boston: Northeastern University Press.

Smith, Elizabeth Dorsey.
  1986.   Infant care review committee and ethical decision making.
                 Nursing Administration Quarterly 10: 44–50.
Smith, George P.
  1984.   The plight of the genetically handicapped newborn: A compar-
                 ative analysis. *Holdsworth Law Review* 9 (2): 164–72.
Smith, George P.
  1985a.   Defective newborns and government intermeddling. *Medicine,
                 Society, and the Law* 25: 44–48.
Smith, George P.
  1985b.   Long day's journeys into night: The tragedy of the handicapped
                 at risk infant. In *Moral issues in mental retardation,* edited by
                 Ronald S. Laura and Adrian F. Ashman. London: Croom
                 Helm.
Smith, Steven R.
  1986.   Disabled newborns and the federal child abuse amendments:
                 Tenuous protection. *Hastings Law Journal* 37: 765–825.
Snider, A. J.
  1974.   Should doctors let deformed babies die? *Science Digest* 75:
                 47–48.
Snowden, Fraser.
  1985.   Bioethical challenges at the dawn of life: An introduction. In
                 Bioethical frontiers in perinatal intensive care, edited by Chan-
                 dice C. Harris and Fraser Snowden. Natchitoches, La.: North-
                 western State University Press.
Solnit, Albert, and Mary H. Stark.
  1961.   Mourning and the birth of a defective child. *Psychoanalytic
                 Study of the Child* 16: 523–37.
Sosnowitz, Barbara G.
  1984.   Managing parents on neonatal intensive care units. *Social Prob-
                 lems* 31: 390–402.
Stahlman, Mildred T.
  1984.   Newborn intensive care: Success or failure? *Pediatrics* 105:
                 162–67.
Stanley, F. J.
  1987.   The changing face of cerebral palsy. *Developmental Medicine
                 and Child Neurology* 29: 263–65.
Stanley, F. J., and S. Atkinson.
  1981.   Impact of neonatal intensive care on cerebral palsy in infants of
                 low-birthweight. *Lancet* 8256 (November 21): 1162.
Starfield, Barbara.
  1985.   *The effectiveness of medical care.* Baltimore: Johns Hopkins
                 University Press.
Starr, Paul.
  1982.   *The social transformation of American medicine.* New York:
                 Basic Books.

Stein, R. E. K., and C. K. Riessman.
   1982.   The development of impact-on-family scale: Preliminary find-
              ings. *Medical Care* 18: 465–72.
Steinbock, Bonnie.
   1985.   Infanticide. In *Moral issues in mental retardation*, edited by
              Ronald S. Laura and Adrian F. Ashman. London: Croom
              Helm.
Steinbock, Bonnie.
   1986.   The logical case for "wrongful life." *Hastings Center Report* 16
              (April): 15–20.
Steinbock, Bonnie.
   1987.   Whatever happened to the Danville Siamese twins? *Hastings
              Center Report* 17 (August): 3–4.
Steinfels, Margaret O.
   1978.   New childbirth technology: A clash of values. *Hastings Center
              Report* 8 (February): 9–12.
Stevenson, David K., Ronald L. Ariagno, Jean S. Kutner, Thomas A.
   Raffin, and Ernle W. D. Young.
   1986.   The "Baby Doe" rule. *Journal of the American Medical Associ-
              ation* 255: 1909–12.
Stewart, Ann L.
   1989.   Outcome. In *The baby under 1000g.*, edited by David Harvey,
              Richard W. I. Cooke, and Gillian A. Levitt. London: Wright.
Stewart, Ann L., E. O. R. Reynolds, and A. P. Lipscomb.
   1981.   Outcome for infants of very low birthweight: Survey of world
              literature. *Lancet* 8228 (May 9): 1038–41.
Stinson, Robert, and Peggy Stinson.
   1979.   On the death of a baby. *Atlantic* 244: 64–72.
Stinson, Robert, and Peggy Stinson.
   1983.   *The long dying of baby Andrew*. Boston: Little, Brown.
Stone, N. W., and B. H. Chesney.
   1976.   Attachment behaviors in handicapped infants. *Mental Retarda-
              tion* 16: 8–12.
Strain, James E.
   1983.   Special report: The American Academy of Pediatrics comments
              on the "Baby Doe II" regulations. *New England Journal of
              Medicine* 309: 443–44.
Strauss, Anselm, Shizuko Fagerhaugh, Barbara Suczek, and Carolyn
   Weiner.
   1987.   The social context of high technology: The case of the intensive
              care nursery. In *Dominant issues in medical sociology*, 2d ed.,
              edited by Howard D. Schwartz. New York: Random House.
Strong, Carson.
   1983.   The tiniest newborns. *Hastings Center Report* 13 (February):
              14–19.
Strong, Carson.
   1984.   The neonatologist's duty to patient and parents. *Hastings Cen-
              ter Report* 14 (August): 10–16.

Sudnow, David.
    1967.   *Passing on: The social organization of dying.* Englewood Cliffs, N.J.: Prentice-Hall.

Superintendent of Belchertown State School v. Saikewiscz.
    1977.   370 NE. 2d, 417.

Survey shows split on issue of treating deformed infants.
    1983.   *New York Times,* June 3, A14.

Svarstad, B., and H. Lipton.
    1976.   Informing parents about mental retardation: A study of professional communication and parental acceptance. Paper presented at the annual meeting of the Pacific Sociological Association, San Diego.

Swinyard, Chester A., ed.
    1978.   *Decision making and the defective newborn.* Springfield, Ill.: Charles C. Thomas.

Sykes, Gresham, and David Matza.
    1957.   Techniques of neutralization: A theory of delinquency. *American Sociological Review* 22: 664–70.

Taylor, Stuart.
    1986a.   Abortion is affirmed, but in a lower voice. *New York Times,* June 15, E1.

Taylor, Stuart.
    1986b.   High court upsets U.S. intervention on infants' lives. *New York Times,* June 10, 1.

Thomas, Emily H., Kathleen S. Andersen, and Jane E. Franz.
    1986.   Treating handicapped newborns: Suggestions for institutional policy. *Journal of Health Politics, Policy, and Law* 11: 297–303.

Thomas, Lewis.
    1971.   Notes of a biology watcher: The technology of medicine. *New England Journal of Medicine* 285: 1366–68.

Tiefel, Hans O.
    1985.   Care and treatment of severly handicapped newborns. In *Questions about the beginning of life: Christian appraisals of seven bioethical issues,* edited by Edward D. Schneider. Minneapolis: Augsburg.

Todres, I. David.
    1985.   "Infant Doe": Federal regulations of the newborn nursery are born. In *Genetics and the law,* vol. 3, edited by Audrey Milunsky and George J. Annas. New York: Plenum.

Todres, I. David, D. Krane, and M. C. Howell.
    1977.   Pediatricians' attitudes affecting decision-making in defective newborns. *Pediatrics* 60: 197–201.

Tooley, Michael.
    1972.   Abortion and infanticide. *Philosophy in Public Affairs* 2: 37–65.

Tooley, Michael.
    1978.   Infanticide: A philosophical perspective. In *Encyclopedia of bioethics,* vol. 2, edited by Warren T. Reich. New York: Free Press.

Tooley, Michael.
1979.   Decisions to terminate life and the concept of person. In *Ethical issues relating to life and death,* edited by John Ladd. New York: Oxford University Press.
Tooley, William, and Roderick Phibbs.
1976.   Neonatal intensive care: The state of the art. In *Ethics of newborn intensive care,* edited by Albert R. Jonsen and Michael Garland. Berkeley: Institute of Governmental Studies.
Treating the defective newborn: A survey of physicians' attitudes.
1976.   *Hastings Center Report* 6 (April): 2.
Turnbull, H. Rutherford.
1986.   Incidence of infanticide in America: Public and professional attitudes. *Issues in Law and Medicine* 1 (5): 363–89.
Twombly, Renée.
1990.   Saving young lives. *Technology Review* 93: 18–19.
U.S. Department of Health and Human Services.
1982.   Discrimination against the handicapped by withholding treatment or nourishment: Notice to health care providers. *Federal Register* 47 (116): 26027.
U.S. Department of Health and Human Services.
1983.   Nondiscrimination on the basis of handicap in the provision of health care to handicapped infants: Notice of court order declaring rule invalid. *Federal Register* 48 (80): 17588.
U.S. Department of Health and Human Services.
1986.   Procedures relating to health care for handicapped infants: Notice. *Federal Register* 52 (20): 3011–12.
Usher, R. H.
1981.   The special problems of the premature infant. In *Neonatology: Pathophysiology and management of the newborn,* edited by Gordon B. Avery. Philadelphia: J. B. Lippincott.
Usher, R. H.
1982.   Clinical implications of perinatal mortality statistics. *Clinics in Obstetrics and Gynecology* 14: 885–925.
Veatch, Robert M.
1977.   The technical criteria fallacy. *Hastings Center Report* 7 (August): 15–16.
Veatch, Robert M.
1978.   Abnormal newborns and the physician's role: Models of physician decision making. In *Decision making and the defective newborn,* edited by Chester A. Swinyard. Springfield, Ill.: Charles C. Thomas.
Visscher, Maurice, ed.
1972.   *Humanistic perspectives in medical ethics.* Buffalo, N.Y.: Prometheus.
Vitiello, Michael.
1985.   On letting seriously ill minors die: A review of Louisiana's Natural Death Act. *Loyola Law Review* 31: 67–91.

Vitiello, Michael.
1986.   Baby Jane Doe: Stating a cause of action against the officious intermeddler. *Hastings Law Journal* 37 (5): 863–908.
Wakefield-Fisher, Mary.
1987.   Balancing wishes with wisdom: Sustaining infant life. *Nursing and Health Care* 8 (9): 517–20.
Waldman, W. H.
1976.   Medical ethics and the hopelessly ill child. *Journal of Pediatrics* 88: 890–95.
Walker, C. H. M., and A. G. M. Campbell.
1988.   Officiously to keep alive. *Archives of Disease in Childhood* 63 (5): 560–66.
Walker, Donna-Jean, Allan Feldman, B. R. Vohr, and William Oh.
1984.   Cost-benefit analysis of neonatal intensive care for infants weighing less than 1000 grams at birth. *Pediatrics* 74: 20–25.
Walker, Donna-Jean, and H. Simpson.
1982.   Mortality rates and neonatal intensive care for very small babies. *Archives of Disease in Childhood* 57: 112–16.
Walker, Donna-Jean, B. R. Vohr, and William Oh.
1985.   Economic analysis of regionalized neonatal care for very low-birth-weight infants in the State of Rhode Island. *Pediatrics* 76: 69–74.
Wallace, Cynthia.
1983.   Outcry over "Baby Doe" may revive little-used hospital ethics committee. *Modern Healthcare,* June, 79–80.
Wallace, H. M.
1979.   Selected aspects of perinatal casualties. *Clinical Pediatrics* 18: 213–23.
Wallis, Claudia.
1983.   The stormy legacy of Baby Doe. *Time,* September 26, 58.
Walters, James W.
1988.   Approaches to ethical decision making in the neonatal intensive care unit. *American Journal of Diseases of Children* 142 (8): 825–30.
Warren, Mary Ann.
1977.   Do potential people have moral rights? *Canadian Journal of Philosophy* 7: 275–89.
Watchko, Jon F.
1983.   Decision making on critically ill infants by parents. *American Journal of Diseases of Children* 137: 795–98.
Weil, William B.
1986.   The Baby Doe regulations: Another view of change. *Hastings Center Report* 16 (April): 12–13.
Weir, Robert F.
1983.   Sounding board: The government and selective nontreatment of handicapped infants. *New England Journal of Medicine* 309: 661–63.

Weir, Robert F.
   1984.   *Selective nontreatment of handicapped newborns: Moral dilemmas in neonatal medicine.* New York: Oxford University Press.
Weir, Robert F.
   1985.   Selective nontreatment—one year later: Reflections and a response. *Social Science and Medicine* 20 (11): 1109–17.
Weir, Robert F., ed.
   1986.   *Ethical issues in death and dying,* 2d ed. New York: Columbia University Press.
Weir, Robert F.
   1987.   Pediatric ethics committees: Ethical advisers or legal watchdogs? *Law, Medicine, and Health Care* 15 (3): 99–109.
Weisberg, Robert W.
   1980.   *Memory, thought, and behavior.* New York: Oxford University Press.
Weitz, J.
   1983.   *Improvements for maternity and infant care.* Washington, D.C.: Children's Defense Fund.
Wertilman, M.
   1981.   Medical constraints to optimal psychological development. In *Preterm birth and psychological development,* edited by S. Freidman and M. Sigman. New York: Academic Press.
Wertz, Richard W., ed.
   1973.   *Readings on ethical and social issues in biology and medicine.* Englewood Cliffs, N.J.: Prentice-Hall.
Wertz, Richard W., and Dorothy C. Wertz.
   1979.   *Lying in: A history of childbirth in America.* New York: Schocken Books.
West, Candace.
   1979.   Against our will: Male interruption of females in cross-sexed conversations. *Annals of the New York Academy of Sciences* 327: 81–97.
West, Candace.
   1983.   Ask me no questions: An analysis of queries and replies in physician-patient dialogues. In *The social organization of doctor-patient communication,* edited by Sue Fisher and Alexandra Dundas Todd. Washington, D.C.: Center for Applied Linguistics.
Whiteford, Linda M., and Marilyn L. Poland, eds.
   1989.   *New approaches to human reproduction: Social and ethical dimensions.* Boulder, Colo.: Westview.
Whitelaw, Andrew.
   1986.   Death as an option in neonatal intensive care. *Lancet* 8502 (August 9): 328–31.
Williams, Preston.
   1973.   *Ethical issues in biology and medicine.* Cambridge: Schenkman.

Williams, R. L.
  1979.   Measuring the effectiveness of perinatal medical care. *Medical
               Care* 17: 95.
Williams, R. L., and P. M. Chen.
  1982.   Identifying the sources of the recent decline in perinatal mortal-
               ity rates in California. *New England Journal of Medicine* 306:
               207–14.
Williamson, Laila.
  1978.   Infanticide: An anthropological analysis. In *Infanticide and the
               value of life,* edited by Marvin Kohl. Buffalo, N.Y.: Prome-
               theus.
Wilson, Ann L., Lawrence R. Wellman, Lawrence J. Fenton, and Donald B.
  Witzke.
  1983.   What physicians know about the prognosis of preterm new-
               borns. *American Journal of Diseases of Children* 137: 551–54.
Winslade, William J., and Judith Wilson Ross.
  1986.   *Choosing life or death: A guide for patients, families, and
               professionals.* New York: Free Press.
Wolinsky, Fredric D.
  1988.   *The sociology of health,* 2d ed. Belmont, Calif.: Wadsworth.
Wood, Amy Tranckino.
  1985.   Withholding lifesaving treatment from defective newborns: An
               equal protection analysis. *St. Louis Law Journal* 29: 853–79.
Wortis, H., and J. Margolis.
  1955.   Parents of children with cerebral palsy. *Medical Social Work* 4:
               110.
York, Glyn Y., Robert M. Gallarno, and Reginald O. York.
  1990.   Baby Doe regulations and medical judgment. *Social Science and
               Medicine* 30 (6): 657–64.
Young, Ernle W. D.
  1983.   Caring for disabled infants. *Hastings Center Report* 13 (Au-
               gust): 15–18.
Youngner, Stuart J., ed.
  1986.   *Human values in critical care medicine.* New York: Praeger.
Yu, V. Y. H., and B. Bajuk.
  1981.   Medical expenses of neonatal intensive care for very low birth-
               weight infants. *Australian Paediatric Journal* 17: 183–85.
Yu, V. Y. H., P. Y. Wong, B. Bajuk, A. A. Orgill, and J. Astbury.
  1986.   Outcome of extremely low birthweight infants. *British Journal
               of Obstetrics and Gynaecology* 93: 162–70.
Zachary, R. B.
  1968.   Ethical and social aspects of the treatment of spina bifida.
               Lancet 7562 (August 3): 274–76.
Zachary, R. B.
  1977.   Life with spina bifida. *British Medical Journal* 2: 1460–62.
Zaner, Richard M.
  1987.   Soundings from uncertain places: Difficult pregnancies and

imperiled infants. In *Ethics of dealing with persons with severe handicaps: Toward a research agenda*, edited by Paul R. Dokecki and Richard M. Zaner. Baltimore: Paul H. Brookes.

Zeskind, Philip Sanford.
     1984.   Effects of maternal visitation to preterm infants in the neonatal intensive care unit. *Child Development* 55: 1887–93.

Index

Compositor: ComCom
Text: Sabon
Display: Centaur
Printer and Binder: Haddon Craftsmen